Pediatric Urology

Guest Editor

THOMAS F. KOLON, MD, FAAP

UROLOGIC CLINICS OF NORTH AMERICA

www.urologic.theclinics.com

May 2010 • Volume 37 • Number 2

SAUNDERS an imprint of ELSEVIER, Inc.

W.B. SAUNDERS COMPANY
A Division of Elsevier Inc.

1600 John F. Kennedy Blvd. • Suite 1800 • Philadelphia, PA 19103-2899

http://www.theclinics.com

UROLOGIC CLINICS OF NORTH AMERICA Volume 37, Number 2
May 2010 ISSN 0094-0143, ISBN-13: 978-1-4377-1917-8

Editor: Kerry Holland

Urologic Clinics of North America (ISSN 0094-0143) is published quarterly by Elsevier Inc., 360 Park Avenue South, New York, NY 10010-1710. Months of issue are February, May, August, and November. Business and Editorial Offices: 1600 John F. Kennedy Blvd., Suite 1800, Philadelphia, PA 19103-2899. Periodicals postage paid at New York, NY and additional mailing offices. Subscription prices are $291.00 per year (US individuals), $463.00 per year (US institutions), $333.00 per year (Canadian individuals), $568.00 per year (Canadian institutions), $414.00 per year (foreign individuals), and $568.00 per year (foreign institutions). Foreign air speed delivery is included in all *Clinics* subscription prices. All prices are subject to change without notice. **POSTMASTER:** Send address changes to *Urologic Clinics of North America*, Elsevier Health Sciences Division, Subscription Customer Service, 3251 Riverport Lane, Maryland Heights, MO 63043. Customer Service: 1-800-654-2452 (US). From outside the United States, call 1-314-447-8871. Fax: 1-314-447-8029. E-mail: JournalsCustomerServiceusa@elsevier.com (for print support) and JournalsOnlineSupport-usa@elsevier.com (for online support).

Reprints. For copies of 100 or more, of articles in this publication, please contact the Commercial Reprints Department, Elsevier Inc., 360 Park Avenue South, New York, New York 10010-1710. Tel.: 212-633-3813; Fax: 212-462-1935; E-mail: reprints@elsevier.com.

Urologic Clinics of North America is covered in MEDLINE/PubMed (*Index Medicus*), *Excerpta Medica, Current Contents/ Clinical Medicine, Science Citation Index,* and *ISI/BIOMED*.

Printed and bound in the United Kingdom
Transferred to Digital Print 2011

GOAL STATEMENT

The goal of *Urologic Clinics of North America* is to keep practicing urologists and urology residents up to date with current clinical practice in urology by providing timely articles reviewing the state of the art in patient care.

ACCREDITATION

The *Urologic Clinics of North America* is planned and implemented in accordance with the Essential Areas and Policies of the Accreditation Council for Continuing Medical Education (ACCME) through the joint sponsorship of the University of Virginia School of Medicine and Elsevier. The University of Virginia School of Medicine is accredited by the ACCME to provide continuing medical education for physicians.

The University of Virginia School of Medicine designates this educational activity for a maximum of 15 *AMA PRA Category 1 Credits*™ for each issue, 60 credits per year. Physicians should only claim credit commensurate with the extent of their participation in the activity.

The American Medical Association has determined that physicians not licensed in the US who participate in this CME activity are eligible for a maximum of 15 *AMA PRA Category 1 Credits*™ for each issue, 60 credits per year.

Credit can be earned by reading the text material, taking the CME examination online at http://www.theclinics.com/home/cme, and completing the evaluation. After taking the test, you will be required to review any and all incorrect answers. Following completion of the test and evaluation, your credit will be awarded and you may print your certificate.

FACULTY DISCLOSURE/CONFLICT OF INTEREST

The University of Virginia School of Medicine, as an ACCME accredited provider, endorses and strives to comply with the Accreditation Council for Continuing Medical Education (ACCME) Standards of Commercial Support, Commonwealth of Virginia statutes, University of Virginia policies and procedures, and associated federal and private regulations and guidelines on the need for disclosure and monitoring of proprietary and financial interests that may affect the scientific integrity and balance of content delivered in continuing medical education activities under our auspices.

The University of Virginia School of Medicine requires that all CME activities accredited through this institution be developed independently and be scientifically rigorous, balanced and objective in the presentation/discussion of its content, theories and practices.

All authors/editors participating in an accredited CME activity are expected to disclose to the readers relevant financial relationships with commercial entities occurring within the past 12 months (such as grants or research support, employee, consultant, stock holder, member of speakers bureau, etc.). The University of Virginia School of Medicine will employ appropriate mechanisms to resolve potential conflicts of interest to maintain the standards of fair and balanced education to the reader. Questions about specific strategies can be directed to the Office of Continuing Medical Education, University of Virginia School of Medicine, Charlottesville, Virginia.

The faculty and staff of the University of Virginia Office of Continuing Medical Education have no financial affiliations to disclose.

The authors/editors listed below have identified no professional or financial affiliations for themselves or their spouse/partner:
Richard A. Ashley, MD; J. Christopher Austin, MD; Nathaniel K. Ballek, MD; Julia S. Barthold, MD; Laurence S. Baskin, MD; Richard Bellah, MD; Douglas A. Canning, MD; Michael C. Carr, MD, PhD; Pasquale Casale, MD; Curtis J. Clark, MD; Christopher S. Cooper, MD; Kassa Darge, MD, PhD; Steven G. Docimo, MD; Fernando A. Ferrer, Jr., MD; Patricio C. Gargollo, MD, Lance J. Hampton, MD; Jeffrey C. Hellinger, MD; Kerry K. Holland (Acquisitions Editor); Nicolas Kalfa, MD, PhD; William A. Kennedy II, MD; Thomas F. Kolon, MD (Guest Editor); Harry P. Koo, MD; Kate H. Kraft, MD; Sarah M. Lambert, MD; John H. Makari, MD, MHA, MA; Patrick H. McKenna, MD; Michael C. Ost, MD; Puneeta Ramachandra, MD; William G. Reiner, MD; Pooja Renjen, MD; Aileen P. Schast, PhD; Aseem R. Shukla, MD; Marc C. Smaldone, MD; Warren T. Snodgrass, MD; William Steers, MD (Test Author); Charles Sultan, MD, PhD; and Eric J.N. Vilain, MD, PhD.

The authors/editors listed below identified the following professional or financial affiliations for themselves or their spouse/partner:
Steve S. Kim, MD's wife is employed by and owns stock in Johnson & Johnson.
Samuel P. Robinson, MD is employed by VCUHS.
Linda D. Shortliffe, MD is on the Advisory Committee/Board of and holds stock options with Vivus.

Disclosure of Discussion of Non-FDA Approved Uses for Pharmaceutical Products and/or Medical Devices.
The University of Virginia School of Medicine, as an ACCME provider, requires that all faculty presenters identify and disclose any off-label uses for pharmaceutical and medical device products. The University of Virginia School of Medicine recommends that each physician fully review all the available data on new products or procedures prior to clinical use.

TO ENROLL

To enroll in the Urologic Clinics of North America Continuing Medical Education program, call customer service at 1-800-654-2452 or visit us online at www.theclinics.com/home/cme. The CME program is available to subscribers for an additional fee of $207.00.

Contributors

GUEST EDITOR

THOMAS F. KOLON, MD, FAAP
Pediatric Urology Fellowship Program Director,
Associate Professor, Department of Urology,
The Children's Hospital of Philadelphia,
University of Pennsylvania School of Medicine,
Philadelphia, Pennsylvania

AUTHORS

RICHARD A. ASHLEY, MD
Pediatric Urology Fellow,
Nemours/Alfred I. DuPont Hospital
for Children, Wilmington, Delaware

J. CHRISTOPHER AUSTIN, MD
Associate Professor, Division of Pediatric
Urology, Oregon Health and Sciences
University, Portland, Oregon

NATHANIEL K. BALLEK, MD
Resident, Department of Surgery,
Division of Urology, Southern Illinois
University School of Medicine,
Springfield, Illinois

JULIA S. BARTHOLD, MD
Associate Professor, Department
of Urology, Jefferson Medical College,
Philadelphia, Pennsylvania; Department
of Urology, Nemours/Alfred I. DuPont
Hospital for Children, Wilmington, Delaware

LAURENCE S. BASKIN, MD
Department of Pediatric Urology, Center
for the Study and Treatment of Hypospadias,
Parnassus Medical Center, University of
California San Francisco Children's Medical
Center, San Francisco, California

RICHARD BELLAH, MD
Radiology Attending, Director of Ultrasound
and Student Programs, Department of
Radiology, The Children's Hospital of
Philadelphia (CHOP), University of
Pennsylvania, Philadelphia, Pennsylvania

DOUGLAS A. CANNING, MD
Division of Urology, The Children's Hospital of
Philadelphia; Division of Urology, Department
of Surgery, University of Pennsylvania School
of Medicine, Philadelphia, Pennsylvania

MICHAEL C. CARR, MD, PhD
Associate Professor of Urology, Division
of Urology, University of Pennsylvania
School of Medicine; Division of Pediatric
Urology, Children's Hospital of Philadelphia,
Philadelphia, Pennsylvania

PASQUALE CASALE, MD
Director of Minimally Invasive Surgery,
Division of Pediatric Urology, Children's
Hospital of Philadelphia, Philadelphia,
Pennsylvania

CURTIS J. CLARK, MD
Pediatric Urology Fellow, Department of
Urology, Lucile Packard Children's Hospital,
Stanford University Medical Center, Stanford
University School of Medicine, Stanford,
California

CHRISTOPHER S. COOPER, MD
Professor, Department of Urology, Director
of Pediatric Urology, University of Iowa,
Iowa City, Iowa

KASSA DARGE, MD, PhD
Radiology Attending, Chief, Division of Body
Imaging, Department of Radiology, The
Children's Hospital of Philadelphia (CHOP),
University of Pennsylvania, Philadelphia,
Pennsylvania

STEVEN G. DOCIMO, MD
Division of Pediatric Urology, Department of
Urology, Children's Hospital of Pittsburgh,
University of Pittsburgh School of Medicine,
Pittsburgh, Pennsylvania

FERNANDO A. FERRER JR, MD
Associate Professor of Surgery (Urology) and
Pediatrics (Oncology), Division of Urology; Vice
Chairman, Department of Surgery, University
of Connecticut School of Medicine,
Farmington, Connecticut; Surgeon-In-Chief,
Director, Division of Pediatric Urology,
Connecticut Children's Medical Center,
Hartford, Connecticut

PATRICIO C. GARGOLLO, MD
Professor of Urology, Chief Pediatric Urology,
University of Texas Southwestern Medical
Center and Children's Medical Center,
Dallas, Texas

LANCE J. HAMPTON, MD
Assistant Professor of Surgery, Director of
Robotic Urology, Division of Urology, Virginia
Commonwealth University School of Medicine,
Richmond, Virginia

JEFFREY C. HELLINGER, MD
Radiology Attending, Director of Cardiovascular
Imaging and the 3D Laboratory, Department
of Radiology, The Children's Hospital of
Philadelphia (CHOP), University of
Pennsylvania, Philadelphia, Pennsylvania

NICOLAS KALFA, MD, PhD
Service de Chirurgie et Urologie Pédiatrique
and Service d'Hormonologie, Hôpital
Lapeyronie, CHU Montpellier and UM1, France

WILLIAM A. KENNEDY II, MD
Associate Professor of Urology, Department of
Urology, Lucile Packard Children's Hospital,
Stanford University Medical Center, Stanford
University School of Medicine; Associate Chief,
Department of Pediatric Urology, Lucile
Packard Children's Hospital, Stanford
University School of Medicine, Stanford,
California

STEVE S. KIM, MD
Fellow, Division of Urology, University of
Pennsylvania School of Medicine; Division of
Pediatric Urology, Children's Hospital of
Philadelphia, Philadelphia, Pennsylvania

THOMAS F. KOLON, MD, FAAP
Pediatric Urology Fellowship Program Director,
Associate Professor, Department of Urology,
The Children's Hospital of Philadelphia,
University of Pennsylvania School of Medicine,
Philadelphia, Pennsylvania

HARRY P. KOO, MD
Professor and Chairman of Urology, Director of
Pediatric Urology, Division of Urology, Virginia
Commonwealth University School of Medicine,
Richmond, Virginia

KATE H. KRAFT, MD
Fellow, Division of Urology, The Children's
Hospital of Philadelphia, Philadelphia,
Pennsylvania

SARAH M. LAMBERT, MD
Pediatric Urology Fellow, Children's Hospital
of Philadelphia, University of Pennsylvania
School of Medicine, Philadelphia, Pennsylvania

JOHN H. MAKARI, MD, MHA, MA
Assistant Professor of Surgery (Urology), Division
of Urology, Department of Surgery, University of
Connecticut School of Medicine, Farmington,
Connecticut; Attending Surgeon, Division of
Pediatric Urology, Connecticut Children's
Medical Center, Hartford, Connecticut

PATRICK H. MCKENNA, MD, FAAP
Professor of Surgery, Chairman and Program
Director, Department of Surgery, Division
of Urology, Southern Illinois University School
of Medicine, St John's Pavilion, Springfield,
Illinois

MICHAEL C. OST, MD
Division of Pediatric Urology, Department
of Urology, Children's Hospital of Pittsburgh,
University of Pittsburgh School of Medicine,
Pittsburgh, Pennsylvania

PUNEETA RAMACHANDRA, MD
Resident, Division of Urology, University
of Connecticut School of Medicine,
Farmington, Connecticut

WILLIAM G. REINER, MD
Professor, Pediatric Urology and Child and
Adolescent Psychiatry; Director, Psychosexual
Development Clinic; Division of Pediatric
Urology, Department of Urology, University of
Oklahoma Health Sciences Center, Oklahoma
City, Oklahoma

POOJA RENJEN, MD
Radiology Fellow, Department of
Radiology, The Children's Hospital
of Philadelphia (CHOP), Philadelphia,
Pennsylvania

SAMUEL P. ROBINSON, MD
Resident in Urology, Division of Urology,
Virginia Commonwealth University
School of Medicine, Richmond,
Virginia

AILEEN P. SCHAST, PhD
Pediatric Psychologist, Division of Urology,
The Children's Hospital of Philadelphia,
Philadelphia, Pennsylvania

LINDA D. SHORTLIFFE, MD
Professor and Chair of Urology, Department
of Urology, Lucile Packard Children's
Hospital, Stanford University Medical
Center, Stanford University School of
Medicine; Department of Pediatric
Urology, Lucile Packard Children's Hospital,
Stanford University School of Medicine,
Stanford, California

ASEEM R. SHUKLA, MD
Associate Professor, Department of
Urologic Surgery, University of Minnesota
Amplatz Children's Hospital, Minneapolis,
Minnesota

MARC C. SMALDONE, MD
Division of Pediatric Urology, Department of
Urology, Children's Hospital of Pittsburgh,
University of Pittsburgh School of Medicine,
Pittsburgh, Pennsylvania

WARREN T. SNODGRASS, MD
Professor of Urology, Chief Pediatric Urology,
Department of Urology, University of Texas
Southwestern Medical Center and Children's
Medical Center, Dallas, Texas

CHARLES SULTAN, MD, PhD
Service d'Homornologie and Unité
d'Endocrinologie Pédiatrique, Hôpital
Lapeyronie - Arnaud de Villeneuve, CHU
Montpellier and UM1, Montpellier, France

ERIC J.N. VILAIN, MD, PhD
Professor of Human Genetics, Pediatrics,
Urology, David Geffen School of Medicine at
UCLA, Los Angeles, California

Contents

Antenatal sonography has markedly increased the detection of urogenital anomalies, including those conditions that lead to significant morbidity and mortality. Prenatal intervention is feasible to arrest and sometimes reverse the sequelae of
bladder outlet obstruction but not necessarily renal damage. Myelomeningoceles,
the most severe form of spina bifida, can be corrected in utero, with improvements
in hydrocephalus seen along with a decreased incidence of ventricular shunting
postnatally. Medical therapy to prevent virilization associated with congenital adrenal hyperplasia has been successful, with improved ability to detect its presence
prenatally now possible. As further techniques evolve to correct underlying disease
processes, it becomes important to critically assess the therapies, particularly with
long-term outcome data.

Hypospadias is one of the most common congenital defects in humans. The molecular events required in the genitourinary tract for normal development of the external
genitalia are just beginning to be elucidated. Identifying the cause of hypospadias
may be relevant not only in the field of pediatric urology, but also for worldwide public health. This article discusses the possible causes of hypospadias and the genes
and growth factors involved. The potential effects of genetic susceptibility and environmental pollutants are also discussed.

Hypospadias results from abnormal development of the penis that leaves the urethral meatus proximal to its normal glanular position anywhere along the penile shaft,
scrotum, or perineum. A spectrum of abnormalities, including ventral curvature of
the penis (chordee), a hooded incomplete prepuce, and an abortive corpora spongiosum, are commonly associated with hypospadias. Advances in understanding of
the causes of hypospadias and current approaches to the correction of hypospadias
to provide a cosmetically and functionally satisfactory repair are the focus of this
article.

Cryptorchidism is a common genital anomaly diagnosed at birth or during childhood.
Genetic and/or environmental factors that alter expression or function of hormones
crucial for testicular descent, insulin-like 3, and testosterone, may contribute to
cryptorchidism. When identified at birth, surgical treatment is indicated by 6 months
of age if testes fail to descend, or at the time of diagnosis in older children.

A laparoscopic approach is preferred for abdominal testes. Early surgical therapy may reduce the risk of subfertility and/or malignancy.

The evaluation and management of neonates with ambiguous genitalia requires sensitivity, efficiency, and accuracy. The approach to these neonates is facilitated by a multidisciplinary team including urology, endocrinology, genetics, and psychiatry or psychology. Disorders of sex development (DSD) encompass chromosomal DSD, 46,XX DSD, and 46,XY DSD. The 46,XX DSD is the most common DSD and in the majority of these children congenital adrenal hyperplasia is the underlying etiology. The 46,XY DSD is a heterogeneous disorder that often results from a disruption in the production or response to testosterone, dihydrotestosterone, or Mullerian inhibitory substance. Chromosomal DSD includes conditions resulting from abnormal meiosis, including Klinefelter syndrome (47, XXY) and Turner syndrome. The evaluation of children with DSD demands a thorough physical examination, medical history, karyotype, metabolic panel, 17-OH progesterone, testosterone, luteinizing hormone, follicle stimulation hormone, and urinalysis. A radiographic evaluation should begin with an abdominal and pelvic ultrasound but may include magnetic resonance imaging, endoscopy, or laparoscopy.

Initial care of newborns with spina bifida centers on preventing bladder and upper tract damage from detrusor leak point pressure of greater than 40cm H_2O. The authors recommend using urodynamic-based management to select patients with elevated pressures for anticholinergic therapy and intermittent catheterization (CIC), using diapers and observation with biannual renal sonography for the remainder. At the age of toilet training, children who have urodynamic evidence of uninhibited contractions or rising pressure during filling are started on anticholinergics and CIC, or have their dosage increased until pressures less than 40cm H_2O and areflexia are achieved. Sphincter incompetency is diagnosed in incontinent children with pressures less than 40 cm H_2O and areflexia or stress incontinence. Augmentation is indicated in patients with hydronephrosis or reflux and end-filling pressures or DLPP less than 40cm H_2O despite medical management to the point of patient tolerance. A minority of patients, not yet well-defined, will also need augmentation after bladder outlet surgery for similar postoperative indications.

Lower urinary tract syndrome is common in children. Incontinence, urinary tract infection, vesicoureteral reflux, and constipation are commonly associated with this syndrome. Examining the clinical history of the afflicted patient plays a major role in the accurate diagnosis and treatment of lower urinary tract disorder. Along with pharmacologic treatment, pelvic floor muscle retraining, biofeedback therapy, and adaptation of a healthy lifestyle are advocated for rapid recovery of patients.

Urinary tract infection (UTI) is a frequent diagnosis in children who are referred to the urologist. Although most infections will resolve without complication after appropriate treatment, a wide array of potential complicating factors exists, which can make difficult the rapid resolution of a UTI. Clinical scenarios involving these factors require a high index of suspicion and prompt initiation of appropriate therapy.

There has been an emergence of a therapeutic nihilistic attitude about the surgical treatment of vesicoureteral reflux (VUR). Evidence-based reviews have questioned whether surgical treatment is beneficial for children with VUR. Even the use of pro-phylactic antibiotics, which have traditionally been the first-line therapy recommen-ded for virtually all patients with VUR, has come under scrutiny after several randomized controlled trials found them to have no effect on decreasing the risk of urinary tract infections (UTIs) in children with VUR. Grade is the strongest predic-tor of VUR resolution, with high-grade VUR being much less likely to resolve. Other factors that negatively influence resolution include lower bladder volume or pressure at onset of reflux, older age, female sex, bilateral VUR, ureteral duplication, abnormal or scarred kidneys, and bladder dysfunction. These factors can be used, along with grade, in computer models or nomograms to improve the ability to predict sponta-neous resolution.

With miniaturization of instruments and refinement of surgical technique, the man-agement of pediatric stone disease has undergone a dramatic evolution. While shock wave lithotripsy (SWL) is still commonly used to treat upper tract calculi, the use of ureteroscopy (URS) has dramatically increased and is now the proce-dure of choice for upper tract stone burdens less than 1.5cm at centers with sig-nificant experience. Percutaneous nephrolithotomy (PCNL) has replaced open surgical techniques for the treatment of large stone burdens greater than 2 cm, with efficacy and complication rates similar to the adult population. Large institu-tional series demonstrate comparable stone-free and complication rates with SWL, URS, and PCNL, but concerns remain with these techniques regarding renal development and damage to the pediatric urinary tract. Randomized controlled tri-als comparing the efficacy of SWL and URS for upper tract stone burdens are needed to reach consensus regarding the most effective primary treatment modal-ity in children.

A varicocele is a dilatation of the testicular vein and the pampiniform venous plexus within the spermatic cord. Although rare in pediatric populations, the prevalence of varicoceles markedly increases with pubertal development. Varicoceles are pro-gressive lesions that may hinder testicular growth and function over time and are the most common and correctable cause of male infertility. Approximately 40% of men with primary infertility have a varicocele, and more than half of them experience improvements in semen parameters after varicocelectomy. The decision to treat ad-olescents with varicocele is a controversial one. The task for pediatricians and urol-ogists is to identify those adolescents who are at greatest risk for infertility in adulthood, in an effort to offer early surgical intervention to those most likely to benefit.

Urologic Clinics of North America

THE CLINICS ARE NOW AVAILABLE ONLINE!

Access your subscription at:
www.theclinics.com

Preface

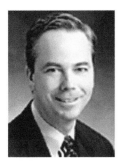

Thomas F. Kolon, MD
Guest Editor

There have been many great advances that have occurred in pediatric urology since the *Urologic Clinics of North America* addressed this topic in 2004. The authors in this issue update readers on the latest research findings and treatment controversies while covering a broad spectrum of topics. It is as equally important for urologists to be knowledgeable of severe bilateral hydronephrosis for an in-depth prenatal visit as they are of daytime wetting. As editor, I am deeply indebted to the distinguished authors, all experts in their fields, who have contributed articles to this undertaking. Any success that this volume may achieve is directly related to their efforts and expertise.

This group of exemplary authors takes us on a journey from the prenatal evaluation and treatment of the hydronephrotic fetus to the most recent recommendations for pediatric urologic oncology. The prenatal/postnatal management of urologic problems includes the latest microinvasive techniques for hydronephrosis, myelomeningocele, and disorders of sex development. Each author provides an insightful approach to the diagnosis of these problems along with state-of-the-art treatment plans that can be practiced by any urologist in a private or academic setting.

Hypospadias and cryptorchidism, the bread and butter of pediatric urology, are updated with discussions of new molecular findings and surgical techniques. The adolescent varicocele is a topic that remains fluid and seems to require a slightly different approach from that for infertility patients seen as adults. How should urologists handle the continually vexing problem of an unstable pediatric bladder? Three sets of authors provide insight into voiding and bowel dysfunction, urinary tract infections, and vesicoureteral reflux. Each year these topics seem to become more complex and harder to treat than in the previous year.

The present and future of internal urologic surgery involves a journey through minimally invasive stone surgery, laparoscopy, and robotics. Oncology is one section of pediatric urology that can be extremely rewarding and terribly discouraging. Articles explore the possibilities and indications for organ-sparing renal and testicular surgery. As a reflection of the most current and relevant topics in pediatric urology, 2 articles address psychology and radiology and how their latest advances are helping to treat urologic patients.

All of the authors deserve hearty thanks for their thoughtful and prompt submissions. I would like to thank my assistant Sharon Brown as well as Kerry Holland and her staff at Elsevier Science for their ever-cheerful, invaluable assistance. I sincerely hope that this issue of *Urologic Clinics of North America* is helpful in daily pediatric urology management and continues the fine tradition of education that this series has provided. As pediatric urologists, we continue to be grateful that the talents that we have received allow us to improve the lives of our patients and their families.

Thomas F. Kolon, MD
Children's Hospital of Philadelphia
Division of Pediatric Urology
39th Street and Civic Center Boulevard
Philadelphia, PA 19104, USA

E-mail address:
KOLON@email.chop.edu

Prenatal Management of Urogenital Disorders

Michael C. Carr, MD, PhD[a,b,*], Steve S. Kim, MD[a,b]

KEYWORDS

- Urogenital disorders • Fetal LUTO
- Prenatal management • Congenital adrenal hyperplasia

With the advent of maternal-fetal screening ultrasonography in the mid-1980s, the ability to identify a variety of congenital anomalies in utero has provided not only an early glimpse into the developmental window of several devastating congenital conditions but also the tantalizing opportunity to intervene at a time that may dramatically alter the long-term prognosis and outcomes. It is estimated that a structural fetal anomaly is detected by antenatal sonography in 1% of all screened pregnancies.[1] Of these anomalies, a fifth are believed to be manifestations of genitourinary origin, second only to those found within the central nervous system. Depending on the sonographic criteria used, anomalies of the genitourinary tract are believed to occur as frequently as 1 out of every 100 pregnancies, with hydronephrosis being the most common finding detected.[2,3]

As prenatal management has evolved, many questions have emerged regarding not only the indications for therapeutic interventions, but more importantly the relative merits of fetal intervention. In this review, the authors provide a historical background of the development of fetal therapeutic interventions and an overview of current fetal interventions for antenatally diagnosed genitourinary tract disorders.

THE DEVELOPMENT OF FETAL INTERVENTION

Significant advances in the past quarter century have moved the concept of therapeutic fetal intervention into the realm of not just what is possible, but even what may be considered by some, routine.

To meet the evolving needs of families facing the dilemma of a fetus diagnosed with a significant structural anomaly, several institutions have established specialized centers dedicated to the comprehensive diagnosis and treatment of fetal anomalies. Today's multidisciplinary team approach to fetal care often includes dedicated providers representing maternal-fetal medicine, pediatric anesthesia, pediatric surgery, pediatric radiology, pediatric urology, and pediatric nursing.

The earliest examples of modern fetal therapeutic intervention included the use of transfusions for erythroblastosis fetalis, the pharmacologic management of fetal cardiac arrhythmias, and the percutaneous drainage of fetal hydrothorax.[4–7] The correction of more complex anatomic defects such as congenital diaphragmatic hernias followed soon after, necessitating the move to the more invasive techniques of direct exposure via hysterotomy and open fetal surgical repair.[8–11]

Early pioneers of open fetal surgery faced several technical and ethical challenges regarding the maternal and fetal risks posed by open fetal surgery using midgestational hysterotomy. The group from the University of California San Francisco (UCSF) proposed the following prerequisites for undertaking open fetal surgery: (1) the natural history of the disease in question must be thoroughly established by careful examination of untreated cases; (2) a strict selection criteria must be developed identifying appropriate candidates for fetal intervention; (3) the pathophysiology and potential benefits of fetal intervention must first be

[a] Division of Urology, University of Pennsylvania School of Medicine, Philadelphia, PA, USA
[b] Division of Pediatric Urology, Children's Hospital of Philadelphia, 34th Street & Civic Center Boulevard, 3rd Floor, Wood Building, Philadelphia, PA 19104-4399, USA
* Corresponding author. Division of Pediatric Urology, Children's Hospital of Philadelphia, 34th Street & Civic Center Boulevard, 3rd Floor, Wood Building, Philadelphia, PA 19104-4399.
E-mail address: carr@email.chop.edu

Urol Clin N Am 37 (2010) 149–158
doi:10.1016/j.ucl.2010.03.015

demonstrated in appropriate animal models; and (4) hysterotomy and open fetal surgery must be accomplished without undue risk to the mother and her future reproductive potential.[11]

The early results of fetal therapy from UCSF included the initial experience with 17 patients who had 1 of 4 indications: (1) bilateral hydronephrosis with presumed lower urinary tract obstruction (LUTO, n = 7); (2) congenital diaphragmatic hernia (CDH, n = 8); (3) sacrococcygeal teratoma (SCT, n = 1); and (4) congenital cystic adenomatoid malformation (CCAM, n = 1). Of the 7 patients with suspected LUTO, 2 died at shortly after birth as a result of complications related to pulmonary hypoplasia, 1 died of septicemia with normal renal function within the first year of life, and 2 were alive at follow-up, although 1 child had manifested renal deterioration. One fetus was removed because of inadequate repair of a coexisting cloacal anomaly and 1 was delivered 12 days following repair when the mother opted to discontinue tocolytics. These early mixed results reinforced the notion that anomalies that may be amenable to correction by hysterotomy and open fetal repair should only be repaired in the context of an acceptable level of risk posed to the mother's health and future reproductive potential. To this end, concerns about maternal risk focused on 3 main areas: (1) the operative risk of general anesthesia and a midgestational hysterotomy; (2) the risk of premature labor following hysterotomy; and (3) the risk of compromising future maternal reproductive potential.[11] The biggest challenge of the early era of fetal surgery was the ability to manage uterine contractions and premature labor following hysterotomy. Despite tocolytic therapy, all mothers developed preterm labor ranging from 25 to 35 week's gestation. In addition, those women who underwent successful hysterotomy and fetal intervention were subsequently committed to delivering by cesarean section, essentially undergoing 2 hysterotomies during the course of a single pregnancy. The fetal therapy team at UCSF cautioned that simply because these procedures were technically feasible did not mean that they should be performed. They further added that it is critical to vigorously examine the efficacy, safety, and cost-effectiveness of fetal therapy compared with conventional conservative treatment. Even as the overall techniques of fetal surgery have improved, these early sentiments are still true today in evaluating the appropriateness of fetal intervention.

ANTENATAL HYDRONEPHROSIS/LUTO

Of the approximately 1% of screened pregnancies that are found to have a genitourinary tract anomaly,

more than 50% represent a diagnosis of antenatal hydronephrosis, making it 1 of the most common fetal anomalies detected.[12] Although antenatal hydronephrosis frequently amounts to little in the way of clinical significance in most cases, it is important to identify the small subset of fetuses that present with a significant LUTO and are at risk for significant postnatal morbidity and mortality.

The identification of antenatal hydronephrosis is made on screening ultrasonography by the demonstration of renal pelvic and calyceal dilatation. Antenatal hydronephrosis does not reflect a singular diagnosis, but rather the clinical manifestation of a heterogeneous group of pathologic and physiologic entities that lead to the appearance of urinary tract dilatation. Potential causes include physiologic dilatation, vesicoureteral reflux, anomalies of the ureteropelvic or ureterovesical junction, primary obstructed megaureters, multicystic dysplastic kidneys, ureteral ectopia, posterior urethral valves, prune-belly syndrome, urethral atresia, and cloacal anomalies.[13] The following list provides a differential diagnosis for the fetus with antenatal hydronephrosis[14]

Anomalous ureteropelvic junction/ureterovesical junction obstruction
Multicystic kidney
Primary obstructive megaureter
Vesicoureteral reflux (bladder may be distended)
Ectopic ureterocele (bladder may be distended)
Ectopic ureter
Physiologic dilatation
Posterior urethral valves (bladder may be distended)
Prune-belly syndrome (bladder may be distended)
Urethral atresia (bladder may be distended)
Hydrocolpos (bladder may be distended)
Pelvic tumor (bladder may be distended)
Cloacal anomaly (bladder may be distended).

Technical issues that may affect the identification of hydronephrosis antenatally include the operator-dependent nature of ultrasonography and the timing of the study with respect to gestational age. Typically, the ability to detect urinary tract dilatation is better later in gestational age because the fetus is not only larger but significant obstructive anomalies are also more readily appreciated with progressive dilatation.[15] The severity of hydronephrosis and the point at which it occurs in gestation may help indicate the likelihood for urinary obstruction and subsequent need for surgical intervention.[16]

Once hydronephrosis has been recognized, management consists of distinguishing clinically significant urinary tract obstruction that poses an imminent risk to the fetus from conditions that may be addressed in the postnatal period. In helping to make this assessment, consideration should be given to the presence of bilateral hydronephrosis, coexisting ureteral and bladder distention, hydronephrosis onset, and the timing and severity of oligohydramnios.

The presence of unilateral hydronephrosis typically requires no specific interventions during the prenatal period beyond close serial imaging. Bilateral hydronephrosis, on the other hand, can be present in the context of clinically significant urinary tract obstruction such as posterior urethral valves or urethral atresia, as well as in nonobstructing entities such as prune-belly syndrome or high-grade vesicoureteral reflux.[17,18] The development of in utero ureteropelvic junction obstruction may compromise renal function depending on timing and severity, but the neonatal kidney often retains a tremendous capacity for improvement following postnatal pyeloplasty.[19] Even in the case of bilateral in utero ureteropelvic junction obstruction, rarely will amniotic fluid volumes be compromised to a degree that would raise concern for the development of pulmonary hypoplasia. The same is true for primary obstructed megaureters. Thus, fetal interventions such as percutaneous drainage of the fetal kidney or early delivery for immediate urologic surgery in these cases are not warranted.

The ominous constellation of bladder distention, impaired bladder emptying, bilateral hydroureteronephrosis, and oligohydramnios represents a significant LUTO that often results in fetal morbidity and mortality. LUTO is predominately associated with male fetuses that are most commonly diagnosed with either posterior urethral valves or urethral atresia. Other causes include prune-belly syndrome, anterior urethral valves, congenital urethral hypoplasia, prolapsing ureteroceles, and cloacal plate anomalies in females. Variable degrees of renal impairment, reduction in amniotic fluid, and subsequent development of pulmonary hypoplasia can be seen depending on the severity and duration of urinary tract obstruction. Progressive renal deterioration manifests as the appearance of fibrous echogenic kidneys and cystic degeneration of fetal kidneys. Animal models support the hypothesis that renal fibrocystic dysplasia occurs in the presence of midgestational urinary tract obstruction as opposed to later in gestation. In humans, the onset of midgestational (second trimester) oligohydramnios is suspected to lead to the development of renal

dysplasia. The resulting reduction in production of amniotic fluid leads to the development of either oligohydramnios, or in the extreme setting, anhydramnios. Reduced amniotic fluid volumes are associated with the development of pulmonary hypoplasia,[20] which represents the leading cause of perinatal mortality in cases of LUTO. Complete obstruction, as seen in urethral atresia, is nearly always fatal because of pulmonary hypoplasia. Prune-belly syndrome, although generally considered nonobstructive in nature, can also lead to the development of renal insufficiency postnatally.

INDICATIONS FOR PRENATAL THERAPY

Over the years, criteria have been established to identify which fetuses with LUTO would benefit from prenatal intervention. The goals were to exclude patients who were unlikely to benefit from therapeutic intervention based on the coexistence of other significant chromosomal or structural anomalies and/or advanced renal fibrocystic dysplasia that would preclude measurable improvement. The selection of candidates for fetal intervention typically includes (1) a fetal karyotype to exclude chromosomal abnormalities, (2) an ultrasound to detect other structural anomalies that may adversely affect prognosis, and (3) serial fetal urine analyses to assess the extent of renal impairment. Reported unfavorable prognostic risk factors include (1) prolonged oligohydramnios,[21,22] (2) presence of renal cortical cysts,[23] (3) urinary sodium level greater than or equal to 100 mEq/L, chloride level more than 90 mEq/L, osmolarity more than 210 mmol/L and increased urinary β2-microglobulin level (>6 mg/L),[24–27] and (4) reduced lung area and/or thoracoabdominal circumference.[28]

More recently, 2 systematic reviews have been conducted evaluating the existing literature on the accuracy of fetal urine analysis and antenatal ultrasonography in predicting poor postnatal renal function. Both reviews are limited by the poor methodological quality of studies available. None of the fetal urine analytes examined yielded clinically significant accuracy in predicting poor postnatal renal function. The 2 most accurate parameters were calcium level greater than 95th percentile for gestation (likelihood ratio [LR]+ 6.65 [0.23,190.96], LR− 0.19 [0.05,0.74]) and sodium level greater than 95th percentile for gestation (LR+ 4.46 [1.71,11.6]; LR− 0.39 [0.17,0.88]).[29] With respect to ultrasonographic findings, the second systematic review and meta-analysis showed that abnormal renal cortical appearance (as defined as echogenicity and/or cystic changes) showed the best predictive accuracy (sensitivity of 0.57 [0.37,0.76], specificity of 0.84 [0.71,0.94], AUC of 0.78, and LR+ 1.29–9.10). The LR+ for severe oligohydramnios was moderately useful ranging from 3.63 to 7.00.[30] Both of these reviews highlight the current limitations in the evidence available to support fetal intervention for LUTO.

THERAPEUTIC OPTIONS

Prenatal management of significant LUTO that compromises renal function and fetal urine production is predicated on establishing adequate drainage between the fetal bladder and the surrounding amniotic space.[31] To date, the mainstay for fetal intervention for LUTO has involved urinary diversion via the placement of a vesicoamniotic shunt. Alternative techniques include open fetal surgery with fetal vesicostomy and/or pyelostomy, or endoscopic management with direct in utero valve ablation using fetal cystoscopy.[32,33] The benefits of the latter would be avoiding the high complication rates of vesicoamniotic shunting and allowing the bladder to cycle and resume some semblance of normal development.

VESICOAMNIOTIC SHUNTING
Technical Considerations

Vesicoamniotic shunting is performed by placement of a specialized double pigtail shunt (Rocket Medical, Washington, UK and Cook Urological, Spencer, IN, USA) under ultrasound guidance between a distended fetal bladder and the surrounding amniotic space (**Fig. 1**). Color-flow Doppler allows visualization of the umbilical arteries, which course laterally to the fetal bladder. Amnioinfusion is performed in the setting of oligohydramnios to allow for a potential space into which the intra-amniotic end of the catheter may be placed. Technical considerations involve low placement of the shunt into the bladder to prevent displacement following bladder decompression. The optimal site for trocar entry is midway between the pubic ramus and the insertion of the umbilical cord.

Outcomes

To date, several small series have reported the initial experience with vesicoamniotic shunting, which is summarized in **Table 1**. Overall perinatal survival following shunt placement was 47% and shunt-related complications occurred in 45% of cases. End-stage renal disease developed in 54% of cases[34] and 56% of fetuses with oligohydramnios did not survive. Failure to restore amniotic fluid volume was associated with 100% mortality. In cases with poor urinary prognosis, postnatal renal insufficiency developed in 87.5% of survivors, and when intervention did improve the chances of survival, it did not substantively alter renal outcomes. Improved survival and lower rates of renal failure are seen by limiting the intervention to only those fetuses with good prognostic parameters.[35] Crombleholme, and colleagues[24] and Freedman and colleagues[36] evaluated outcomes based on prognosis as determined by fetal urine biochemistry. Fetuses with oligohydramnios were separated into those with dysplasia and those with normal renal function. Poor renal function was confirmed in 14 to 16 cases (88%), which were successfully shunted, indicating that diversion rarely preserves/ameliorates function in this subset. In other words, the underlying dysplasia is not reversed with successful intervention. In contrast, 85% of survivors with a good prognosis did have normal renal function. When amniotic fluid returned to normal, pulmonary function was preserved as has been demonstrated in animal studies.[35]

Complications

The early experience with vesicoamniotic shunting was associated with significant complications including shunt blockage, shunt migration, preterm labor, urinary ascites, chorioamnionitis and iatrogenic gastroschisis.[37] In addition, there

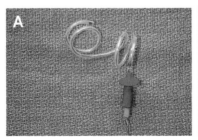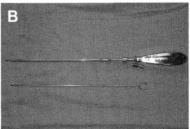

Fig. 1. Double pigtail fetal bladder drainage catheter: (*A*) used through a trocar; (*B*) placed percutaneously using color-flow Doppler imaging.

Table 1
Reports of vesicoamniotic shunts

Author	Number of Patients	Number of Survivors	Oligohydramnios	Normal Renal Function
Elder et al[25]	21	9	9	1 (11)
Crombleholme et al[24]	19	12	17	7 (58)
Manning et al[55]	87	35	69	16 (59)
Lipitz et al[27]	124	6	13	0
Freedman et al[36]	28	17	28	12 (70)
Holmes et al[40]	14	8	14	3 (37)

are times when shunting is not technically possible or is associated with significant procedural complications.[34] The fetal surgery registry documented that only 10% of shunts were placed successfully in various centers during the 1980s. The most significant maternal complication of percutaneous intervention was infection. Maternal life-threatening infections associated with fetal loss were reported in 3/159 cases.[35] Quintero, and colleagues[38] reported on at least 7 intrauterine deaths believed to be caused by shunt placement.

Mechanical complications include shunt displacement from the fetal bladder. This is often caused by a fetal extremity becoming entangled in the distal intra-amniotic segment of the shunt, with subsequent physical displacement of the proximal end out of the fetal bladder. This can result in significant urinary ascites as urine flows through the iatrogenic defect in the bladder wall. This can occasionally lead to massive fetal abdominal distention, diaphragmatic elevation, intra-abdominal and intrathoracic hemodynamic changes and even the subsequent development of hydrops. Shunts may occasionally have to be placed in the fetal abdomen to drain urinary ascites until the defect in the bladder wall heals. Ultimately, reshunting may be necessary when the defect is healed.[35]

FETAL CYSTOSCOPY

The approach of direct valve ablation in the case of posterior urethral valves can potentially obviate many of the complications encountered with vesicoamniotic shunt placement and theoretically restore the concept of normal bladder cycling. In addition, the direct visualization provided by fetal cystoscopy allows for diagnostic confirmation of valves as the cause of significant LUTO. This technique was first described by Quintero and colleagues[38] in the management of fetal obstructive uropathy under maternal general anesthesia.

The indications are similar to those for vesicoamniotic shunting with a midgestation pregnancy during 17 to 20 weeks described as being optimal.

Technical Considerations

Fetal cystoscopy is best performed jointly by the fetal medicine and urologic teams. The fetal cystoscope is introduced via a 14 gauge trocar and cannula through the maternal abdomen, uterus and fetal abdomen into the fetal bladder under ultrasound guidance and antibiotic coverage following local anesthetic infiltration.[35]

As opposed to shunt placement, the fetoscope needs to enter the bladder via the dome so that it can be directed downward in a straight line with the urethra. Color-flow Doppler is, once again, helpful in delineating vascular structures. The semi-rigid fetoscope that is currently used has a 1.3-mm outer diameter and a 1-mm lens diameter with a 0° and 70° field of view (Karl Storz, Ltd, Tuttlinger, Germany). On entry into the fetal bladder, aspirated urine is sent for electrolyte analysis and inspection performed to note presence of bladder trabeculation and hemorrhage. The fetoscope is carefully advanced into the prostatic urethra following visualization of the trigone and bladder neck to appreciate the site of obstruction. Posterior urethral valves appear as a membrane arising from the verumontanum. Once the presence of posterior urethral valve has been confirmed, laser ablation using a 400- to 600-μm yttrium-aluminum-garnet laser fiber, in which 30 to 40 W of successive 0 to 2 second pulses are used to ablate the valves.[39] Direct contact with the valves achieves a more intense effect in a smaller zone of tissue to only ablate the valves and no surrounding tissue. Other techniques that have been experimented with include saline injection to disrupt the membranous valves or insertion of guidewire through the valves to mechanically disrupt them.

Successful ablation can be documented by placing the color Doppler probe over the amniotic cavity and injecting fluid into the bladder; a color Doppler signal seen in the amniotic space indicates successful ablation.

Outcome

The initial series that reported by Quintero and colleagues[38] included 9 fetuses who underwent fetal cystoscopy and laser ablation of posterior urethral valves. Urethral patency was found in only 4 of the 9 cases. Of those with a patent urethra, 2 were viable at birth, 1 had progressive renal damage and was aborted, and 2 were lost to chorioamnionitis. The 2 successful cases ultimately had neonatal demise, 1 at 4 months of age for bronchopneumonia; the second died at 3 months of age from necrotizing enterocolitis.

Agarwal and colleagues[35] reported on 11 fetuses between 16 and 24 weeks's gestation who had fetal cystoscopy. There were no immediate or long-term iatrogenic complications from the procedure. Five of the 11 cases did develop postprocedural urinary ascites that was managed conservatively. Seven out of 11 cases were for diagnosis only with the remainder undergoing therapeutic intervention with either hydroablation (n = 1) or guidewire technique (n = 3). Complete valve ablation was successful once. Two were felt to be partial successes (increase in amniotic fluid volume and decrease in bilateral hydroureteronephrosis during pregnancy) but did require retreatment postnatally. Three of 4 infants had acceptable renal function.

The investigators found the main challenge was in gaining access to the posterior urethra with the cystoscope. This vesicourethral angle can be difficult to negotiate and becomes more acute with advancing gestation. Even if the posterior urethra is entered, valves may not always be visualized. This certainly limits the usefulness of the procedure. Further refinements of the fetoscopes, such as a curved trocar or flexible cystoscope are currently being evaluated.

FUTURE DIRECTIONS

Current practice supports fetal intervention in a male fetus with suspected LUTO, good renal prognosis, and oligohydramnios. The effectiveness of such interventions has been called into question with respect to long-term outcomes. In a series of fetal patients with posterior urethral valves from UCSF, 36 patients with favorable electrolytes and oligohydramnios were treated by 1 of 3 methods in an 18-year period. Of these patients, only 14 (39%) were confirmed to have had posterior urethral valves and only 8 of these (57%) survived. Five of the survivors (63%) developed chronic renal impairment and an equal number required urinary diversion/reconstructive procedures.[40] This would imply that intervention may facilitate a viable infant at birth, but the sequelae of posterior urethral valves has not been reversed. Similar findings were seen in the long-term follow-up of fetal interventions from the combined experience at the Children's Hospital of Philadelphia and the Detroit Medical Center. Although 1-year survival was reported to be 91% (21/23 patients), one-third of patients went on to require either dialysis or renal transplantation. In 2003, a systematic review and meta-analysis by Clark and colleagues[41] reviewed the literature on the effect of prenatal shunting versus conservative management on the primary outcome of perinatal survival. Among the few observational controlled studies that met the inclusion criteria, the pooled estimate of effect suggested an improvement in perinatal survival in the prenatal shunting group (odds ratio [OR] 2.5; 95% confidence interval [CI] 1.1,5.9). However, subgroup analysis revealed that this apparent benefit is largely driven by improvement in those fetuses who were categorized as poor prognosis (OR 8.1; 95% CI 1.2,52.9). Slight trends toward improved perinatal survival in good prognosis subjects was suggested by the meta-analysis (OR 2.8; 95% CI 0.7,10.8). Much like the aforementioned meta-analyses evaluating predictors of postnatal renal function, this meta-analysis also suffered from poor quality studies and significant biases.

As a result of the clear lack of evidence to support fetal intervention for LUTO, a multicenter, randomized controlled trial, the Percutaneous shunting in Lower Urinary Tract Obstruction (PLUTO) trial, is currently underway to assess the benefits and harms of prenatal vesicoamniotic shunting versus conservative therapy on renal outcomes.[42] In addition, the North American Fetal Therapy Network (NAFTNet) is conducting an observational cohort study to collect information on renal, bladder, and pulmonary outcomes in fetuses with lower urinary tract obstruction and normal amniotic fluid volumes.[43] The results of these studies are eagerly awaited in the hope that they will provide the necessary information to better inform decisions on if and when fetal interventions for LUTO are merited.

FETAL MYELOMENINGOCELE REPAIR

The success of dealing with potentially lethal conditions in utero has opened the door for correction of disorders that are not lethal, but cause considerable morbidity. In particular, myelomeningocele is the most common and severe form of spina bifida. This condition affects nearly 1 in 2000 infants born alive. In addition to varying degrees of paralysis, individuals with myelomeningocele are often limited by mental retardation, bowel and bladder dysfunction, and orthopedic disabilities. Hydrocephalus, Arnold-Chiari II malformations, and spinal cord tethering at the site of surgical repair all lead to significant morbidity and mortality. Management of these individuals has previously involved termination of pregnancy following diagnosis or postnatal closure and a lifetime of supportive care.

Experimental work in various animal models proved that the fetal closure of the myelomeningocele can arrest the ongoing damage to the spinal cord as it is exposed to the amniotic fluid. This could potentially preserve function to lower extremities and bowel and bladder. What became apparent with the early experience of human fetal myelomeningocele closure is that the Arnold-Chiari malformation and progressive hydrocephalous are arrested. Thus, given the significant risk of prenatal intervention, the Center for Fetal Diagnosis and Treatment at Children's Hospital of Philadelphia offers this treatment with selected patients who meet strict criteria. The fetus must have an Arnold-Chiari malformation, mild or moderate ventriculomegaly, normal leg movement, no apparent clubbing of the feet, normal karyotype, and no accompanying lethal anomalies. By limiting intervention to those with the Arnold-Chiari malformation, the infants most likely to suffer from hydrocephalus or life-threatening brain stem symptoms and to require frequent postnatal surgical intervention are being offered therapy. The spinal defect is closed between 21 and 25 weeks's gestation, using techniques similar to those of postnatal repair.[44]

The early experience with such a repair demonstrated the arrest of hind brain herniation, decreasing the need for ventricular shunting that was necessary with the Arnold-Chiari II malformation and hydrocephalus.[45,46] This exciting finding requires long-term follow-up to determine whether neurologic function is improved. In addition, the incidence of clubbed feet and other orthopedic anomalies is expected to diminish, thus reducing the need for future surgical intervention.

Bowel and bladder function, which remain lifetime management issues, may be improved with successful in utero repair of the myelomeningocele. To date, Vanderbilt and UCSF have reported on the early urodynamic findings in this group of patients.[47,48] There have not as yet been significant alterations in bladder function as noted with neonatal urodynamic testing. These patients may have had their closure performed at a time when arrest of the progressive spinal cord injury could not have been prevented (beyond 25 weeks's gestation). In addition, assessing bladder function solely on 1 early urodynamic study may be unfounded. Recent work from Sillen and colleagues[49] have shown a changing urodynamic pattern in healthy infants, premature infants,[50] and even toddlers.[51] Preterm infants' voiding pattern is characterized by an increased number of interrupted voidings caused by the immature behavior of the detrusor-sphincter complex. The high number of voidings during sleep underscore the immature pattern for preterm infants. Healthy full term infants void an average of 1 time per hour but generally less than 10% of bladder capacity remaining as mean residual urine. They still manifest an interrupted voiding in which complete voiding consists of 2 or 3 small voidings with an empty bladder only after the final voiding. By age 2 years, the interrupted voiding pattern becomes rare. Voiding during sleep occurs mainly during the first 7 months of life but is rarely seen after 18 months. It will be mandatory to follow these children through their potty training years to understand the effects of the surgery.

A multicenter, prospective, randomized clinical trial, the Management of Myelomeningocele Study (MOMS) trial, was initiated by the National Institute of Child Health and Human Development (NICHD) in 2003 to assess the efficacy of intrauterine repair of fetal myelomeningocele at 19 to 25 weeks on the outcomes of death and need for ventriculoperitoneal shunting by 1 year of life. The study is currently being conducted at the Children's Hospital of Philadelphia, Vanderbilt, and UCSF. Appropriate candidates who met study inclusion criteria were randomized to either fetal repair before 26 weeks's gestation or standard postnatal repair. A total of 100 cases and 100 controls were planned to be recruited and as of early 2009, approximately 150 subjects have been enrolled.

Secondary end points include the development of Arnold-Chiari malformation, neonatal morbidity and mortality, long-term neurologic function, maternal morbidity, and cost. Other important variables being assessed include locomotion, distal somatosensory function, bowel and bladder continence, and the need for subsequent surgical procedures. Currently, a supplemental grant is being proposed to follow these patients for at least 5 years to more accurately assess bowel and bladder issues. As with the PLUTO trial, we eagerly await the results of the MOMS trial to better define the role of intrauterine repair of myelomeningoceles and its overall effect on urinary tract function.

CONGENITAL ADRENAL HYPERPLASIA

A female with congenital adrenal hyperplasia often presents with ambiguous genitalia in the newborn period, with some infants developing life-threatening adrenal insufficiency. The most common enzyme defect is 21-hydroxylase deficiency, resulting in excessive levels of 17-hydroxy progesterone in the amniotic fluid. If the condition is recognized in utero, prenatal therapy can be instituted that will prevent the virilization of the female fetus by adrenal suppression. Appropriate therapy involves the use of dexamethasone given daily to the expectant mother.[52] Because the masculinization occurs early in the first trimester, the therapy needs to be instituted before the gender of the fetus is even known (6–8 weeks's gestation). Subsequent chorionic villous sampling can be safely performed at 9–12 weeks's gestation, so that appropriate measurements of amniotic fluid and now direct DNA analysis of the 21-hydroxylase gene (CYP21) with molecular genetic techniques are performed. Once confirmed, the steroid treatment is then continued for the duration of the pregnancy. If it is found that the fetus is an unaffected male or female, the maternal dexamethasone is discontinued. Although ultimately needed in only 1/8 fetuses with possible congenital adrenal hyperplasia, when properly administered, dexamethasone is effective in preventing ambiguous genitalia in the affected female and has been shown to be safe for the mother and fetus.[52]

The New York Hospital-Cornell Medical Center experience comprised prenatal examination for congenital adrenal hyperplasia as a result of 21-hydroxylase deficiency in 403 pregnancies in the past 15 years. In 280 pregnancies, the diagnosis was made by amniocentesis, in 123, chorionic villous sampling was performed and of late, the rapid allele-specific polymerase chain reaction (PCR) is used for DNA analysis. Eighty-four fetuses were found to be affected with classic 21-hydroxylase deficiency. Fifty-two of these fetuses were female, 36 of whom were treated prenatally with dexamethasone. Dexamethasone administrated before 10 weeks's gestation (23 affected female fetuses) was clearly effective in reducing masculinization. Overall, the average Prader score for affected females treated prenatally was 1.7 (including the partially treated). In contrast, the average score for untreated affected females was 3.9.[53] Current long-term studies of outcome in medical, psychological, gender, behavior, and neuropsychological studies are being conducted in a large cohort of patients who are 12 years and older and who underwent prenatal dexamethasone treatment.[54]

SUMMARY

Fetal therapy has evolved in the past 20 years to include treatment of life-threatening or severely disabling malformations in which postnatal treatment is either too late or inadequate. Less invasive basic procedures are being devised that could potentially decrease the morbidity associated with open fetal surgery. In certain situations, early detection of medical conditions can allow for successful in utero treatment and reverse or prevent devastating sequelae. Critical to the success of such interventions will be ongoing research efforts and ongoing controlled clinical trials that randomize patients to in utero versus conservative therapy and carefully define and follow outcomes long-term. The future prospect of prenatal gene therapy may transform the treatment of an increasing number of devastating inborn errors of metabolism (lysosomal storage diseases), immunodeficiencies (severe combined immunodeficiency syndrome), and hemoglobinopathies (thalassemias and sickle cell anemia).[44] The important points/objectives are: (1) the prenatal detection of hydronephrosis is a common finding and can be the result of such diverse causes as a ureteropelvic junction obstruction, multicystic dysplastic kidney, vesicoureteral reflux, or physiologic dilation; (2) the mainstay of prenatal therapy for bladder outlet obstruction because of posterior urethral valves or urethral atresia is placement of a vesicoamniotic shunt to improve or maintain amniotic fluid volume; (3) the in utero repair of myelomeningocele has decreased the need for postnatal ventriculoperitoneal shunting because of hydrocephalus and may ultimately improve the neurologic function of affected individuals; (4) congenital adrenal hyperplasia, often the result of a 21-hydroxylase deficiency, leads to virilization of the female fetus. These effects can be negated by administering dexamethasone to expectant mothers before 8 weeks's gestation.

REFERENCES

1. Grisoni ER, Gauderer MW, Wolfson RN, et al. Antenatal ultrasonography: the experience in a high risk perinatal center. J Pediatr Surg 1986;21: 358–61.
2. Johnson CE, Elder JS, Judge NE, et al. The accuracy of antenatal ultrasonography in identifying renal abnormalities. Am J Dis Child 1992;146(10):1181–4.

3. Morin L, Cendron M, Crombleholme TM, et al. Minimal hydronephrosis in the fetus: clinical significance and implications for management. J Urol 1996;155(6):2047–9.

4. Harrigan JT, Kangos JJ, Sikka A, et al. Successful treatment of fetal congestive heart failure secondary to tachycardia. N Engl J Med 1981;304(25):1527–9.

5. Dumesic DA, Silverman NH, Tobias S, et al. Transplacental cardioversion of fetal supraventricular tachycardia with procainamide. N Engl J Med 1982;307(18):1128–31.

6. Longaker MT, Laberge JM, Dansereau J, et al. Primary fetal hydrothorax: natural history and management. J Pediatr Surg 1989;24(6):573–6.

7. Rodeck CH, Fisk NM, Fraser DI, et al. Long-term drainage of fetal hydrothorax. N Engl J Med 1988; 319:1135–8.

8. Harrison MR, Langer JC, Adzick NS, et al. Correction of congenital diaphragmatic hernia in utero, V. Initial clinical experience. J Pediatr Surg 1990; 25(1):47–55 [discussion: 56–7].

9. Crombleholme TM, Harrison MR, Langer JC, et al. Early experience with open fetal surgery for congenital hydronephrosis. J Pediatr Surg 1988;23(12):1114–21.

10. Langer JC, Harrison MR, Schmidt KG, et al. Fetal hydrops and death from sacrococcygeal teratoma: rationale for fetal surgery. Am J Obstet Gynecol 1989;160(5 Pt 1):1145–50.

11. Longaker MT, Golbus MS, Filly RA, et al. Maternal outcome after open fetal surgery. A review of the first 17 human cases. JAMA 1991;265(6):737–41.

12. Peters C. Perinatal urology. In: Wein AJ, Kavoussi LR, Novick AC, et al, editors. Campbell-Walsh urology. 9th edition. Philadelphia: Saunders Elsevier; 2007.

13. Stocks A, Richards D, Frentzen B, et al. Correlation of prenatal renal pelvic anteroposterior diameter with outcome in infancy. J Urol 1996;155(3):1050–2.

14. Elder JS. Antenatal hydronephrosis. Fetal and neonatal management. Pediatr Clin North Am 1997;44(5):1299–321.

15. Fugelseth D, Lindemann R, Sande HA, et al. Prenatal diagnosis of urinary tract anomalies: the value of two ultrasound examinations. Acta Obstet Gynecol Scand 1994;73(4):290–3.

16. Thomas DF, Madden NP, Irving HC, et al. Mild dilatation of the fetal kidney: a follow-up study. Br J Urol 1994;74(2):236–9.

17. Cendron M, Elder JS, Duckett JW. Perinatal urology. In: Gillenwater JY, Grayhack JT, Howards SS, et al, editors. Adult and pediatric urology. 3rd edition. St. Louis (MO): Mosby Year-Book; 1996. p. 2075.

18. Mandell J, Lebowitz RL, Peters CA, et al. Prenatal diagnosis of the megacystis-megaureter association. J Urol 1992;148(5):1487–9.

19. King LR, Coughlin PW, Bloch EC, et al. The case for immediate pyeloplasty in the neonate with ureteropelvic junction obstruction. J Urol 1984; 132(4):725–8.

20. Adzick NS, Harrison MR, Glick PL, et al. Experimental pulmonary hypoplasia and oligohydramnios: relative contributions of lung fluid and fetal breathing movements. J Pediatr Surg 1984;19(6):658–65.

21. Elder JS, Hladky D, Selzman AA. Outpatient nephrectomy for nonfunctioning kidneys. J Urol 1995;154(2 Pt 2):712–4 [discussion: 714–5].

22. Mandell J, Peters CA, Estroff JA, et al. Late onset severe oligohydramnios associated with genitourinary abnormalities. J Urol 1992;148(2 Pt 2):515–8.

23. Mahony BS, Filly RA, Callen PW, et al. Fetal renal dysplasia: sonographic evaluation. Radiology 1984;152(1):143–6.

24. Crombleholme TM, Harrison MR, Golbus MS, et al. Fetal intervention in obstructive uropathy: prognostic indicators and efficacy of intervention. Am J Obstet Gynecol 1990;162(5):1239–44.

25. Elder JS, O'Grady JP, Ashmead G, et al. Evaluation of fetal renal function: unreliability of fetal urinary electrolytes. J Urol 1990;144(2 Pt 2):574–8.

26. Johnson MP, Bukowski TP, Reitelman C, et al. In utero surgical treatment of fetal obstructive uropathy: a new comprehensive approach to identify appropriate candidates for vesicoamniotic shunt therapy. Am J Obstet Gynecol 1994;170(6):1770–6.

27. Lipitz S, Ryan G, Samuell C, et al. Fetal urine analysis for the assessment of renal function in obstructive uropathy. Am J Obstet Gynecol 1993; 168(1 Pt 1):174–9.

28. Yoshimura S, Masuzaki H, Gotoh H, et al. Ultrasonographic prediction of lethal pulmonary hypoplasia: comparison of eight different ultrasonographic parameters. Am J Obstet Gynecol 1996;175(2): 477–83.

29. Morris RK, Quinlan-Jones E, Kilby MD, et al. Systematic review of accuracy of fetal urine analysis to predict poor postnatal renal function in cases of congenital urinary tract obstruction. Prenat Diagn 2007;27:900–11.

30. Morris RK, Malin GL, Khan KS, et al. Antenatal ultrasound to predict postnatal renal function in congenital lower urinary tract obstruction: systematic review of test accuracy. BJOG 2009;116: 1290–9.

31. Golbus MS, Harrison MR, Filly RA, et al. In utero treatment of urinary tract obstruction. Am J Obstet Gynecol 1982;142(4):383–8.

32. Quintero RA, Hume R, Smith C, et al. Percutaneous fetal cystoscopy and endoscopic fulguration of posterior urethral valves. Am J Obstet Gynecol 1995;172(1 Pt 1):206–9.

33. Quintero RA, Johnson MP, Romero R, et al. In-utero percutaneous cystoscopy in the management of fetal lower obstructive uropathy. Lancet 1995; 346(8974):537–40.

34. Coplen DE. Prenatal intervention for hydronephrosis. J Urol 1997;157(6):2270–7.

35. Agarwal SK, Fisk NM. In utero therapy for lower urinary tract obstruction. Prenat Diagn 2001;21(11):970–6.

36. Freedman AL, Johnson MP, Smith CA, et al. Long-term outcome in children after antenatal intervention for obstructive uropathies. Lancet 1999;354(9176):374–7.

37. Elder JS, Duckett JW Jr, Snyder HM. Intervention for fetal obstructive uropathy: has it been effective? Lancet 1987;2(8566):1007–10.

38. Quintero RA, Johnson MP, Munoz H. In utero endoscopic treatment of posterior urethral valves: preliminary experience. Prenat Neonatal Med 1998;3:208–16.

39. Agarwal SK, Fisk N, Welsh A. Endoscopic management of fetal obstructive uropathy. J Urol 1999;161:108.

40. Holmes N, Harrison MR, Baskin LS. Fetal surgery for posterior urethral valves: long-term postnatal outcomes. Pediatrics 2001;108(1):E7.

41. Clark TJ, Martin WL, Divakaran TG, et al. Prenatal bladder drainage in the management of fetal lower urinary tract obstruction: a systematic review and meta-analysis. Obstet Gynecol 2003;102:367–82.

42. PLUTO Trial. University of Birmingham website. Available at: http://www.pluto.bham.ac.uk. Accessed March 6, 2010.

43. North American Fetal Therapy Network (NAFTnet) website. Available at: http://www.naftnet.org. Accessed March 6, 2010.

44. Walsh DS, Adzick SN. Fetal intervention: where we are, where we're going. Contemp Pediatr 2000;17(6):33–58.

45. Bruner JP, Tulipan N, Paschall RL, et al. Fetal surgery for myelomeningocele and the incidence of shunt-dependent hydrocephalus. JAMA 1999;282(19):1819–25.

46. Sutton LN, Adzick NS, Bilaniuk LT, et al. Improvement in hindbrain herniation demonstrated by serial fetal magnetic resonance imaging following fetal surgery for myelomeningocele. JAMA 1999;282(19):1826–31.

47. Holzbeierlein J, Pope JC IV, Adams MC, et al. The urodynamic profile of myelodysplasia in childhood with spinal closure during gestation. J Urol 2000;164(4):1336–9.

48. Holmes NM, Nguyen HT, Harrison MR, et al. Fetal intervention for myelomeningocele: effect on postnatal bladder function. J Urol 2001;166(6):2383–6.

49. Holmdahl G, Hanson E, Hanson M, et al. Four-hour voiding observation in healthy infants. J Urol 1996;156(5):1809–12.

50. Sillen U, Solsnes E, Hellstrom AL, et al. The voiding pattern of healthy preterm neonates. J Urol 2000;163(1):278–81.

51. Jansson UB, Hanson M, Hanson E, et al. Voiding pattern in healthy children 0 to 3 years old: a longitudinal study. J Urol 2000;164(6):2050–4.

52. Mercado AB, Wilson RC, Cheng KC, et al. Prenatal treatment and diagnosis of congenital adrenal hyperplasia owing to steroid 21-hydroxylase deficiency. J Clin Endocrinol Metab 1995;80(7):2014–20.

53. New MI. Prenatal treatment of congenital adrenal hyperplasia. The United States experience. Endocrinol Metab Clin North Am 2001;30(1):1–13.

54. Nimkarn S, New MI. Prenatal diagnosis and treatment of congenital adrenal hyperplasia due to 21-hydroxylase deficiency. Mol Cell Endocrinol 2009;300:192–6.

55. Manning FA. The fetus with obstructive uropathy: the fetal surgery registry. In: Harrison MR, Golbus MS, Filly RA, editors. The unborn patient: prenatal diagnosis and treatment. Philadelphia: WB Saunders; 1991. p. 394–8.

Hypospadias: Etiology and Current Research

Nicolas Kalfa, MD, PhD[a,b], Charles Sultan, MD, PhD[a,b],
Laurence S. Baskin, MD[c],*

KEYWORDS

- Hypospadias • Etiology • Genetics
- Sex differentiation disorders • Receptors
- Androgen • Environment

Hypospadias is one of the most common congenital defects in humans. The molecular events required in the genitourinary tract for normal development of the external genitalia are just beginning to be elucidated. A cause is identified in approximately 20% of hypospadias, mainly in severe forms, but remains unknown in a vast majority of cases. *ATF3* and mastermind-like domain-containing 1 gene (*MAMLD1*, formerly *CXorf6*) are new candidate genes that have been recently identified. *ATF3*, an estrogen responsive gene implicated in the stress response, has its expression increased in hypospadiac boys and exhibits genetic variants. *MAMLD1*, which is expressed in the gonad during sex differentiation and interacts with SF-1, is also mutated in patients with isolated hypospadias or disorder of sex differentiation.

Penile and urethral development is a fragile process requiring a correct genetic program, hormonal action (mainly testosterone and its 5α reduced form, dihydrotestosterone [DHT]), time- and space-adapted cellular differentiation, and complex tissue interactions. A failure of these regulatory processes may induce a defect in the development of the ventral aspect of the penis and an ectopic opening on the urethral meatus.

This congenital malformation, often considered as a lack of virilization of male external genitalia, is the second most frequent genital malformation in newborn males after cryptorchidism. Its incidence ranges from 1 in 1000 to 1 in 100,[1–3] with significant variations according to ethnic origin.

Management of hypospadias is based on surgery to ensure an acceptable cosmetic aspect, a good urinary function without obstruction or fistula, and a correction of the ventral curvature, which is frequent in severe forms of hypospadias and which may impair future sexual life if left uncorrected. There has been a recent effort to better elucidate the cause of hypospadias. First, several investigators have reported increasing trends in birth prevalence of hypospadias from 1960s to 1990s,[4–6] even if recent reports cast doubt upon them.[7–9] Second, hypospadias may be a smaller component of a much larger disease group (including reproductive disorder, testicular cancer, and cryptorchidism) and may reflect current exposure to environmental pollutants and a subsequent testicular dysgenesis.[10] Identifying the cause of hypospadias may thus be relevant not only in the field of pediatric urology but also for worldwide public health.

Supported by Grant DK058105 from the National Institutes of Health, Washington, DC, USA, and by PHRC UF8270 from University Hospital of Montpellier, France.

a Service de Chirurgie et Urologie Pédiatrique, Hôpital Lapeyronie, 371 Avenue Giraud, 34295 Montpellier Cedex 5, CHU Montpellier, France

b Service d'Hormonologie, Hôpital Lapeyronie, 371 Avenue Giraud, 34295 Montpellier Cedex 5, CHU Montpellier, France

c Department of Pediatric Urology, Center for the Study and Treatment of Hypospadias, Parnassus Medical Center, University of California San Francisco Children's Medical Center, 400 Parnassus Avenue, A 640, San Francisco, CA 94143, USA

* Corresponding author.
E-mail address: lbaskin@urology.ucsf.edu

Urol Clin N Am 37 (2010) 159–166
doi:10.1016/j.ucl.2010.03.010
0094-0143/10/$ – see front matter © 2010 Published by Elsevier Inc.

CLASSIC CAUSES OF HYPOSPADIAS: A DEVELOPMENTAL FETAL STORY

The role of fetal androgens is crucial, especially during the first trimester of pregnancy. Two steps are required to reach well-masculinized genitalia: sexual determination with testicular formation and sexual differentiation based on an effective hormonal biosynthesis and action.This hormonal factor has to interact with a normal genital tubercle (GT) and implicate the presence and action of penile developmental genes.

Hypospadias and Testicular Differentiation

Heterozygous mutations of WT1 (Wilms tumor 1 gene implicated in male gonadal determination) are associated with severe hypospadias and other genital abnormalities. In animals, knockout of WT1 induces anorchidism, defective GT development along with bilateral renal agenesis.[11–16] In humans, mutations of WT1 are associated with syndromic hypospadias.[17] SRY (sex-determining region of the Y chromosome) and its targets (SOX9, DMRT1, GATA4) encode a transcriptional activator that acts immediately before the differentiation of the gonad into testis. Testicular dysgenesis and secondary hypospadias have been described along with mutations of these genes.[18–21]

Hypospadias and Androgen Biosynthesis and Action

Androgenic steroids, synthesized by the Leydig cells of the testes, are first seen just before the onset of androgen-induced genital differentiation. 5α-Reductase type 2 is highly expressed in the mesenchymal stroma surrounding the urethra,[22] and androgen receptor (AR) gene is expressed in the epithelium of the urethra.[22] Mutations of these 2 genes may induce hypospadias. Mutations of 5α-reductase have been identified in severe variants of hypospadias in combination with other genital abnormalities.[19,23,24] Mutations of AR gene have been mainly found in patients with severe forms of hypospadias,[25] that is, perineal-scrotal hypospadias[26,27] and hypospadias associated with cryptorchidism[28] and micropenis.[29,30] The phenotype is variable in partial androgen insensitivity syndrome,[29,31] and a mutation in one of the 8 exons is found in less than 10% of cases.

Hypospadias and Penile Development

Homeobox A (HOXA) and homeobox D (HOXD) genes are expressed in the fetal urogenital structures and are implicated in penile development in a non–endocrine-dependant manner. These genes induce the expression of fibroblast growth factor (FGF) 8 and bone morphogenetic protein 7.[32] In mice, heterozygosity of HOXA13 genes is associated with a defect in penile development and in penile patterning.[33] In humans, mutations of HOXA13 are associated with genital abnormalities, including hypospadias in males[34,35] and the hand-foot-genital syndrome. Beside this nonendocrine action, HOXA13 also acts in AR gene expression and mediates glans vascularization.[36]

ACTIVE RESEARCH TO ELUCIDATE THE CAUSE OF HYPOSPADIAS
MAMLD1

A recent candidate gene that is critical for the development of the male genitalia is MAMLD1 (formerly CXorf6). This gene was discovered in the course of identifying the gene responsible for X-linked myotubular myopathy, MTM1, which maps to proximal Xq28.[37,38] Myopathic individuals with intragenic mutations of MTM1 have normal sexual development, whereas those with microdeletions of MTM1 extending to the CXorf6 locus exhibit abnormal external genitalia.[39–42] Subsequent studies have demonstrated that CXorf6 is mutated in 46,XY disorders of sexual development (46,XY DSD). Fukami and colleagues[43] have identified 3 nonsense mutations in 4 individuals with 46XY, DSD, including micropenis, bifid scrotum, and penoscrotal hypospadias. The authors show that mutations are also present in almost 10% of patients with isolated hypospadias.[44] Mutation 1295T→C (V432A) was found in a patient with a proximal hypospadias. Two deletions at the beginning of the first translated exon were also identified (E109fsX121). A CAG repeat amplification of the second polyglutamine domain of the protein was found in a boy with an isolated subcoronal hypospadias ($CAG_{10} \rightarrow CAG_{13}$). None of these mutations were noted in the control group.

The mechanism by which MAMLD1 mutations induce hypospadias is under study, and these mutations may impair or interfere with androgen metabolism. In situ hybridization studies indicate that MAMLD1 is expressed in fetal Sertoli and Leydig cells during the critical period for sex development.[43,45] Moreover, MAMLD1 is coexpressed with adrenal 4 binding protein/steroidogenic factor 1 (Ad4bp/Sf-1) in mouse. SF-1 is known to regulate multiple genes involved in sex development by binding to specific DNA sequences.[46–48] Fukami and colleagues[49] further showed that MAMLD1 harbors a putative SF-1 binding sequence in introns 1 and 2. Luciferase assays confirmed that SF-1 binds to the putative target sequence and exerts a transactivation function. These findings suggest that *MAMLD1* is regulated by SF-1. Finally, knockdown analysis with small interfering RNAs of m-*CXorf6* using mouse Leydig tumor cells showed reduced capability of testosterone production and responsiveness after human chorionic gonadotropin stimulation.[49]

ATF3

A previous microarray study of the foreskin of normal and hypospadiac patients found 3 upregulated genes, the most prominent being activation transcription factor 3 (ATF3).[50] ATF3 is a transcription factor whose expression is induced in a variety of cell types by many stress signals, including peripheral nerve injury, nutrient deprivation, and DNA damaging agents, as well as mitogenic agents and cytokines,[51,52] suggesting that ATF3 is a key regulator in cellular stress responses. Although induction of ATF3 is neither tissue specific nor stimulus specific, one common theme of all the signals that induce ATF3 is that they also induce cellular damage.[53] ATF3 may be a part of the cellular response that leads to detrimental outcomes. Transgenic mice expressing ATF3 in selective tissues have malfunction in the target tissues. For instance, increased expression of ATF3 in the liver or pancreas of transgenic mice results in reduced expression of gluconeogenic genes[54] and insulin-dependent diabetes mellitus,[54] respectively. Therefore, ATF3 appears to be a part of the cellular response that leads to detrimental outcomes.

Several studies argue for a major role of this gene and protein in hypospadias in the urethra. As discussed earlier, microarray analysis of tissues from normal and hypospadiac patients revealed upregulation of this gene in hypospadias.[50] This result was confirmed by immunohistochemical analysis of human foreskin showing 86% of the hypospadias samples to be positive for expression of ATF3, whereas only 13% of those from normal penises were positive.[55] ATF3 expression and promoter activity in foreskin fibroblasts were responsive to in vitro exposure to ethinyl estradiol.[55] It is noteworthy that this aberrant expression of ATF3 is mainly present on the pathologic hypospadiac part of the urethra in human fetuses.[56]

Hypospadias and Defects in Urethral Patterning and Structuring

Appropriate cell-cell interactions between mesenchyme and urothelium are necessary during male genital organogenesis to achieve the complete closure of the urethral plate. Sonic Hedgehog (Shh), a secreted signaling factor that regulates cell function and fate in development and adulthood,[57,58] is implicated in the interaction between mesenchyme and urothelium. Urothelium-derived Shh has been shown to orchestrate the induction of fetal mouse bladder differentiation and patterning.[59] Shh was thus suspected to participate in penile patterning and urethral development in a similar manner. In mice, Shh is expressed in the endodermally derived urethral plate epithelium situated along the ventral side of the GT and is required for outgrowth and patterning of the GT.[60,61] Mice with a targeted deletion of Shh have penile and clitoral agenesis, consistent with the crucial role of Shh in genital development.[62,63] No mutations have yet been reported in children with hypospadias.

Growth factors

Growth factors also participate in the development of genital structures. The FGF family is linked to genital development. FGF receptor 2 gene (FGFR2) is a transcriptional target of AR.[64] Knockout of FGF10 is associated with hypospadias.[61] Genetic variants of FGF8, FGF10, and FGFR2 increase the risk of hypospadias.[32,64] Another group of growth factors strongly suspected to participate in the urethral tube development is the transforming growth factor (TGF) β family. In mice, genes involved in the TGF-β pathway, as well as in Wnt-Frizzled and thrombospondin 4 (a member of a cell-migration molecule family) pathways, exhibit increased expression profiles in GT during urethral tube development at ED 14, ED 15, ED 16, and ED 17.[65] Immunohistochemical analysis confirms expression of TGF-β1 and TGF-β receptor III in urethral epithelia from ED 14 to ED 17. In the same manner that proteins of the TGF-β signaling pathway are involved in regulation of palate fusion in mammals, it could regulate the ventral closure of urethra.[66]

More interestingly, the TGF-β signaling pathway could be connected to the ATF3 hypothesis. First, the most upregulated estrogen responsive genes are *ATF3* and *CTGF* (which encodes connective tissue growth factor),[67,68] and *CTGF* is part of the TGF-β signaling pathway.[69] Second, ATF3 responds to signals in epithelial cells via the TGF-β pathway.[70–72] ATF3 lies at the center of interactions between the TGF-β signaling pathway and steroid hormone receptors[73] and may play a central role in the well-coordinated epithelial-mesenchymal interactions during the male GT development.[74]

Environment Acting on a Genetic Susceptibility

Multiple chemical substances found in the environment can potentially interfere with male genital development because of their similarity to hormones. Such substances are called endocrine disruptors and have both estrogenic and antiandrogenic activities.[73,75] It has been proposed that hypospadias and other disorders of the otherwise androgen-dependent male sexual development may occur as a result of androgen-estrogen imbalances. This is suggested by subtle developmental defects of the genital masculinization such as the genital distance, a witness of male reproductive tract development, which is reduced in children with hypospadias and in case of prenatal exposure to phthalates.[76,77]

More recently, the concept of individual susceptibility, whereby different individuals may not react in the same manner after a toxic exposure, emerged. Genetic background could be the main basis of individual susceptibility to environment. Polymorphisms of hormone responsive genes have been investigated in a hypospadiac population and compared with controls. Genomic variants of the ATF3 genes were identified in 10% of boys with hypospadias.[56] None of these genomic variants were present in controls. A missense variant (L23 M, a highly conserved amino acid) was identified in a boy with anterior hypospadias. Three genomic variants (C53070T, C53632A, Ins53943A) were found in or close to exon 6 in patients with perineal, penoscrotal, and anterior hypospadias. This important exon includes splice sites for an alternative transcript that codes for a regulating isoform, ATF3ΔZip, which regulates the function of ATF3.[78] The authors hypothesize that these genomic defects impair the regulation of ATF3 function and release its cell cycle suppression effect. Beleza-Meireles and colleagues[70] also identified that 3 common single nucleotide polymorphisms (SNPs), spanning a region of about 16 kb in intron 1 of ATF3, are associated with hypospadias. The authors note that these SNPs are not linked, their effects are independent, and the combination of the 3 risk SNPs yields the highest significance. Functional studies remain to be performed to confirm the cell cycle suppression effect of these polymorphisms.

Genomic variants of the androgen and estrogen signaling pathways are also under study. There is an increased number of GGN trinucleotide repeats in the AR gene, which reduce the transcriptional activity of the gene in hypospadiac patients.[79,80] But the role of amplification of the CAG repeats remains to be determined.[81] The V89L variant of the SRD5A2 gene is a risk factor for hypospadias (Maimoun L, personal data, 2010).[82] The polymorphisms of estrogen receptor (ESR) may also facilitate the deleterious effects of xenoestrogen because their effects are mainly mediated through this receptor. AGAGA haplotype of ESR 1 gene is strongly associated with hypospadias.[83] The ESR1 C-A haplotype, for ESR1 XbaI and ESR2 2681-4A>G, respectively, also increases the risk of malformation.[84] Increased number of CA repeats (and subsequent increased ESR activity) also increases the risk of malformation.[85]

The interaction between genes and environment is not limited to genomic variants modulating the response to toxic substances. The expression of genital development genes also varies according to the exposition to estrogenlike substances. Using a mouse model of steroid hormone–dependent GT development, ATF3 messenger RNA (mRNA) levels were found to be elevated in all estrogen-exposed fetal GTs compared with controls.[86] Di-(2-ethylhexyl) phthalate (DEHP), the most common plasticizer, has been suspected to contribute to hypospadias of male offspring of pregnant women exposed to it. In a fetal murine model, DEHP activates ATF3 both at the mRNA and protein levels in GT with an apoptosis dysregulation.[87] Exogenous administration of estrogens results in an increased expression of ESR α (but not of ESR β).[88] Endocrine disruptors also modulate expression of TGF-β1. Reverse-transcription polymerase chain reaction and Western blot studies showed that the expression of TGF-β1 is upregulated in DEHP-treated mice along with a significant inhibition of male fetal genital tubercule.[87]

These data about environment should nevertheless be interpreted with caution. The undisputable proof of detrimental effects of environment is still pending, and some studies provide contradictory results in similar fashion to epidemiologic studies that provide inconclusive evidence on temporal trends in hypospadias. Some recent reports describe an increased incidence,[89,90] whereas others showed no trend over time.[9,91,92] Epidemiologic studies on maternal exposition are also inconclusive. Three studies report the possible relationship between exposure to pesticides and hypospadias. Kristensen and colleagues[93] published a moderate increase of odds ratio (OR) for hypospadias in individuals exposed to farm chemicals (OR, 1.5%). Weidner and colleagues[94] stated that maternal farming or gardening led to a low risk of hypospadias (OR, 1.27). More recently, studies on occupational exposures to phthalates and hair spray suggest that antiandrogenic endocrine-disrupting chemicals may play a role in hypospadias.[95] In contrast, Longnecker and colleagues[96] did not confirm any significant risk of hypospadias (OR, 1.2) when mothers were exposed to dichlorodiphenyltrichloroethane. No relationship was identified between exposure to polybrominated biphenyl[97] or polychlorinated biphenyls[98] and hypospadias. A recent meta-analysis indicates only a modestly increased risk for hypospadias associated with pesticide exposure.[99] Although several xenoestrogens consistently induce hypospadias in murine male offspring exposed in utero, extrapolation to humans may not be comparable.

Overall, the proportion of hypospadias cases for which a precise and undisputed cause is detected varies according to studies, but it remains the minority, especially for less severe cases. The occurrence of hypospadias remains unexplained in most cases. A multifactorial explanation and the implication of genetic susceptibility and environmental pollutants remain a plausible working hypothesis.

REFERENCES

1. Stevenson AC, Johnston HA, Stewart MI, et al. Congenital malformations. A report of a study of series of consecutive births in 24 centres. Bull World Health Organ 1966;34(Suppl):9–127.
2. Sweet RA, Schrott HG, Kurland R, et al. Study of the incidence of hypospadias in Rochester, Minnesota, 1940–1970, and a case-control comparison of possible etiologic factors. Mayo Clin Proc 1974; 49(1):52–8.
3. Avellan L. The incidence of hypospadias in Sweden. Scand J Plast Reconstr Surg 1975;9(2):129–39.
4. Czeizel A, Toth J, Czvenits E. Increased birth prevalence of isolated hypospadias in Hungary. Acta Paediatr Hung 1986;27(4):329–37.
5. Paulozzi LJ, Erickson JD, Jackson RJ. Hypospadias trends in two US surveillance systems. Pediatrics 1997;100(5):831–4.
6. Canning DA. Hypospadias trends in two US surveillance systems. Rise in prevalence of hypospadias. J Urol 1999;161(1):366.
7. Ahmed SF, Dobbie R, Finlayson AR, et al. Prevalence of hypospadias and other genital anomalies among singleton births, 1988–1997, in Scotland. Arch Dis Child Fetal Neonatal Ed 2004;89(2):F149–51.
8. Carmichael SL, Shaw GM, Nelson V, et al. Hypospadias in California: trends and descriptive epidemiology. Epidemiology 2003;14(6):701–6.
9. Fisch H, Lambert SM, Hensle TW, et al. Hypospadias rates in New York state are not increasing. J Urol 2009;181(5):2291–4.
10. Main KM, Skakkebaek NE, Toppari J. Cryptorchidism as part of the testicular dysgenesis syndrome: the environmental connection. Endocr Dev 2009;14: 167–73.
11. Pritchard-Jones K, Fleming S, Davidson D, et al. The candidate Wilms' tumour gene is involved in genitourinary development. Nature 1990;346(6280):194–7.
12. van Heyningen V, Bickmore WA, Seawright A, et al. Role for the Wilms tumor gene in genital development? Proc Natl Acad Sci USA 1990;87(14):5383–6.
13. Pelletier J, Bruening W, Li FP, et al. WT1 mutations contribute to abnormal genital system development and hereditary Wilms' tumour. Nature 1991; 353(6343):431–4.
14. Shimamura R, Fraizer GC, Trapman J, et al. The Wilms' tumor gene WT1 can regulate genes involved in sex determination and differentiation: SRY, Mullerian-inhibiting substance, and the androgen receptor. Clin Cancer Res 1997;3(12 Pt 2):2571–80.
15. Gao F, Maiti S, Alam N, et al. The Wilms tumor gene, Wt1, is required for Sox9 expression and maintenance of tubular architecture in the developing testis. Proc Natl Acad Sci USA 2006;103(32): 11987–92.
16. Kohler B, Delezoide AL, Boizet-Bonhoure B, et al. Co-expression of Wilms' tumor suppressor 1 (WT1) and androgen receptor (AR) in the genital tract of human male embryos and regulation of AR promoter activity by WT1. J Mol Endocrinol 2007;38(5):547–54.
17. Kaltenis P, Schumacher V, Jankauskiene A, et al. Slow progressive FSGS associated with an F392L WT1 mutation. Pediatr Nephrol 2004;19(3):353–6.
18. Huang B, Wang S, Ning Y, et al. Autosomal XX sex reversal caused by duplication of SOX9. Am J Med Genet 1999;87(4):349–53.
19. Wang Y, Li Q, Xu J, et al. Mutation analysis of five candidate genes in Chinese patients with hypospadias. Eur J Hum Genet 2004;12(9):706–12.
20. Maciel-Guerra AT, de Mello MP, Coeli FB, et al. XX maleness and XX true hermaphroditism in SRY-negative monozygotic twins: additional evidence for a common origin. J Clin Endocrinol Metab 2008;93(2):339–43.
21. Leipoldt M, Erdel M, Bien-Willner GA, et al. Two novel translocation breakpoints upstream of SOX9 define borders of the proximal and distal breakpoint cluster region in campomelic dysplasia. Clin Genet 2007;71(1):67–75.
22. Kim KS, Liu W, Cunha GR, et al. Expression of the androgen receptor and 5 alpha-reductase type 2 in the developing human fetal penis and urethra. Cell Tissue Res 2002;307(2):145–53.
23. Ocal G, Adiyaman P, Berberoglu M, et al. Mutations of the 5alpha-steroid reductase type 2 gene in six Turkish patients from unrelated families and a large pedigree of an isolated Turkish village. J Pediatr Endocrinol Metab 2002;15(4):411–21.
24. Nicoletti A, Baldazzi L, Balsamo A, et al. SRD5A2 gene analysis in an Italian population of under-masculinized 46, XY subjects. Clin Endocrinol (Oxf) 2005;63(4):375–80.
25. Sultan C, Paris F, Terouanne B, et al. Disorders linked to insufficient androgen action in male children. Hum Reprod Update 2001;7(3):314–22.

26. Kaspar F, Cato AC, Denninger A, et al. Characterization of two point mutations in the androgen receptor gene of patients with perineoscrotal hypospadia. J Steroid Biochem Mol Biol 1993;47(1–6):127–35.

27. Holterhus PM, Werner R, Struve D, et al. Mutations in the amino-terminal domain of the human androgen receptor may be associated with partial androgen insensitivity and impaired transactivation in vitro. Exp Clin Endocrinol Diabetes 2005;113(8):457–63.

28. Hiort O, Klauber G, Cendron M, et al. Molecular characterization of the androgen receptor gene in boys with hypospadias. Eur J Pediatr 1994;153(5): 317–21.

29. Sultan C, Lumbroso S, Poujol N, et al. Mutations of androgen receptor gene in androgen insensitivity syndromes. J Steroid Biochem Mol Biol 1993;46(5): 519–30.

30. Li Q, Li SK, Xu JJ, et al. [Study of genic mutations of androgen receptor in hypospadias]. Zhonghua Zheng Xing Wai Ke Za Zhi 2004;20(6):421–4.

31. Deeb A, Mason C, Lee YS, et al. Correlation between genotype, phenotype and sex of rearing in 111 patients with partial androgen insensitivity syndrome. Clin Endocrinol (Oxf) 2005;63(1):56–62.

32. Beleza-Meireles A, Lundberg F, Lagerstedt K, et al. FGFR2, FGF8, FGF10 and BMP7 as candidate genes for hypospadias. Eur J Hum Genet 2007; 15(4):405–10.

33. Morgan EA, Nguyen SB, Scott V, et al. Loss of Bmp7 and Fgf8 signaling in Hoxa13-mutant mice causes hypospadia. Development 2003;130(14):3095–109.

34. Mortlock DP, Innis JW. Mutation of HOXA13 in hand-foot-genital syndrome. Nat Genet 1997;15(2): 179–80.

35. Frisen L, Lagerstedt K, Tapper-Persson M, et al. A novel duplication in the HOXA13 gene in a family with atypical hand-foot-genital syndrome. J Med Genet 2003;40(4):e49.

36. Gearhart J, Rink R, Garrett R, et al. Hypospadias. In: Gearhart J, Rink R, Mouriquand P, editors. Pediatric urology. Philadelphia: W.B. Saunders; 2001. p. 713–28.

37. Laporte J, Kioschis P, Hu LJ, et al. Cloning and characterization of an alternatively spliced gene in proximal Xq28 deleted in two patients with intersexual genitalia and myotubular myopathy. Genomics 1997;41(3):458–62.

38. Laporte J, Guiraud-Chaumeil C, Vincent MC, et al. Mutations in the MTM1 gene implicated in X-linked myotubular myopathy. ENMC International Consortium on Myotubular Myopathy. European Neuro-Muscular Center. Hum Mol Genet 1997;6(9): 1505–11.

39. Bartsch O, Kress W, Wagner A, et al. The novel contiguous gene syndrome of myotubular myopathy (MTM1), male hypogenitalism and deletion in Xq28: report of the first familial case. Cytogenet Cell Genet 1999;85(3–4):310–4.

40. Bates PA, Kelley LA, MacCallum RM, et al. Enhancement of protein modeling by human intervention in applying the automatic programs 3D-JIGSAW and 3D-PSSM. Proteins 2001;S5(Suppl 5):39–46.

41. Biancalana V, Caron O, Gallati S, et al. Characterisation of mutations in 77 patients with X-linked myotubular myopathy, including a family with a very mild phenotype. Hum Genet 2003;112(2):135–42.

42. Hu LJ, Laporte J, Kress W, et al. Deletions in Xq28 in two boys with myotubular myopathy and abnormal genital development define a new contiguous gene syndrome in a 430 kb region. Hum Mol Genet 1996;5(1):139–43.

43. Fukami M, Wada Y, Miyabayashi K, et al. CXorf6 is a causative gene for hypospadias. Nat Genet 2006;38(12):1369–71.

44. Kalfa N, Liu B, Klein O, et al. Mutations of CXorf6 are associated with a range of severities of hypospadias. Eur J Endocrinol 2008;159(4):453–8.

45. O'Shaughnessy PJ, Baker PJ, Monteiro A, et al. Developmental changes in human fetal testicular cell numbers and messenger ribonucleic acid levels during the second trimester. J Clin Endocrinol Metab 2007;92(12):4792–801.

46. Morohashi KI, Omura T. Ad4BP/SF-1, a transcription factor essential for the transcription of steroidogenic cytochrome P450 genes and for the establishment of the reproductive function. FASEB J 1996;10(14): 1569–77.

47. Parker KL, Schimmer BP. Steroidogenic factor 1: a key determinant of endocrine development and function. Endocr Rev 1997;18(3):361–77.

48. Ozisik G, Achermann JC, Jameson JL. The role of SF1 in adrenal and reproductive function: insight from naturally occurring mutations in humans. Mol Genet Metab 2002;76(2):85–91.

49. Fukami M, Wada Y, Okada M, et al. Mastermind-like domain-containing 1 (MAMLD1 or CXorf6) transactivates the Hes3 promoter, augments testosterone production, and contains the SF1 target sequence. J Biol Chem 2008;283(9):5525–32.

50. Wang Z, Liu BC, Lin GT, et al. Up-regulation of estrogen responsive genes in hypospadias: microarray analysis. J Urol 2007;177(5):1939–46.

51. Hunt D, Hossain-Ibrahim K, Mason MR, et al. ATF3 upregulation in glia during Wallerian degeneration: differential expression in peripheral nerves and CNS white matter. BMC Neurosci 2004;5:9.

52. Wolfgang CD, Liang G, Okamoto Y, et al. Transcriptional autorepression of the stress-inducible gene ATF3. J Biol Chem 2000;275(22):16865–70.

53. Chen BP, Wolfgang CD, Hai T. Analysis of ATF3, a transcription factor induced by physiological stresses and modulated by gadd153/Chop10. Mol Cell Biol 1996;16(3):1157–68.

54. Allen-Jennings AE, Hartman MG, Kociba GJ, et al. The roles of ATF3 in glucose homeostasis. A

transgenic mouse model with liver dysfunction and defects in endocrine pancreas. J Biol Chem 2001; 276(31):29507–14.

55. Liu B, Wang Z, Lin G, et al. Activating transcription factor 3 is up-regulated in patients with hypospadias. Pediatr Res 2005;58(6):1280–3.

56. Kalfa N, Liu B, Klein O, et al. Genomic variants of ATF3 in patients with hypospadias. J Urol 2008; 180(5):2183–8 [discussion: 2188].

57. Ericson J, Muhr J, Placzek M, et al. Sonic hedgehog induces the differentiation of ventral forebrain neurons: a common signal for ventral patterning within the neural tube. Cell 1995;81(5):747–56.

58. Ericson J, Muhr J, Jessell TM, et al. Sonic hedgehog: a common signal for ventral patterning along the rostrocaudal axis of the neural tube. Int J Dev Biol 1995;39(5):809–16.

59. Shiroyanagi Y, Liu B, Cao M, et al. Urothelial sonic hedgehog signaling plays an important role in bladder smooth muscle formation. Differentiation 2007;75(10):968–77.

60. Digilio MC, Marino B, Giannotti A, et al. Specific congenital heart defects in RSH/Smith-Lemli-Opitz syndrome: postulated involvement of the sonic hedgehog pathway in syndromes with postaxial polydactyly or heterotaxia. Birth Defects Res A Clin Mol Teratol 2003;67(3):149–53.

61. Yucel S, Liu W, Cordero D, et al. Anatomical studies of the fibroblast growth factor-10 mutant, Sonic Hedge Hog mutant and androgen receptor mutant mouse genital tubercle. Adv Exp Med Biol 2004; 545:123–48.

62. Haraguchi R, Mo R, Hui C, et al. Unique functions of Sonic hedgehog signaling during external genitalia development. Development 2001;128(21): 4241–50.

63. Perriton CL, Powles N, Chiang C, et al. Sonic hedgehog signaling from the urethral epithelium controls external genital development. Dev Biol 2002;247(1):26–46.

64. Petiot A, Perriton CL, Dickson C, et al. Development of the mammalian urethra is controlled by Fgfr2-IIIb. Development 2005;132(10):2441–50.

65. Li J, Willingham E, Baskin LS. Gene expression profiles in mouse urethral development. BJU Int 2006;98(4):880–5.

66. Kaartinen V, Voncken JW, Shuler C, et al. Abnormal lung development and cleft palate in mice lacking TGF-beta 3 indicates defects of epithelial-mesenchymal interaction. Nat Genet 1995;11(4):415–21.

67. Pedram A, Razandi M, Aitkenhead M, et al. Integration of the non-genomic and genomic actions of estrogen. Membrane-initiated signaling by steroid to transcription and cell biology. J Biol Chem 2002; 277(52):50768–75.

68. Inoue A, Yoshida N, Omoto Y, et al. Development of cDNA microarray for expression profiling of estrogen-responsive genes. J Mol Endocrinol 2002;29(2):175–92.

69. Rageh MA, Moussad EE, Wilson AK, et al. Steroidal regulation of connective tissue growth factor (CCN2; CTGF) synthesis in the mouse uterus. Mol Pathol 2001;54(5):338–46.

70. Beleza-Meireles A, Tohonen V, Soderhall C, et al. Activating transcription factor 3: a hormone responsive gene in the etiology of hypospadias. Eur J Endocrinol 2008;158(5):729–39.

71. Valcourt U, Kowanetz M, Niimi H, et al. TGF-beta and the Smad signaling pathway support transcriptomic reprogramming during epithelial-mesenchymal cell transition. Mol Biol Cell 2005;16(4):1987–2002.

72. Kang Y, Chen CR, Massague J. A self-enabling TGFbeta response coupled to stress signaling: smad engages stress response factor ATF3 for Id1 repression in epithelial cells. Mol Cell 2003;11(4):915–26.

73. Willingham E, Baskin LS. Candidate genes and their response to environmental agents in the etiology of hypospadias. Nat Clin Pract Urol 2007;4(5):270–9.

74. Yamada G, Satoh Y, Baskin LS, et al. Cellular and molecular mechanisms of development of the external genitalia. Differentiation 2003;71(8):445–60.

75. Paris F, Balaguer P, Terouanne B, et al. Phenylphenols, biphenols, bisphenol-A and 4-tert-octylphenol exhibit alpha and beta estrogen activities and antiandrogen activity in reporter cell lines. Mol Cell Endocrinol 2002;193(1–2):43–9.

76. Swan SH, Main KM, Liu F, et al. Decrease in anogenital distance among male infants with prenatal phthalate exposure. Environ Health Perspect 2005; 113(8):1056–61.

77. Hsieh MH, Breyer BN, Eisenberg ML, et al. Associations among hypospadias, cryptorchidism, anogenital distance, and endocrine disruption. Curr Urol Rep 2008;9(2):137–42.

78. Chen BP, Liang G, Whelan J, et al. ATF3 and ATF3 delta Zip. Transcriptional repression versus activation by alternatively spliced isoforms. J Biol Chem 1994;269(22):15819–26.

79. Aschim EL, Nordenskjold A, Giwercman A, et al. Linkage between cryptorchidism, hypospadias, and GGN repeat length in the androgen receptor gene. J Clin Endocrinol Metab 2004;89(10):5105–9.

80. Radpour R, Rezaee M, Tavasoly A, et al. Association of long polyglycine tracts (GGN repeats) in exon 1 of the androgen receptor gene with cryptorchidism and penile hypospadias in Iranian patients. J Androl 2007;28(1):164–9.

81. Muroya K, Sasagawa I, Suzuki Y, et al. Hypospadias and the androgen receptor gene: mutation screening and CAG repeat length analysis. Mol Hum Reprod 2001;7(5):409–13.

82. Thai HT, Kalbasi M, Lagerstedt K, et al. The valine allele of the V89L polymorphism in the 5-alpha-reductase gene confers a reduced risk for

hypospadias. J Clin Endocrinol Metab 2005;90(12):6695–8.

83. Watanabe M, Yoshida R, Ueoka K, et al. Haplotype analysis of the estrogen receptor 1 gene in male genital and reproductive abnormalities. Hum Reprod 2007;22(5):1279–84.

84. Ban S, Sata F, Kurahashi N, et al. Genetic polymorphisms of ESR1 and ESR2 that may influence estrogen activity and the risk of hypospadias. Hum Reprod 2008;23(6):1466–71.

85. Beleza-Meireles A, Kockum I, Lundberg F, et al. Risk factors for hypospadias in the estrogen receptor 2 gene. J Clin Endocrinol Metab 2007;92(9):3712–8.

86. Liu B, Agras K, Willingham E, et al. Activating transcription factor 3 is estrogen-responsive in utero and upregulated during sexual differentiation. Horm Res 2006;65(5):217–22.

87. Liu X, He DW, Zhang DY, et al. Di (2-ethylhexyl) phthalate (DEHP) increases transforming growth factor-beta1 expression in fetal mouse genital tubercles. J Toxicol Environ Health A 2008;71(19):1289–94.

88. Agras K, Willingham E, Shiroyanagi Y, et al. Estrogen receptor-alpha and beta are differentially distributed, expressed and activated in the fetal genital tubercle. J Urol 2007;177(6):2386–92.

89. Lund L, Engebjerg MC, Pedersen L, et al. Prevalence of hypospadias in Danish boys: a longitudinal study, 1977–2005. Eur Urol 2009;55(5):1022–6.

90. Sun G, Tang D, Liang J, et al. Increasing prevalence of hypospadias associated with various perinatal risk factors in chinese newborns. Urology 2009;73(6):1241–5.

91. Aho M, Koivisto AM, Tammela TL, et al. Is the incidence of hypospadias increasing? Analysis of Finnish hospital discharge data 1970–1994. Environ Health Perspect 2000;108(5):463–5.

92. Martinez-Frias ML, Prieto D, Prieto L, et al. Secular decreasing trend of the frequency of hypospadias among newborn male infants in Spain. Birth Defects Res A Clin Mol Teratol 2004;70(2):75–81.

93. Kristensen P, Irgens LM, Andersen A, et al. Birth defects among offspring of Norwegian farmers, 1967–1991. Epidemiology 1997;8(5):537–44.

94. Weidner IS, Moller H, Jensen TK, et al. Risk factors for cryptorchidism and hypospadias. J Urol 1999;161(5):1606–9.

95. Ormond G, Nieuwenhuijsen MJ, Nelson P, et al. Endocrine disruptors in the workplace, hair spray, folate supplementation, and risk of hypospadias: case-control study. Environ Health Perspect 2009;117(2):303–7.

96. Longnecker MP, Klebanoff MA, Brock JW, et al. Maternal serum level of 1,1-dichloro-2,2-bis(p-chlorophenyl)ethylene and risk of cryptorchidism, hypospadias, and polythelia among male offspring. Am J Epidemiol 2002;155(4):313–22.

97. Small CM, DeCaro JJ, Terrell ML, et al. Maternal exposure to a brominated flame retardant and genitourinary conditions in male offspring. Environ Health Perspect 2009;117(7):1175–9.

98. McGlynn KA, Guo X, Graubard BI, et al. Maternal pregnancy levels of polychlorinated biphenyls and risk of hypospadias and cryptorchidism in male offspring. Environ Health Perspect 2009;117(9):1472–6.

99. Rocheleau CM, Romitti PA, Dennis LK. Pesticides and hypospadias: a meta-analysis. J Pediatr Urol 2009;5(1):17–24.

Hypospadias

Kate H. Kraft, MD[a], Aseem R. Shukla, MD[b],
Douglas A. Canning, MD[a,c],*

KEYWORDS

- Hypospadias • Urethral meatus • Urogenital folds
- Human chorionic gondadotropin

Hypospadias results from abnormal development of the penis that leaves the urethral meatus proximal to its normal glanular position anywhere along the penile shaft, scrotum, or perineum (**Fig. 1**). A spectrum of abnormalities, including ventral curvature of the penis (chordee), a hooded incomplete prepuce, and an abortive corpus spongiosum, are commonly associated with hypospadias.

Hypospadiology is a term coined by John W. Duckett, Jr., the former chief of the Division of Urology at the Children's Hospital of Philadelphia (CHOP) and a pioneer in hypospadias repairs. Hypospadiology encompasses a continuously evolving and expanding discipline. Although modern experiments have only recently begun to yield a deeper understanding of the genetic, hormonal, and environmental basis of hypospadias, the quest for a surgical procedure that consistently results in a straight penis with a normally placed glanular meatus has occupied surgeons for more than two centuries. Advances in understanding of the causes of hypospadias and current approaches to the correction of hypospadias to provide a cosmetically and functionally satisfactory repair are the focus of this article.

ETIOLOGY

In normal development, the urogenital folds fuse to form the penile urethra. A small region of the distal urethra in the glans is formed by the invagination of a surface epithelial tag (**Fig. 2**). Hypospadias results from partial or complete failure of urethral folds to form throughout their normal length or a failure of the folds to close distally if they have formed. The extent of the closure determines the position of the urethral orifice.

A unifying etiology for hypospadias remains elusive and is likely multifactorial. The hypospadiac anatomy appears consistent with incomplete embryologic development due to (1) abnormal androgen production by the fetal testis, (2) limited androgen sensitivity in target tissues of the developing genitalia, or (3) premature cessation of androgenic stimulation due to early atrophy of the Leydig cells of the testes.[1]

Endocrine Factors

Several investigators have suggested that hypospadias represents a mild disorder of sex

[a] Division of Urology, The Children's Hospital of Philadelphia, 3rd Floor, Wood Building, 34th Street and Civic Center Boulevard, Philadelphia, PA 19104-4399, USA
[b] Department of Urologic Surgery, University of Minnesota Amplatz Children's Hospital, 420 Delaware Street SE, Suite B435, Minneapolis, MN 55455, USA
[c] Division of Urology, Department of Surgery, University of Pennsylvania School of Medicine, 3rd Floor, Wood Building, 34th Street and Civic Center Boulevard, Philadelphia, PA 19104-4399, USA
* Corresponding author. Division of Urology, The Children's Hospital of Philadelphia, 3rd Floor, Wood Building, 34th Street and Civic Center Boulevard, Philadelphia, PA 19104-4399.
E-mail address: canning@email.chop.edu

Urol Clin N Am 37 (2010) 167–181
doi:10.1016/j.ucl.2010.03.003
0094-0143/10/$ – see front matter © 2010 Published by Elsevier Inc.

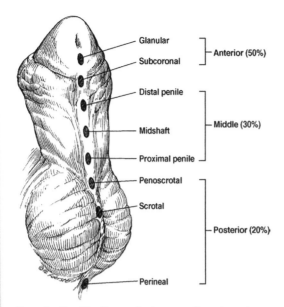

Fig. 1. Classification of hypospadias based on anatomic location of the urethral meatus. Anterior, or distal, hypospadias is the most commonly encountered variant. (*From* Duckett JW. Successful hypospadias repair. Contemp Urol 1992;4:42–55; with permission.)

development (DSD). It could represent one end of a spectrum, the other of which is a completely feminized male.[2] Hypospadias may result from an endocrinopathy in which there is a disruption in the synthetic biopathway of androgens. A qualitative androgen receptor (AR) abnormality or defects at a postreceptor level may explain the defect in some of boys with hypospadias. For example, the blunted response to hCG injections seen in many boys with hypospadias may suggest a mutation in the luteinizing hormone receptor in the testis or perhaps an increase in receptor numbers as a consequence of the previous stimulation.[3] In a study by Allen and Griffin[3] of 15 boys (< 4 years of age) with severe hypospadias, 11 boys were diagnosed with a total of 6 distinct endocrine-related abnormalities. The most consistent finding was a subnormal testosterone response to hCG stimulation in 7 boys. The investigators postulated that their findings may represent a delay in the maturation of the hypothalamic-pituitary-testicular axis.

Genetic Factors

Hypospadias is believed to have a complex genetic background with gene expression acting in concert with environmental factors. The familial rate of hypospadias is approximately 7%, reflecting

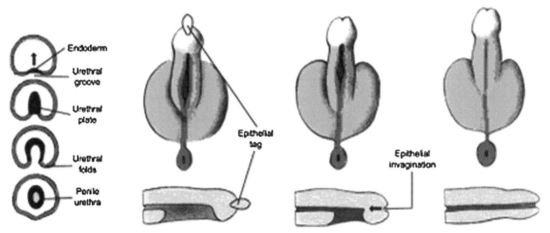

Fig. 2. The urogenital folds fuse and the genital tubercle elongates to form the penile shaft and glans. A small region of the distal urethra in the glans is formed by the invagination of surface epithelial tag. The fused labioscrotal folds give rise to the scrotum. (*Modified from* Park JM. Normal development of the genitourinary system. In: Walsh PC, Retik AB, Vaughan ED Jr, et al, editors. Campbell's Urology. Philadelphia: Saunders; 2007. p. 3119 [Fig. 106–25].)

a nonfamilial, sporadic finding in most cases. Recent studies have suggested a role for müllerian inhibiting substance (MIS) in the etiology of hypospadias. There is an inverse relationship between MIS and testosterone and this may be related to the MIS inhibition of cytochrome P450c17 (CYP17), the enzyme that catalyzes the committed step in testosterone synthesis.[4] MIS may directly inhibit testosterone production by suppressing the CYP17 gene.[5] Abnormalities of other genes, such as fibroblast growth factor 10, have also been shown to result in hypospadias.[6]

Normal sexual differentiation depends on testosterone and its metabolites as well as functional ARs. Despite a correlation of certain clear defects in the androgen metabolism pathway and hypospadias, as in the 5α-reductase defect (mutation in SRD5A2 gene on chromosome 2), such associations have been limited to few cases—underlining the importance of seeking other genetic explanations for this congenital defect.[7]

Environmental Factors

Some experts believe that the incidence of hypospadias is on the rise worldwide. One possible explanation is environmental contamination. It is well known that insecticides, pharmaceuticals, and plant estrogens contain estrogenic ingredients and that metal cans used in the canned food industry are coated internally with plastics known to contain estrogenic substances.[6] These substances are ultimately present in the fresh and seawater in trace amounts that are bioaccumulated and concentrated in higher organisms of the food chain. For this reason, predators at the top of the food chain, such as large fish, birds, sea mammals, and humans, accumulate high levels of estrogenic environmental contaminants. Thus, humans and wild animals are constantly exposed to estrogenic compounds known to disrupt reproduction—the so-called endocrine disrupters.[6] Antiandrogens interfere with testosterone function in many ways, including a conformational change within the AR, increasing AR degradation, or blocking the release of heat shock proteins from AR.[8] Additionally, environmental factors coupled with maternal stress may increase the risk of hypospadias, as has been shown in an animal model.[9]

Maternal Factors

In 1967, Goldman and Bongiovanni[10] suggested a role for maternal progestin exposure in the development of hypospadias. These researchers produced hypospadias in male rats by experimentally inducing congenital adrenal hyperplasia. A disturbance in the maternal-fetal hormonal milieu as a causative factor in humans was substantiated when male offspring conceived by in vitro fertilization requiring progestin therapy had a markedly increased incidence of hypospadias.[11,12] Fredell and colleagues[13] associated low birth weight with hypospadias in discordant monozygotic twins. Recent evidence suggests that a diet lacking in meat and fish results in a more than 4-fold increased risk of hypospadias.[14] Advanced maternal age may also predispose male infants to more severe forms of hypospadias.[15]

Future Areas of Research

Studies that elucidate the role of cellular signals other than testosterone and dihydrotestosterone in normal phallic development and hypospadias, endocrine disrupters, and mesenchymal-epithelial interaction may hold the key to explaining the etiology of hypospadias.[6] Research in the areas of homeobox (Hox) gene may also open new avenues toward increased understanding of the cause of hypospadias.

EPIDEMIOLOGY

The incidence of hypospadias is rising and varies geographically. Prevalence ranges from 0.26 per 1000 births (male and female births) in Mexico to 2.11 in Hungary and 2.6 per 1000 live births in Scandinavia.[16] A recent study found the rate of hypospadias in a two-year prospective study to be 38 per 10,000 live births in Netherlands, a number six times higher than previously recorded.[17] Sweet and colleagues[18] reported a much lower incidence in Sweden of 1 in 1250 live male births.

In 1997, 2 independent surveillance systems in United States, the nationwide Birth Defects Monitoring Program (BDMP) and the Metropolitan Atlanta Congenital Defects Program (MACDP), reported a nearly doubling of rate of hypospadias when compared with immediately preceding decades.[19] The incidence of all types of hypospadias increased from 20.2 to 39.7 per 10,000 live male births during the period from 1970–1993 (ie, 1 in every 250 live male births was a boy with hypospadias [measured by BDMP]). MACDP reported a rise in severe hypospadias rate of between 3-fold and 5-fold. These rising trends, however, may reflect earlier diagnosis or an increase in reporting to registries of congenital defects. The increased reporting of more proximal than distal hypospadias cases, however, refutes the argument that these findings represent more frequent reporting of minor cases.[20]

Recent studies have linked the rising rate of hypospadias in boys born prematurely and small for gestational age, boys with low birth weight, and boys born to mothers over 35 years of age.[21–23] Roberts and Lloyd[24] noted an 8.5-fold increase in hypospadias in one of monozygotic male twins compared with singleton live male births. This may suggest a discrepancy in the supply of hCG to the fetus where a single placenta is unable to meet the requirements of two developing male fetuses.

CHORDEE

Ventral penile curvature (previously known as chordee) accompanies hypospadias in some cases. It is seen more commonly in severe cases of hypospadias but can also occur independent of hypospadias. Study of penile development via examination of fetal specimens has led to the understanding that chordee is a normal stage in penile development and that significant variation in the severity of chordee was noted at all stages of embryogenesis.

If curvature is an arrest of normal embryologic development analogous to failure of descent of the testicle, it is no surprise that fibrosis is conspicuously absent in some clinical cases of chordee.[25,26] Snodgrass and colleagues[27] further supported this by studying subepithelial biopsies of urethral plate examined under a microscope. They demonstrated well-vascularized connective tissue comprised of smooth muscle and collagen without evidence of fibrous bands or dysplastic tissue.[27] Baskin and colleagues[28] found well-vascularized connective tissue under the epithelial surface of the urethral plate in a 33-week fetus with distal hypospadias.

In some patients, curvature is present without hypospadias. Devine and Horton[29] described three types of chordee without hypospadias. In class I, the most severe defect, the corpus spongiosum is deficient from the site at which the chordee begins, up to the glans, whereas the urethra has a thin tube of mucous membrane. In class II, the urethra has

a normal corpus spongiosum with abnormal Buck's fascia and dartos fascia layers. In class III, only the dartos fascia layer alone is abnormal.

ASSOCIATED FINDINGS
Cryptorchidism and Inguinal Hernia

Between 8% and 10% of boys with hypospadias have a cryptorchid testicle and 9% to 15% have an associated inguinal hernia.[18,30,31] In boys with more proximal hypospadias, cryptorchidism may occur as frequently as 32%.[32] This strong association between proximal hypospadias and undescended testis further suggests that this clinical entity may represent one end of a spectrum of endocrinopathy. The incidence of chromosomal anomaly in these groups of patients is much higher (22%) than hypospadias (5%–7%) or cryptorchidism (3%–6%) occurring alone.[33,34] In a series of more than 600 cases of hypospadias, the authors found that children with associated cryptorchidism and midshaft to distal hypospadias had a much higher complication rate when corrected. It is not certain why this occurs but it may be that a change in the endocrine milieu with the associated cryptorchidism may make the tissues less amenable to correction.[35]

Disorders of Sex Development

Hypospadias and disorders of sex development (DSD) may represent two ends of a spectrum.[2] The more severe the hypospadias, the more likely a DSD state exists.[36] Rajfer and Walsh[37] reported DSD in 27.3% of boys with a normal-sized phallus, cryptorchidism, and hypospadias. Presence of severe hypospadias and nonpalpable testes with otherwise normal-looking phallus requires that the urologist test for the presence of a DSD state.[36]

Partial androgen insensitivity, chromosomal abnormalities, Smith-Lemli-Opitz syndrome, 5α-reductase deficiency, Denys-Drash syndrome, and other conditions can also occur in association with hypospadias.

Prostatic Utricle

The prostatic utricle is an elementary structure developing from the müllerian ducts cranially and from the wolffian ducts and the urogenital sinus caudally.[38] Boys with hypospadias often have enlargement of the prostatic utricle with resultant urinary tract infections, stone formation, pseudoincontinence, and, often, difficult catheterization.[39–41] Devine and colleagues[42] reported that 57% of patients with perineal hypospadias and

10% with penoscrotal hypospadias had prostatic utricle enlargement demonstrated on urethroscopy. The overall incidence of utricle enlargement in patients with hypospadias was 14% in this series of 44 patients. Utricular enlargement in itself does not indicate a DSD but is seen with increased frequency in patients with 46 XY DSD.[42]

PRESENTATION

The abnormal dorsal prepuce and ventral glans tilt of the newborn penis usually signifies the presence of hypospadias. Further examination of the penis typically reveals the proximally displaced urethral orifice that is often stenotic in appearance but rarely obstructive. An exception is the megameatus variant of hypospadias. In this unusual case (6% of all distal hypospadias presentations), an intact prepuce is present. The diagnosis is usually not made until after a routine neonatal circumcision is completed.[43]

The anatomic location of the meatus and extent of ventral curvature, or chordee, should be determined. In some instances, multiple pinpoint dimples may be present on the surface of the urethral plate in addition to the hypospadiac urethral meatus. The meatus is always the most proximal of these defects. Meatal position may be classified as anterior (distal), middle, or posterior (proximal) with more anatomically specific subgroups further applied (see **Fig. 2**). The meatus is located on the glans or distal shaft of the penis in approximately 70% to 80% of all boys with hypospadias. Twenty percent to 30% of boys with hypospadias have the meatus located in the middle of the shaft of the penis. The remainder of boys with hypospadias has more severe defects with the urethral meatus located in the scrotum or even more proximally on the perineum.[44]

Increased understanding of the endocrinologic origins of hypospadias has corroborated the clinical association of hypospadias with DSD states.[37,45] Boys with severe proximal hypospadias and those with hypospadias and cryptorchidism should undergo karyotype analysis and a DSD evaluation as indicated. The unilaterality or bilaterality of cryptorchidism concomitant with hypospadias does not predict the diagnosis of a DSD state.

A complete penile examination requires independent evaluation of penile length. If the stretched penile length is significantly below the third percentile for age or if inadequate phallic size precludes surgical repair of hypospadias, then androgen stimulation as pretreatment should be considered. Androgenic pretreatment with hCG has been shown to increase penile length and may also move the meatus to a relatively more distal position as the shaft elongates in response to the hCG.[46]

SURGICAL REPAIR

The goal of hypospadias surgery is a functional sexual organ that is free of curvature. Equally important is a glanular urethral meatus that allows a boy to void with a laminar flow while standing. A cosmetically sound penis requires a cone-shaped glans and supple penile shaft skin.

Timing of Surgery

Historically, the American Academy of Pediatrics has stated that the ideal age for genital surgery is between 6 and 12 months of age.[47] This age range seems to insulate most children from the psychological, physiologic, and anesthetic trauma associated with hypospadias surgery. The authors prefer, however, to perform the repair at the age of 4 months in infant boys with an adequately sized phallus and without medical problems. Surgery even earlier may be effective in boys with adequate glans volume. Healing seems to occur quickly, with less intense scarring, and young infants overcome the stress of surgery more easily.

Instruments

Increasing experience has demonstrated the applicability of the principles of plastic surgery to hypospadiology. Instruments, such as fine scissors, 0.5-mm tooth forceps, and Castroviejo needle holders, are standard. Fine absorbable 6-0, 7-0, or 8-0 sutures work well for suturing with precision. Considerable variation exists among surgeons as to the choice of suture material. The authors prefer polyglycolic suture material for construction of the neourethra and for buried sutures and continue to use a glanular stay suture to minimize tissue handling during repair. The authors do not recommend polydiaxanone suture for urethral repair due to its extended absorption time interval and increased urethral stricture rate.[48]

Hemostasis

Adequate hemostasis may be achieved by a variety of techniques in hypospadias surgery. A tourniquet placed at the base of the penis that is removed every 15 to 30 minutes alone or combined with needlepoint spot and bipolar electrocoagulation is often used to control blood loss that may occlude the surgical field. The authors avoid the use of electrocautery to minimize the potential for tissue damage caused by cautery dispersal and continue to inject 1:100,000 epinephrine in 1% lidocaine along the proposed incision line in the glans. In the authors' experience, this injection affords the twin benefits of adequate local hemostasis while hydrodissecting a reliable dissection plane between the skin and dartos fascia.

Dressing and Urinary Diversion

An ideal posthypospadias repair dressing should provide adequate but pliable compression and be easily removable within 48 hours in most cases. Many variations in type and style of dressing have been proposed, although even no dressing at all is a viable alternative.[49,50] The authors continue to prefer the sandwich-type dressing preferred by Duckett that compresses the penis against the lower abdominal wall by placing a Telfa (Kendall, Mansfield, MA, USA) pad and a folded gauze sponge on top of the penis followed by a bioocclusive dressing such as Tegaderm (3M, St Paul, MN, USA).

Urinary diversion is often preferred after proximal and midshaft hypospadias repairs, yet its usefulness in distal repairs is based on surgeon preference rather than proved benefit. A multicenter experience reported by Hakim and colleagues[51] revealed similar results for distal repairs with or without postoperative urethral diversion. The authors use a 6 French (F) hydrophilic Kendall catheter placed through the neourethra and sutured to the glans with a prolene suture anchored to the inner aspect of the meatus to avoid scarring of the glans. Because the rate of urinary infection is no different between an open and closed system, the authors allow the open end of the Kendall tube to passively drain into the outer of two diapers and prescribe chemoprophylaxis.[52]

TYPES OF HYPOSPADIAS REPAIRS

Because hypospadias repair is so challenging, a plethora of surgical options, from those representing truly novel approaches to modifications of known procedures, have been described for various presentations of hypospadias. The surgical technique that is most appropriate for a given case is based on anatomic factors, previous surgical descriptions, and, of course, a surgeon's personal experience.

Historically, hypospadias repairs were categorized as primary closures, meatal-based flaps, dorsally based flaps, and free grafts. Conceptual advances, such as recognition of the urethral plate and its potential for incision and preservation, have profoundly affected the approach to hypospadias repair today. This article describes the techniques implemented at the authors' institution for hypospadias repair with an understanding that these descriptions are truly templates that are constantly modified, amplified, and reinvented—a practice that is the basis of evolution in hypospadiology.

DISTAL HYPOSPADIAS
Meatal Advancement and Glanuloplasty

The meatal advancement and glanuloplasty (MAGPI) offers reliable cosmesis and long-term success when applied to repair glanular and selected coronal hypospadias. Presence of urethral mobility and a rounded glans along with the absence of significant chordee ensure an ideal outcome and avoid meatal regression.

The MAGPI begins with a circumferential incision 6 to 8 mm proximal to the corona of the glans and proximal to the meatus. Penile shaft skin is dissected in a drop-back fashion with extreme care exercised ventrally over the corpus spongiosum to avoid urethral injury. Residual chordee or penile torsion may be corrected at this point. A longitudinal incision from the dorsal distal edge of meatus is carried to the distal glans groove as it transects the transverse bridge of tissue that is often present. The incised tissue edges are approximated in a Heineke-Mikulicz fashion with 7-0 absorbable suture to effectively advance the meatus distally. The medial edge of the ventral meatus is then pulled distally and the exposed glans edges are trimmed and anastamosed to leave the glans with a cosmetically sound, rounded appearance. The dorsal hood foreskin is trimmed in the midline as Byars flaps allow adequate ventral skin transfer, and skin is approximated to the glans with absorbable, subcuticular suture to complete the repair.

The authors are using the MAGPI repair less and less. The tubularized incised plate urethroplasty (TIP) has become the standard for all but the most distal repairs.

Tubularized Incised Plate Urethroplasty

Recognition that surgical repair of a hypospadias based on a flat urethral plate resulted in a horizontal, recessed meatus in contrast to the

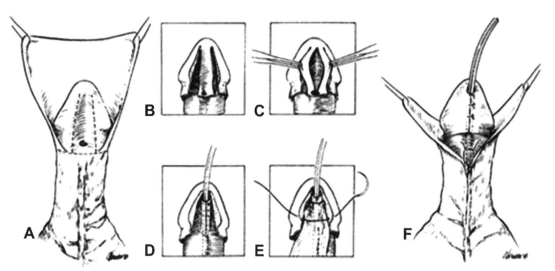

Fig. 3. Tubularized, incised plate hypospadias repair as described by Snodgrass. (*A*) Horizontal dotted line indicating circumscribing incision approximately 2 mm proximal to the meatus. Vertical dotted lines indicate the junction of the urethral plate to the glans wings. (*B*) Urethral plate is separated from the glans wings, which are then mobilized laterally. (*C*) The key step of the operation is a deep, midline incision into the urethral plate extending from within the meatus to its distal margin, but not continuing into the glans apex. (*D*) The plate is tubularized over a small stent leaving a generous, oval meatus. (*E*) The neourethra is covered by a dartos flap and then glansplasty begins at the coronal margin. (*F*) Glans wings, mucosal collar, and ventral shaft skin are closed. (*From* Snodgrass W. Tubularized incised plate hypospadias repair: indications, technique, and complications. Urology 1999;54:6; with permission.)

cosmetically superior results when repairing a deeply grooved plate led Rich and colleagues[53] to propose the "hinging of the urethral plate" by incising it distally. Snodgrass[54] extended this concept by incising the plate deeply through the entire urethral plate to the corporal bodies followed by a Thiersch-Duplay tubularization. A multicenter experience supported the concept and was followed by the application of TIP to proximal hypospadias repairs.[55,56]

A circumscribing skin incision is carried ventrally to 1 to 2 mm proximal to the urethral meatus and followed by skin drop-back to the penoscrotal junction (**Fig. 3**A). Penile curvature is resolved and corrected by dorsal midline plication, if necessary. Two parallel longitudinal incisions in the glans allow lateral mobilization of the glans wings as care is taken not to undermine the vascularity of the urethral plate (see **Fig. 3**B).

The critical step in this repair involves a midline relaxing incision from within the meatus to the end of the urethral plate (see **Fig. 3**C). The incidence of meatal stenosis is reduced by limiting the incision to the actual plate and not incising

the rim of the glans at the distal margin of the plate.[57] A 6F stent is passed into the bladder and a 2-layer running subepithelial closure tubularizes the plate and creates a neourethra (see **Fig. 3**D). Subepithelial 6-0 polyglactin sutures approximate the glans wings beginning at the corona to complete a glansplasty (see **Fig. 3**E). The glans wings, mucosal collar, and ventral shaft skin are closed (see **Fig. 3**F). The inherent disadvantage of superimposed suture lines with this closure may be countered by developing a dartos pedicle from dorsal shaft skin that is buttonholed and transposed to the ventrum.

More proximal hypospadias cases are approached for a TIP repair by first incising the proximal plate and leaving the distal plate intact. If the urethral plate increases in width, as expected, then incising the distal plate continues the repair. Snodgrass and Yucel[58] have reported success of the TIP repair for proximal hypospadias, with significantly improved outcomes when using a 2-layer polyglactin subepithelial closure. Overall complication rate was 25%, and the incidence of fistula formation was 10%.

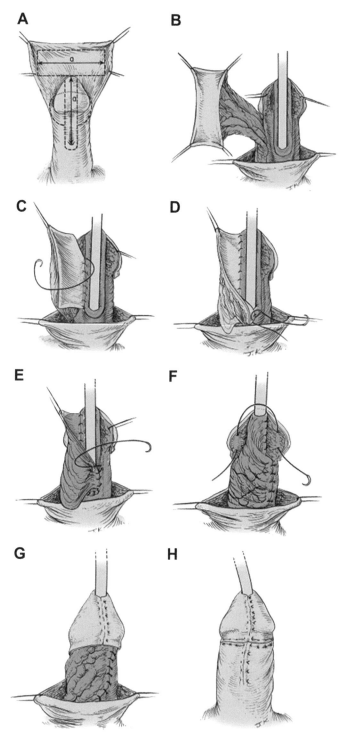

Fig. 4. Island onlay flap repair. (*A*) Proposed incisions for urethral plate and preputial skin onlay. (*B*) Pedicled preputial skin onlay with stay sutures. (*C*) Initial full-thickness suture approximation of onlay flap and urethral plate. (*D*) Approximation at proximal extent. (*E*) Completion of anastomosis with running subcuticular technique. (*F*) Inferolateral border of onlay pedicle has been advanced as a second layer coverage of proximal and longitudinal suture lines. (*G*) Approximated glans. (*H*) Completed repair. (*Reprinted from* Atala A, Retik AB. Hypospadias. In: Libertino JA, editor. Reconstructive urologic surgery. 3rd edition. St. Louis [MO]: Mosby-Year Book; 1998. p. 467.)

MIDDLE AND PROXIMAL HYPOSPADIAS OR DISTAL HYPOSPADIAS WITH CHORDEE

The authors are getting more and more aggressive with the TIP repair for more proximal hypospadias, but still use island onlay repair in cases with concern about the width of the urethral plate. If significant curvature exists, flap-based repairs continue to be used.

Island Onlay Hypospadias Repair

Van Hook introduced the concept of a preputial flap based on a vascular pedicle to repair proximal hypospadias in 1896.[59] Asopa and colleagues[60] developed the effective use of inner preputial skin for a substitution urethroplasty and Duckett furthered this technique by describing a transverse preputial island flap repair in 1980.[61,62] The island onlay flap evolved from the transverse preputial island flap as experience demonstrated that repair of the chordee with hypospadias can be accomplished by dissection of the subcutaneous tissue and dorsal midline plication and that division of the urethral plate is required in only 10% of cases.[62] The concept that spongiosum consists of vascularized tissue and smooth muscle bundles that may be used in a hypospadias repair evolved during the 1980s after histologic examination.[27,63] In the past, the onlay island flap was used for more than 90% of the authors' patients with subcoronal hypospadias. The authors currently use it less in favor of the TIP repair, but it still remains an important part of the hypospadias portfolio.

The circumferential incision begins dorsally 6 to 8 mm proximal to the corona and is carried ventrally just proximal to the meatus (**Fig. 4**A). The incision is then carried further proximally to split ventral shaft skin in the midline to the penoscrotal junction. Parallel incisions 5 mm wide or narrower are then made along the urethral plate distally to the glans tip at a point where the flat ventral surface of the glans begins to curve around the meatal groove. Care is taken to keep these incisions superficial to avoid injury to underlying spongiosum. The skin and dartos fascia are dropped back as residual chordee is released. Dissection of the skin should avoid entering a plane into the intrinsic vascularity of the skin to preserve its viability as a preputial flap. As is commonly the case, if dissection of the penile ventrum reveals thinned spongiosal tissue that is nearly transparent, the urethra is incised proximally to what seems to be normal spongiosum. The urethral plate need not be more than 2 mm wide before the onlay transfer.

The island onlay flap is outlined on the inner preputial skin surface with interrupted 5-0 polypropylene sutures that are also used as stay sutures (see **Fig. 4**B). The sutures are grasped so that the fold of tissue between the inner and outer prepuce is accentuated. An 8- to 10-mm segment of this epithelium is sharply divided with the initial incision just beneath the skin at the junction between the inner and outer preputial faces of foreskin. The combined width of the preserved plate and the flap should be approximately 10 mm and no wider at the anastomosis than at the urethral meatus.

The freeing of the vascular pedicle begins at the midshaft where it is most easily separated from the blood supply to the dorsal penile shaft skin. This approach to the harvest of the flap easily identifies the proper plane and assures preservation of blood supply to the flap (**Fig. 5**D). The splitting of ventral foreskin completed during the initial circumcising skin incision, in the authors' experience, releases the base of the dorsal vascular pedicle and allows for wider mobilization of preputial foreskin for flap isolation. The flap is then rotated ventrally or, more commonly, transferred by creating a window in the vascular mesentery through which the glans is passed and then tapered proximally and distally (see **Fig. 4**C). Experience has shown that too wide a neourethra may lead to kinking or diverticulum formation. The appropriately designed flap is then sutured into place using lubricated interrupted 7-0 polyglactic suture at the proximal meatus and then in a interrupted subepithelial fashion along the lateral edges of the plate (see **Fig. 4**D, E). The flap is no longer closed over a feeding tube. The authors prefer to place the tube at the conclusion of the construction of the neourethra. The 8F feeding tube then serves as a spacer to assure an adequately sized glansplasty. The glansplasty is completed by medial rotation of mobilized glans wings with 6-0 polyglyconate sutures placed parallel to the cut edge of the glans wing beginning at the urethral meatus (see **Fig. 4**F, G). A 6F Kendall urethral stent is placed and the dorsal preputial skin is split in the midline and rotated ventrally to afford adequate circumferential skin coverage (see **Fig. 4**H).

Transverse Island Tube Repair

The transverse island tube repair remains a preferred option at CHOP for proximal hypospadias cases that remain amenable to a one-stage repair even after division of the urethral plate to release persistent, severe penile curvature. This

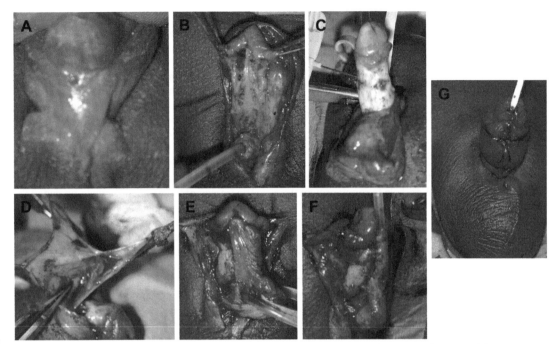

Fig. 5. Island tube hypospadias repair. (*A*) Preoperative appearance. Note shiny ventral tissue. This appearance suggests thinning of the ventral spongiosum and likely curvature. (*B*) Release of urethral plate with urethral meatus cannulated with feeding tube. (*C*) Artificial erection after placating sutures dorsally documents penile straightening after correction of curvature. (*D*) Dissection of dorsal preputial island flap from dorsal penile skin. (*E*) One suture line completed on midline. (*F*) Second suture line. (*G*) Completed repair. (*From* Mattei P, editor. Fundamentals of pediatric surgery [in press]; with permission.)

procedure incorporates inner preputial skin, as in the onlay technique, to be rolled completely into a neourethra without use of the urethral plate as a vascularized template. A bulky glansplasty, penile torque and an oval rather than slit-like meatal result have, however, hampered popular use of the island tube. Incorporating excessive preputial skin into a neourethra has also raised concern for forming a urethral diverticulum and turbulent flow. The authors describe recent modifications to this classic procedure that have addressed these cosmetic and functional problems.

Skin incisions facilitate penile degloving to the penopubic junction dorsally and into the penoscrotal junction ventrally. The urethra is opened proximally to healthy vascularized spongiosum as in the onlay repair. The urethral plate is then transected at the corona and dissected off of the corporal tissue (see **Fig. 5**B). An artificial erection delineates the extent of residual penile curvature and a Heineke-Mikulicz incision made vertically and closed horizontally straighten the penis (see **Fig. 5**C).

A segment of inner preputial tissue is harvested dorsally as described for the island onlay (see **Fig. 5**D). The pedicled flap is buttonholed and then ventrally transposed. Rather then rolling the tissue into a tube at this point, as described previously, the medial margin of the flap is first anchored to the urethra proximally. This maneuver allows the flap to be optimally tailored by stretching the skin to the opposite, anchored edge of the flap (see **Fig. 5**E). The tube can be fashioned to properly align the anastamosis to the native urethra and to construct a tube of ideal caliber. A second interrupted suture line then rolls the tube effectively into the glans (see **Fig. 5**F).

A glansplasty is completed with 6-0 polyglyconate sutures placed parallel to the cut edge of the glans as a horizontal mattress to cover the distal edge of the tube. A 6F urethral stent is placed and dorsal preputial skin is fashioned to provide adequate skin coverage as in all hypospadias repairs (see **Fig. 5**G).

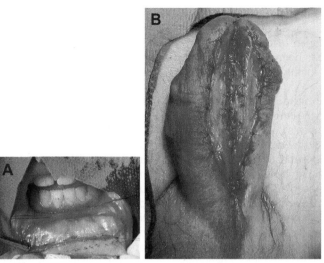

Fig. 6. Staged buccal mucosa repair for failed hypospadias. (*A*) Lip harvest site for graft. (*B*) Graft sutured into place along midline of strictured urethral plate.

Two-Stage Repair

The authors rarely, but occasionally, encounter challenging cases where severe chordee and a proximal meatus limit the applicability of a one-stage tube repair. In a few cases, injury to the vascular pedicle of the onlay tube during harvest requires that the repair be staged. Anecdotal and reported experience maintains that the two-stage technique offers overall fewer complications and better cosmetic results than the single-stage repair for select cases.[64,65] In cases where curvature is a great challenge and there is concern that the success of the repair needs to be monitored, the authors have elected to stage the repair. In anecdotal experience, however, there is a similar fistula rate after the second stage of a two-stage repair to that after a one-stage island onlay or tube repair.

A two-stage repair often involves a scrotoplasty with an aggressive attempt to relieve penile curvature, including transection and proximal removal of the plate. A dermal graft or tunica vaginalis may be interpositioned, although rarely in the authors' experience, to bridge any defect in the ventral tunica albuginea surface. Preputial skin at the dorsum is then split to rotate the resultant flaps ventrally. These flaps are allowed to settle into place and represent the future urethral plate.

The second stage is planned after an interval of approximately 6 months. At that point, parallel vertical incisions 12 to 15 mm apart are mapped distally beginning at the meatus and including the glans. Glans wings are mobilized as in the Thiersch-Duplay repair and, if also needed, the glans may be incised in the midline as with the TIP repair. Incisions are completed and a neourethra is then tubularized to complete the repair using a standard Thiersch-Duplay technique. The repair is aggressively covered with dartos tissue or in some cases with processus vaginalis flaps taken adjacent to the spermatic cord on one side or the other. In some cases, placement of the suture line into the scrotum facilitates healing. The penis is then mobilized from the scrotal flaps in a third stage, usually 3 to 12 months later.

Free Grafts

Severe proximal hypospadias and repeat hypospadias repairs may incorporate free grafts to construct a neourethra or augment an existing plate. The versatility of most primary hypospadias repairs using preputial skin or the urethral plate, however, has obviated free grafts for primary hypospadias repairs. In the past, at the authors' institution, this technique was reserved only for re-operations or rare instances where a paucity of local tissue is evident.[66] Free skin, bladder mucosa, tunica vaginalis, and buccal mucosa have variously been described as appropriate tissue for free graft use.[67–69]

The authors' experience has been that bladder mucosa is less pliable than buccal mucosa, with the latter less likely to shrink and requiring a 1:1 ratio for harvest compared with the defect to be repaired. The authors prefer buccal mucosa also as thick epithelium, tensile strength, and high levels of type IV collagen favor graft take.[70] Use of bladder mucosa has been abandoned in favor the buccal mucosa in the rare cases requiring a free graft.

The authors prefer to harvest buccal mucosa from the lower lip, although the inner cheek may be used with care to avoid Stensen's duct (**Fig. 6**A). The graft is placed on a scaffold to tailor it for onlay. This involves freeing all adipose tissue to expose the sub-epithelium and creating multiple perforations in the graft with an 18-gauge needle. This creates a surface that optimizes graft take and allows evacuation of accumulated fluid or blood, thereby preventing hematoma formation and subsequent disruption of the graft. The graft is trimmed to size if used as an onlay or tailored to be wrapped into a neourethra, without allowing for contracture in the case of buccal mucosa (see **Fig. 6**B). The edges of the graft epithelium are sutured to the surrounding shaft skin, and several plicating sutures are placed to approximate the graft directly to the base and facilitate neovascularization. The authors stent repairs completed with free grafts for 10 to 21 days depending on location and length. First-stage repairs with grafts are dressed with glycerin-soaked cotton secured with nonabsorbable suture followed by a sandwich dressing. In most cases a suprapubic catheter is placed into the bladder under cystoscopic guidance to divert the urinary stream from the fresh graft.

Metro and colleagues[66] and Hensle and colleagues[71] have reported long-term results for buccal mucosal grafts in complex hypospadias re-operations. Overall complication rates between 32% and 57% were reported with graft stricture and meatal stenosis most common. All complications were evident by 11 months in both groups and were seen less commonly as the surgical experience widened. Buccal mucosa remains a viable nongenital tissue alternative for a select subgroup of patients requiring urethral reconstruction.

COMPLICATIONS
Urethrocutaneous Fistula

The postoperative appearance of a urethrocutaneous fistula remains one of the most frustrating, although increasingly rare, complications of hypospadias surgery today. Adaptations in technique, including strict adherence to the principles of plastic surgery in tissue handling, avoiding suture line overlap, and the transposition of additional tissue layers, have cumulatively contributed to minimizing the incidence of failure. The team at CHOP has previously reported a less than 5% fistula rate for the island onlay hypospadias repair.[72]

When a fistula is diagnosed as a perioperative or delayed complication, at least 6 months (more if an older boy) should be allowed to elapse before repeat surgical intervention. This interval allows inflammation and edema to resolve and enables an accurate assessment of the viability and suitability of local tissue to be incorporated during re-operation. Although a small proximal fistula may be approached by excising the fistula tract to the urethra and performing an inverting closure with additional adjacent tissue, a larger fistula or multiple small fistulae often require a preputial or dartos-based skin flap for an onlay closure. Transposition of considerable dorsal tissue to the ventrum with an originally completed onlay repair provides enough tissue for a primary closure at re-operation. The authors have found that the smaller, distal fistulae represent a deceptively more complex problem, because repair often requires an onlay to ensure adequate coverage as well as a reconstruction of the distal glansplasty.

In complex hypospadias patients with urethrocutaneous fistula or severe stricture disease, excision of all abnormal tissue with onlay of buccal mucosa in a two-stage repair has proved successful in the authors' experience. Hosseini and colleagues[73] describe a 78.6% overall success rate with use of buccal mucosa grafts in patients who developed fistulae after previous hypospadias repair. Evaluation of staged repairs with buccal mucosal grafts in hypospadias cripples suggests that this approach provides good results.[74]

Use of buccal mucosa grafts in complex hypospadias patients can result in complications, however, with rates of meatal stenosis as high as 12.5%, urethral stricture in 31%, and urethrocutaneous fistula in up to 25%.[75] These data are based on small patient cohorts with short follow-up intervals, however, and further investigation is mandated.

Urethral Diverticula and Meatal Stenosis

Urethral diverticula may occur as an independent complication or as a secondary consequence of meatal stenosis. Incorporating excessive tissue in a primary closure or incomplete tailoring of an onlay flap increases the likelihood of diverticula formation. The diverticulum may be trimmed followed by closure and the overlay of local tissue. The authors are cautious about overzealous narrowing of the diverticulum. The tissue that makes up the diverticulum is less distensible laterally. Aggressive narrowing of the urethroplasty, particularly if the defect is long, may result in higher voiding pressures and flattened micturition curves. The authors prefer to wait up to one year to repair diverticula after an onlay or tube repair because local revascularization of the flap in that interval allows for transection of the pedicle if required at the time of reoperation.

Urethral meatal stenosis occurs if blood supply to the distal urethra is compromised after hypospadias repair. Several technical modifications have sought to limit its occurrence. Limiting the involvement of the very distal urethral plate during a TIP or MAGPI procedure and avoiding an excessively tight glansplasty are now understood to be important measures to avoid meatal stenosis.

REFERENCES

1. Devine CJ Jr, Horton CE. Hypospadias repair. J Urol 1977;118:188–93.
2. Willis RA. Pathology of tumors. London: Butterworth; 1948.
3. Allen TD, Griffin JE. Endocrine studies in patients with advanced hypospadias. J Urol 1984;131:310–4.
4. Austin PF, Siow Y, Fallat ME, et al. The relationship between mullerian inhibiting substance and androgens in boys with hypospadias. J Urol 2002;168:1784–8.
5. Teixeira J, Maheswaran S, Donahoe PK. Mullerian inhibiting substance: an instructive developmental hormone with diagnostic and possible therapeutic applications. Endocr Rev 2001;22:657.
6. Baskin LS, Erol A, Li YW, et al. Hypospadias and urethral development. J Urol 2000;163:951–6.
7. Silver RI, Russell DW. 5 alpha-reductase type 2 mutations are present in some boys with isolated hypospadias. J Urol 1999;162:1142–5.
8. Wang MH, Baskin LS. Endocrine disruptors, genital development, and hypospadias. J Androl 2008;29: 499–505.
9. Drake AJ, van den Driesche S, Scott HM, et al. Glucocorticoids amplify dibutyl phthalate-induced disruption of testosterone production and male reproductive development. Endocrinology 2009; 150:5055–64.
10. Goldman AS, Bongiovanni AM. Induced genital anomalies. Ann N Y Acad Sci 1967;142:755–67.
11. Macnab AJ, Zouves C. Hypospadias after assisted reproduction incorporating in vitro fertilization and gamete intrafallopian transfer. Fertil Steril 1991;56: 918–22.
12. Silver RI, Rodriguez R, Chang TS, et al. In vitro fertilization is associated with an increased risk of hypospadias. J Urol 1999;161:1954–7.
13. Fredell L, lichenstein P, Pedersen NL, et al. Hypospadias is related to birth weight in discordant monozygotic twins. J Urol 1998;160:2197–9.
14. Akre O, Boyd HA, Ahlgren M, et al. Maternal and gestational risk factors for hypospadias. Environ Health Perspect 2008;116:1071–6.
15. Carlson WH, Kisely SR, MacLellan DL. Maternal and fetal risk factors associated with severity of hypospadias: a comparison of mild and severe cases. J Pediatr Urol 2009;5:283–6.
16. Kallen B. Case control study of hypospadias, based on registry information. Teratology 1988;38:45.
17. Pierik FH, Burdorf A, Nijman JMR, et al. A high hypospadias rate in Netherlands. Hum Reprod 2002; 17(4):1112–5.
18. Sweet RA, Schrott HG, Kurlan R, et al. Study of the incidence of hypospadias in Rochester, Minnesota, 1940–1970, and a case-controlled comparison of possible etiological factors. Mayo Clin Proc 1974; 49:52.
19. Paulozzi LJ, Erickson JD, Jackson RJ. Hypospadias trends in two US surveillance systems. Pediatrics 1997;100:831.
20. Dolk H. Rise in prevalence of hypospadias. Lancet 1998;351:770.
21. Gatti JM, Kirsch AJ, Troyer WA, et al. Increased incidence of hypospadias in small-for-gestational age infants in a neonatal intensive care unit. BJU Int 2001;87(6):548–50.
22. Fredell L, Kockum I, Hansson E, et al. Heredity of hypospadias and the significance of low birth weight. J Urol 2002;167(3):1423–7.
23. Fisch H, Golden RJ, Libersen GL, et al. Maternal age as a risk factor for hypospadias. J Urol 2001;165(3): 934–6.
24. Roberts CJ, Lloyd S. Observations on the epidemiology of simple hypospadias. Br Med J 1973;1:768–70.
25. Kaplan GW, Lamm DL. Embryogenesis of chordee. J Urol 1975;114:769–72.
26. Glenister JW. The origin and fate of the urethral plate in man. J Anat 1954;288:413–8.
27. Snodgrass W, Patterson K, Plaire JC, et al. Histology of the urethral plate: implications for hypospadias repair. J Urol 2000;164:988–90.
28. Baskin LS, Erol A, Li YW, et al. Anatomical studies of hypospadias. J Urol 1998;160:1108–15.
29. Devine CJ Jr, Horton CE. Chordee without hypospadias. J Urol 1973;110:264–71.
30. Khuri FJ, Hardy BE, Churchill BM. Urologic anomalies associated with hypospadias. Urol Clin North Am 1981;8:565–71.
31. Sorber M, Feitz WF, De Vries JD. Short and mid-term outcome of different types of one-stage hypospadias corrections. Eur Urol 1997;32:475–9.
32. Cerasaro TS, Brock WA, Kaplan GW. Upper urinary tract anomalies associated with congenital hypospadias: is screening necessary? J Urol 1986;135:537–8.
33. Yamaguchi T, Kitada S, Osada Y. Chromosomal anomalies in cryptorchidism and hypospadias. Urol Int 1991;147:60–3.
34. Moreno-Garcia M, Miranda EB. Chromosomal anomalies in cryptorchidism and hypospadias. J Urol 2002;168(5):2170–2.

35. Chang AY, Fan J, Kim SS, et al. Complications of hypospadias surgery are higher in boys with cryptorchidism. Presented at the American Urological Association Annual Meeting, Orlando (FL), May 17–22, 2008.

36. Kaefer M, Diamond D, Hendren WH, et al. The incidence of intersexuality in children with cryptorchidism and hypospadias: stratification based on gonadal palpability and meatal position. J Urol 1999;162(3-II):1003–6.

37. Rajfer J, Walsh PC. The incidence of intersexuality in patients with hypospadias and cryptorchidism. J Urol 1976;116:769–70.

38. Glenister TW. The development of the utricle and of the so called "middle" or "median" lobe of the human prostate. J Anat 1962;96:443.

39. Shima H, Ikoma F, Terakawa T, et al. Testicular function in patients with hypospadias associated with enlarged prostatic utricle. Br J Urol 1992;69:192.

40. Ikoma F, Shima H, Yabumoto H. Classification of enlarged prostatic utricle in patients with hypospadias. Br J Urol 1985;57:334.

41. Ikoma F, Shima H, Yabumoto H, et al. Surgical treatment of enlarged prostatic utricle and vagina masculina in patients with hypospadias. Br J Urol 1986;58:423.

42. Devine CJ Jr, Gonzales-Serva L, Stecker JF Jr, et al. Utricle configuration in hypospadias and intersex. J Urol 1980;123:407.

43. Duckett JW, Baskin LS. Hypospadias. In: Gillenwater JY, Grayhack JT, Howards SS, et al, editors. Adult and pediatric urology. 3 edition. St. Louis (MO): Mosby; 1996. p. 2549–91.

44. Duckett JW. Hypospadias. In: Walsh PC, Retik AB, Vaughan ED Jr, et al, editors, In: Campbell's urology, vol. 2. Philadelphia: WB Saunders; 1998. p. 2093–119.

45. Aarskog D. Clinical and cytogenetic studies in hypospadias. Acta Paediatr Scand Suppl 1970;203:1–61.

46. Koff SA, Jayanthi VR. Preoperative treatment with human chorionic gonadotropin in infancy decreases the severity of proximal hypospadias and chordee. J Urol 1999;162:1435–9.

47. Kass E, Kogan SJ, Manley C. Timing of elective surgery on the genitalia of male children with particular reference to the risks, benefits, and psychological effects of surgery and anesthesia. Pediatrics 1996;97:590–4.

48. DiSandro M, Palmer JM. Stricture incidence related to suture material in hypospadias surgery. J Pediatr Surg 1996;31:881–4.

49. Cromie WJ, Bellinger MF. Hypospadias dressings and diversion. Urol Clin North Am 1981;8:545–8.

50. Van Savage JG, Palanca LG, Slaughenhoupt BL. A prospective randomized trial of dressings versus no dressings for hypospadias repair. J Urol 2000;164:981–3.

51. Hakim S, Merguerian PA, Rabinowitz R, et al. Outcome analysis of the modified Mathieu hypospadias repair: comparison of stented and unstented repairs. J Urol 1996;156:836–8.

52. Montagnino B, Gonzales ET Jr, Roth DR. Open catheter drainage after urethral surgery. J Urol 1988;140:1250.

53. Rich MA, Keating MA, Snyder HM, et al. Hinging the urethral plate in hypospadias meatoplasty. J Urol 1989;142:1551–3.

54. Snodgrass W. Tubularized, incised plate urethroplasty for distal hypospaidas. J Urol 1994;151:464.

55. Snodgrass W, Koyle M, Manzoni G, et al. Tubularized incised plate hypospadias repair for proximal hypospadias: results of a multicenter experience. J Urol 1996;156:839.

56. Snodgrass W, Koyle M, Manzoni G, et al. Tubularized incised plate hypospadias repair for proximal hypospadias. J Urol 1998;159:2129.

57. Snodgrass W, Nguyen MT. Current technique of tubularized incised plate hypospadias repair. Urology 2002;60:157.

58. Snodgrass W, Yucel S. Tubularized incised plate for mid shaft and proximal hypospadias repair. J Urol 2007;177:698–702.

59. Horton CE, Devine CJ, Baran N. Pictorial history of hypospadias repair techniques. In: Horton CE, editor. Plastic and reconstructive surgery of the genital area. Boston: Little Brown; 1973. p. 237–48.

60. Asopa HS, Elhence IP, Atri SP, et al. One stage correction of penile hypospadias using a foreskin tube. Int Surg 1971;55:435.

61. Duckett JW. Transverse preputial island flap technique for repair of severe hypospadias. Urol Clin North Am 1980;7:423.

62. Baskin LS, Duckett JW, Ueoka K, et al. Changing concepts of hypospadias curvature lead to more onlay island flap procedures. J Urol 1994;151:191–6.

63. Avellan L, Knuttson F. Microscopic studies of curvature-causing structures in hypospadias. Scand J Plast Reconstr Surg 1980;14:249–58.

64. Retik AB, Bauer SB, Mandell J, et al. Management of severe hypospadias with a stage repair. J Urol 1994;152:749.

65. Gershbaum MD, Stock JA, Hanna MK. A case for 2-stage repair of perineoscrotal hypospadias with severe chordee. J Urol 2002;168:1727.

66. Metro MJ, Wu HY, Snyder HM. Buccal mucosal grafts: lessons learned from an 8-year experience. J Urol 2001;166:1459.

67. Hendren WH, Keating MA. Use of a dermal graft and free urethral graft in penile reconstruction. J Urol 1988;140:1259–64.

68. Baskin LS, Duckett JW. Mucosal grafts in hypospadias and stricture management. American Urological Association Update Series 1994;13:270.

69. Duckett JW, Coplen D, Ewalt D, et al. Buccal mucosal urethral replacement. J Urol 1995;153:1660.

70. Baskin LS, Duckett JW. Buccal mucosa grafts in hypospadias surgery. Br J Urol 1995;76:23.

71. Hensle TW, Kearney MC, Bingham JB. Buccal mucosa grafts for hypospadias surgery: long-term results. J Urol 2002;168:1734.

72. Cooper CS, Noh PH, Snyder HM. Preservation of urethral plate spongiosum: technique to reduce hypospadias fistulas. Urology 2001;57:351.

73. Hosseini J, Kaviani A, Mohammadhosseini M, et al. Fistula repair after hypospadias surgery using buccal mucosal graft. Urol J 2009;6:19–22.

74. Sripathi V, Satheesh M, Shubha K. Salvage hypospadias repairs. J Indian Assoc Pediatr Surg 2008;13:132–6.

75. Irani D, Hekmati P, Amin-Sharifi A. Results of buccal mucosal graft urethroplasty in complex hypospadias. Urol J 2005;2:111–4.

Cryptorchidism: Pathogenesis, Diagnosis, Treatment and Prognosis

Richard A. Ashley, MD[a], Julia S. Barthold, MD[a],
Thomas F. Kolon, MD[b],*

KEYWORDS

- Cryptorchidism • Testis • Pathogenesis • Diagnosis

Cryptorchidism or undescended testis is the most common disorder of the male endocrine glands in children. Up to one-third of boys with true cryptorchidism have bilaterally cryptorchid testes.[1,2] The main reasons for treatment of cryptorchidism include increased risks of progressive infertility, testicular malignancy, torsion, and/or associated inguinal hernia, and because of cosmetic concerns. The current standard of therapy in the United States is orchidopexy, or surgical repositioning of the testis within the scrotal sac; hormonal therapy has fewer advocates.[3] However, successful relocation of the testis may reduce but does not prevent these potential long-term sequelae in susceptible individuals.

EPIDEMIOLOGY/PATHOGENESIS

The incidence of cryptorchidism is 1% to 4% in full-term newborns and in up to 45% of preterm male babies.[4] A small increase in the prevalence of cryptorchidism in prepubertal boys has been reported by several investigators but is not consistent in all populations.[1,5,6] This condition is an associated finding in hundreds of clinical syndromes, with the ratio of nonsyndromic to syndromic cryptorchidism reported to be greater than 6:1.[7] However, confounding factors such as variations in diagnosis of cryptorchidism between observers, in study populations, and in study design complicate estimates of true prevalence.[4] Advanced maternal age, maternal obesity, maternal diabetes, family history of cryptorchidism, preterm birth, low birth weight or small for gestational age, breech presentation, and consumption of cola-containing drinks during pregnancy have all been suggested as possible risk factors for cryptorchidism.[8,9]

Spontaneous testicular descent in infancy may occur as a result of the normal gonadotropin surge (luteinizing hormone [LH] and follicle-stimulating hormone [FSH]) that occurs around 60 to 90 days of life.[10–13] Gendrel and colleagues[11] and Job and colleagues[13] reported blunting of this surge in boys with cryptorchidism that remain undescended in the first year of life. They reported a significant difference in the polynomial regression curves comparing the testosterone levels of persistently cryptorchid testes with those having delayed spontaneous descent. However, the positive predictive value that bilateral cryptorchidism will have abnormally low testosterone levels is only about 23%.[13] Subsequent studies have been inconsistent, with reduced[14] or normal[15,16] serum testosterone levels and normal[14,15] or relatively increased[16] LH levels, when comparing patients with cryptorchidism and controls.

Studies have suggested genetic susceptibility for cryptorchidism does exist, but this is likely

[a] Nemours/Alfred I. DuPont Hospital for Children, Division of Pediatric Urology, 1600 Rockland Road, Wilmington, DE 19803-3607,USA
[b] Children's Hospital of Philadelphia, Division of Pediatric Urology, 39th Street and Civic Center Boulevard, Philadelphia, PA 19104, USA
* Corresponding author.
E-mail address: kolon@email.chop.edu

Urol Clin N Am 37 (2010) 183–193
doi:10.1016/j.ucl.2010.03.002

polygenic and multifactorial. In a recent population-based study by Schnack and colleagues[17] more than 1 million male births were reviewed. Risk ratios for cryptorchidism were 10.1 in twins, 3.5 in brothers, and 2.3 in offspring of fathers who had an undescended testis. Previous data on this subject suggested a 5-fold increased risk in offspring of affected fathers and a 7- to 10-fold increased risk in those with an affected brother compared with patients with no family history of the disorder.[18–20]

The possibility that environmental chemicals alter normal reproductive tract development has been debated in the recent literature. There is significant potential concern that endocrine-disrupting chemicals that may be linked to the testicular dysgenesis syndrome, described as linked male reproductive tract anomalies, including cryptorchidism, that may have a common cause.[21,22] Concerns about a connection between an endocrine-disrupting chemical and cryptorchidism developed because of a reported higher risk related to early maternal exposure to diethylstilbestrol.[23] However, only indirect correlations and suggestive data have been found correlating exposure to endocrine-disrupting chemicals such as pesticides, flame retardants, and phthalates and the occurrence of cryptorchidism.[24–28] Some question whether epidemiologic data truly support the existence of a clinical testicular dysgenesis syndrome.[29]

The hormonal pathways that are crucial for testicular descent were largely elucidated by studies of animal models. The obvious anatomic differences between human and rodent has incited controversy as to how to interpret the data from such research. Nonetheless, some observers believe the species have sufficient similarity to warrant translational studies of these models.[30] Based on murine models, Hutson and Hasthorpe[31] have proposed that testicular descent occurs in 2 phases. The initial transabdominal descent accompanied by enlargement of the gubernaculum is controlled by the Leydig cell hormone, insulin-like 3 (INSL3).[32,33] Transgenic mice with deletion of *Insl3* are viable but show a severe cryptorchidism phenotype[34,35] suggesting the crucial nature of INSL3 in the process of testicular descent. In addition, these mice have developmental abnormalities of the gubernaculum, abnormal spermatogenesis, and infertility. In human fetuses, Leydig cell production of INSL3 peaks at 15 to 17 weeks' gestation just after the peak in testosterone production at 14 to 16 weeks' gestation.[36,37] In vitro, these hormones cause proliferation of gubernacular cells.[33,38] Animal models suggest that inguinoscrotal descent is

androgen mediated, via the genitofemoral nerve (GFN) and/or by activation of androgen receptors in the gubernaculum.[31,32] The GFN releases calcitonin gene-related peptide (CGRP) on stimulation to produce rhythmical contractions of the murine gubernaculum, which aids migration of the testis and gubernaculum into the scrotum. In addition, androgens may also alter the composition of the gubernaculum resulting in the appropriate swelling and elasticity that promotes testicular descent through the masculinized inguinal canal.[32] Indeed, cryptorchidism has been noted in rodent models exposed to androgen receptor blockade,[39] with defective innervation (the cryptorchid TS rat)[40] and/or with altered muscle-specific gene expression in the gubernaculum (the Long-Evans orl rat).[41]

Androgen Receptor Signaling

The role for androgens in testicular descent is readily observed in clinical human correlates. Cryptorchidism is a common component of complete or partial androgen insensitivity syndrome (CAIS, PAIS) caused by mutations of the androgen receptor (*AR*) gene.[42] The role of *AR* gene mutations in isolated forms of hypospadias or cryptorchidism is less clear. Analysis of this gene in boys with isolated cryptorchidism suggests that longer alleles of the GGN (polyglycine) repeat polymorphism are more common in cases compared with controls but no association of cytosine-adenosine-guanine (CAG) repeat length or variants in other *AR* exons with isolated cryptorchidism.[43–48]

INSL3/RXFP2 Signaling

Several investigators have examined the role of genetic variants of *INSL3* and its receptor, *RXFP2* (relaxin/insulin-like family peptide receptor 2, also known *LGR8* and *GREAT*) in the etiology of cryptorchidism. Binding of the INSL3 protein to RXFP2, which is highly expressed in the gubernaculum, results in increased cAMP production and downstream signaling important in gubernacular development.[49] Several genetic studies have examined the INSL3-RXFP2 pathway to determine the frequency of mutations in either gene in patients with cryptorchidism. The available data suggest that variants of 1 of these genes exist in 3% of cases of cryptorchidism.[50] However, it is not clear at present which genetic variants are functionally significant.[51–53] As yet unidentified genetic and/or environmental factors could also alter expression of INSL3 and/or RXFP2 protein during a critical period of testicular descent. Indeed, a recent study suggests that levels of

INSL3 are reduced in cord blood of boys with persistent cryptorchidism after birth.[54] Further studies are needed to elucidate the role of this important signaling pathway in the pathogenesis of cryptorchidism in man.

Other Genetic Risk Factors for Isolated Undescended Testis

Two posterior HOX genes have been identified as possible candidates for cryptorchidism from murine genetic knockout phenotypes because loss of either Hoxa10 or Hoxa11 is associated with a nonsyndromic cryptorchid phenotype in transgenic mice.[55,56] However, no variants of these genes are consistently associated with cryptorchidism in human studies.[57–59] Similarly, mixed results were obtained in studies of the association of the estrogen receptor alpha (ESR1) gene in clinical cryptorchidism.[60–63]

DIAGNOSIS

Traditionally, testicular position at birth was used to determine the presence or absence of undescended testis. However, in recent decades new evidence supports the concept that some testes that are documented as descended at birth are no longer intrascrotal at a subsequent time.[64] This situation is frequently called acquired cryptorchidism, but it more likely represents primary failure of complete testicular descent, and is associated with similar histopathology to that observed in cases discovered at birth.[65] Although the incidence of acquired maldescent in the general population of boys with normally positioned testes at birth seems to be low in longitudinal studies,[66,67] the risk in boys with retractile testes is 7% to 45%.[68–71]

History and Physical Examination

Potential risk factors include prematurity, birth weight, breech presentation, maternal diabetes, maternal use/exposure to exogenous hormones (estrogens), lesions of the central nervous system (myelomeningocele or cerebral palsy), and previous inguinal surgery. Family history of cryptorchidism or other genital anomalies, congenital syndromes, infertility, and consanguinity are relevant. It is also important to note if the testes were ever palpable in the scrotum at the time of birth or within the first year of life.

Classification is based on testicular location, either along the normal line of descent (abdomen, inguinal canal, external ring, prescrotal, upper scrotal) or in an ectopic position (usually in the superficial inguinal pouch or perineal; rarely perirenal). An important distinction is whether or not the testis is palpable, and whether the cryptorchidism is isolated or a component of a syndrome, as these classifications may affect treatment plans and provide further direction to evaluate for other associated urologic conditions. It is important to document associated findings such as hernia, hydrocele, penile size, and meatal position.

The patient should be examined supine with legs abducted initially. With warmed hands, check the size, location, and texture of the contralateral descended testis. Begin examination of the undescended testis at the anterior superior iliac spine and sweep the groin from lateral to medial with the nondominant hand. Once the testis is palpated, grasp it with the dominant hand and continue to sweep the testis toward the scrotum with the other hand. Assess testicular mobility, size, consistency, and spermatic cord tension. Maintain the position of the testis in the scrotum for a minute, so that the cremaster muscle is fatigued. Release the testis, and if it remains in place for a short time but then retracts, it is considered retractile. The key to distinguishing a retractile from an undescended testis is success of delivery and stability of the testis within the scrotum. The retractile testis will remain intrascrotal after overstretching of the cremaster muscle, whereas a low cryptorchid testis will return to its undescended position after being released. If there is any question, a follow-up examination is indicated. An experienced examiner should evaluate patients with retractile testes on a yearly basis.

For patients who are difficult to examine because of obesity, lack of cooperativity, and/or a hyperactive cremasteric reflex, the cross-legged or baseball catcher's position can also help relax the cremaster muscle. Wetting the fingers of the nondominant hand with lubricating jelly or soap can increase the sensitivity of the fingers in palpating the small mobile testis. Usually the cryptorchid testis is palpable (~80%), as reported in large contemporary series.[72,73]

When the testis is truly nonpalpable, possible findings include complete testicular atrophy (vanishing testis or testicular regression syndrome), an abdominal or peeping (in and out of the internal ring) testis and extra-abdominal location but not palpable because of patient factors or small testicular size.[72,74–77] A vanishing testis can be found anywhere along the normal path to the scrotum. The cause is prenatal vascular thrombosis or torsion because of the frequent identification of hemosiderin associated with the testicular remnant.[78] Hypertrophy of the contralateral descended testis (>1.8–2 mL) in combination with a palpable scrotal nubbin and absence of palpable scrotal appendages (sac, gubernaculums, or cord structures) indicates a high likelihood of monorchism as a result of testicular regression.[79] If abnormal penile and/or urethral development occurs with unilateral or bilateral cryptorchidism, further diagnostic studies may be indicated to evaluate for hypogonadism or disorders of sexual differentiation.[80,81]

Imaging and Laboratory Tests

The use of imaging studies to aid in the diagnosis in cases of nonpalpable testis is controversial. Ultrasound (US), computed tomography (CT) scan and magnetic resonance imaging (MRI) have been applied in this clinical scenario but the accuracy of these studies in identifying intra-abdominal testes may be low. Hrebinko and Bellinger[82] found that the most reliable mode of examination has been the physical examination by a pediatric urologist (84%) compared with a referring physician (53%). The accuracy of imaging studies in this series was 44% and imaging did not influence management decisions in any of the cases. Similarly, Elder[83] reported that US has limited usefulness when an experienced surgeon examines a patient with cryptorchidism. In contrast, other studies suggest that if an experienced surgeon evaluates a child and determines the testis to be nonpalpable, the sensitivity of US can be as high as 95% to 97% for an inguinal testis, and even identify an abdominal testis in certain cases.[84,85] Thus, US may be useful in certain cases of nonpalpable testes to aid in planning for either laparoscopic or inguinal approaches. Furthermore, MRI may be useful in identifying an ectopic abdominal testis, if not found by laparoscopy or open exploration. Yeung and colleagues[86] identified 100% of canalicular and 96% of intra-abdominal testes using gadolinium-enhanced MR angiography. However, this technique is expensive, requires sedation, and the results have not been reproduced.[87]

In boys with bilateral nonpalpable testes or associated hypospadias, chromosomal and endocrine evaluation may be useful. In infants with bilateral nonpalpable testes, the postnatal testosterone surge is absent if anorchia is present. After 3 months of age, a human chorionic gonadotropin (hCG) stimulation test can aid in the diagnosis of anorchia, most frequently showing a low serum testosterone level and increased LH and FSH levels.[88] However, in mid-childhood low baseline gonadotropin levels and poor response to hCG may occur in anorchia.[89] Serum levels of anti-Müllerian hormone (AMH) or inhibin B can also document the presence of testicular tissue.[90]

TREATMENT
Hormonal Therapy

Primary hormonal therapy with hCG or gonadotropin-releasing hormone (GnRH or LH-releasing hormone [LHRH]) have been used for many years, especially in Europe. The exact mechanism of action of gonadotropin on postnatal testicular descent is not known but may involve effects on the spermatic cord and/or cremaster muscle. Divergent results have been reported likely because of suboptimal study design, differences in patient age and treatment schedules, possible inclusion of retractile testes, and variable follow-up. However, several meta-analyses of this published literature suggest that the effectiveness of primary hormonal therapy in cryptorchidism is less than 20%.[91–93] A recent consensus statement discourages use of hormone therapy for cryptorchidism.[3]

Some data suggest that spermatogonia/tubule (S/T) ratios may improve after treatment with low dose LHRH analogue therapy.[94,95] However, caution is advised when evaluating these data because of retrospective, nonrandomized study design and patient heterogeneity.[96]

Surgery

Palpable testis

Standard inguinal orchidopexy involves several steps after repeat examination under anesthesia to reconfirm testicular location. A transverse inguinal incision is made along Langer lines and Scarpa fascia is incised with care to avoid injury to a testis in the superficial inguinal pouch. The testis is mobilized after incision of the gubernacular remnant. The cremasteric muscle fibers are transected and the hernia sac isolated, transected, mobilized to the internal inguinal, and ligated. After division of lateral fascial bands, the testis is placed in the scrotum in a subcutaneous or subdartos pouch without transcapsular sutures.

A primary scrotal approach to orchidopexy is described in cases in which the testis is palpable and is either close to the scrotum or can be easily drawn into the sac.[97–103] Successful mobilization of the testis and ligation of the hernia sac at the level of the external or internal ring is described; alternatively a secondary inguinal incision is made if needed. Many series report use of testicular fixation sutures within the dartos pouch to maintain the testis in a dependent scrotal position. Testicular retraction or atrophy has been reported at 0% to 2%, and postoperative hernia has been noted in 2% to 3% of cases with follow-up in these series ranging from 1 month to 3 years. Thus, this approach may be a viable option in select cases of cryptorchidism when testes are distal to the external ring.

Further maneuvers may be used to obtain adequate length of a high inguinal testis. Passing the testis behind the inferior epigastric artery and vein after opening the transversalis fascia (the Prentiss maneuver) allows more medial positioning of the cord. Dividing the internal oblique muscles with lengthening the incision as needed allows further opening of the internal ring and additional dissection of the lateral spermatic fascia in the retroperitoneal space.

A Fowler-Stephens orchiopexy, or division of the internal spermatic artery, can be performed if extensive dissection between the vas and cord has not occurred, as testicular survival then relies on the deferential and external spermatic blood supply. An alternative for the high testis is microvascular autotransplantation to the ipsilateral inferior epigastric artery and vein.

Rarely, a 2-stage orchidopexy may be used without division of the spermatic vessels when the Prentiss maneuver and cord dissection fail to provide adequate length. The testis is anchored in its most dependent position or the spermatic cord may be wrapped in a protective sheath[104] for ease of the second stage, generally 6 to 12 months later.

Nonpalpable testis

Exploration for a nonpalpable testis may occur through an extended inguinal incision, an abdominal incision, or, more commonly, via diagnostic laparoscopy. At the time of exploration, the most likely findings are intra-abdominal or peeping testis just at the internal ring (25%–50%), vanishing testis most commonly distal to the internal ring (15%–40%) or cord structures (vessels and vas) that enter the internal ring in the presence of a viable testis that is nonpalpable because of the size of the testis or patient's body habitus.[72,74–77] Absence of visible spermatic vessels warrants further full exploration of the retroperitoneum to document testicular agenesis, which is extremely rare. The finding of cord vessels entering the ring warrants inguinal exploration for identification of a distal viable or vanishing testis. Some surgeons use a primary transscrotal approach when a palpable scrotal nubbin is present and confirm the diagnosis of vanishing testis by visualizing a black area containing hemosiderin.[105,106] However, if findings are questionable using this approach, laparoscopy is warranted. Although controversial, fixation of the solitary testis should be considered to protect against the theoretic risk of torsion.

Options for treatment of an intra-abdominal testis are varied depending on the patient's age,

testis size, contralateral testis, and the skills of the surgeon, but laparoscopic orchidopexy is often the procedure of choice with high success rates reported. Goals are to mobilize all structures extending distal to the internal ring, transect the peritoneum lateral to the spermatic vessels and distal to the vas, and to mobilize these vessels proximally while maintaining collateral blood supply with the vas should a Fowler-Stephens maneuver be required. Adequate length is defined by mobilization of the testis to the contralateral internal ring. A new hiatus is created by retrograde passage of a clamp or port at the level of the medial umbilical ligament. Formal closure of the dissected internal ring is not necessary.[107,108] If dissection does not allow for adequate length to reach the scrotum, the spermatic vessels are clipped, followed by a 1- or 2-stage operation to bring the testis into the scrotum. The typical success rates of contemporary series for standard, 1-stage and 2-stage Fowler-Stephens laparoscopic orchiopexy are 90% to 100%, 71% to 97% and 84% to 96%, respectively.[77,107,109–117]

PROGNOSIS

Although most patients with unilateral cryptorchidism do not present with complaints of infertility, spermatogenic function is reduced to some extent in the most men with a history of undescended testis. Moreover, the risk of tumor formation exists in affected and to a lesser extent contralateral descended testes. These long-term risks exist even after completion of successful treatment, although there is evidence to suggest that earlier orchidopexy may reduce the frequency of these complications.

Fertility

The most consistent finding in histologic evaluation of the cryptorchid testis is abnormal germ cell development. Normally, primordial germ cells migrate into the testicular cords and differentiate into gonocytes; some degenerate by apoptosis, whereas others attach to the basement membrane and give rise to type A spermatogonia during the third to fifth months of life (**Fig. 1**). Although several spermatogonial subtypes exist, the adult dark (Ad) cells likely represent spermatogonial stem cells.[118] Type B spermatogonia and primary spermatocytes appear during the fourth year and spermatogenesis arrests at this stage until puberty.

The total number of germ cells (GC) and Leydig cells in the cryptorchid testis is within the normal range during the first 6 months of life.[119] However, the number of spermatogonia remains low in many cases and does not increase with time. Although

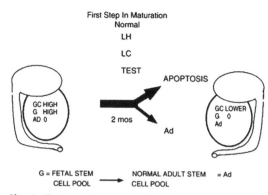

Fig. 1. First steps to germ cell maturation.

the ratio of gonocytes to spermatogonia seems normal in cryptorchid testes at about 1.5 months of age, by 7.5 months, the ratio of persistent gonocytes is greater than that observed in scrotal testes at a mean of 10 months of age.[12] Thus, observations of arrested development of spermatogonia is a common finding in cryptorchid testes and has been recognized for more than 40 years.[120] Low S/T ratios are associated with increased risk for infertility.[121,122] However, failure to establish an adequate Ad spermatogonia population in cryptorchid testes seems to correlate more closely with sperm counts in adulthood than total S/T count alone.[123,124] A reduced number of Leydig/interstitial cells in undescended compared with contralateral descended testis[119] and with increasing age at orchidopexy[125] is also reported. In addition, there is disruption of morphology, failure of maturation at puberty and evidence for reduced number of Sertoli cells after 4 months of age in the cryptorchid testis.[126–129]

Abnormal semen quality is common, with reduced sperm counts reported in 75% to 100% and 18% to 43% of men with bilateral and unilateral cryptorchidism, respectively.[130–133] However, paternity rates are higher in these groups than would be predicted solely by sperm counts. In a review of case-control studies, Lee[134] reported paternity rates of 65%, 90%, and 93% in bilaterally and unilaterally ex-cryptorchid and matched controls, respectively, with no significant difference between unilateral cases and controls. Testicular position or size did not correlate with paternity rate in the unilateral group, and the frequency of abnormal sperm counts was similar to data reported previously (81% and 17%, respectively). Moreover, earlier orchidopexy was associated with higher inhibin B and lower FSH levels. Lee notes that there is large overlap in semen and hormonal findings in these patients and a relative paucity of information regarding

the outcome of men with a history of bilateral cryptorchidism. Further studies are required to better predict prognosis for fertility in this common disease.

Testicular Malignancy

The increased risk of germ cell tumor (GCT) arising in a cryptorchid testis may be related to persistence of gonocytes, which as precursors of testicular carcinoma in situ (CIS) may then evolve into frank GCT.[135] Recent analyses by Wood and Elder[136] critically evaluated several concerns surrounding the topic of cryptorchidism and testicular cancer. They determined from their review that previous estimates of cancer risk in cryptorchid testes were too high (at 26–40 times greater risk) and are more likely 2.5 to 8 overall, with a decreased relative risk of 2 to 3 if prepubertal orchidopexy is performed. In their review of the risk of malignancy in contralateral descended testes, they noted that studies suggesting such a risk demonstrated significant flaws in study design, such as use of patient recall to determine if previous cryptorchidism was present, and the total number of cancer cases reviewed were rarely in the testis not affected by maldescent. In contrast, in their recent meta-analysis Akre and colleagues[137] derived a significantly increased relative risk of tumor in the contralateral testis of 1.7 (95% confidence interval [CI] 1.01–2.98) in men with a history of unilateral cryptorchidism.

Recent data suggest that risk of malignant degeneration may be 2 to 6 times higher in men who underwent orchidopexy after puberty compared with those having surgery at an earlier age.[138,139] Orchiectomy is the best option for postpubertal men up to age 50 years because these gonads have poor fertility potential and increased risk, whereas nonoperative treatment is recommended in men older than 50 years because their cancer risk has never been defined.[136] The malignant tumor developing in persistently cryptorchid testes is most commonly seminoma (74%); after orchidopexy two-thirds of malignancies are non-seminoma.[136] In summary, every cryptorchid testis carries some risk for cancer. As a result, patients with a history of cryptorchidism should be taught testicular self-examination. Parents should be made aware that orchidopexy enables early detection but does not necessarily decrease risk for testicular cancer.

SUMMARY

Ongoing research has begun to define the possible molecular and environmental factors contributing to the risk of cryptorchidism.

Increasing evidence suggests that early orchidopexy may be beneficial for testicular function and reduced risk of tumor, although normal fertility is expected in unilateral cases. Laparoscopy is preferred for diagnosis and treatment of abdominal testes, with high success rates reported.

REFERENCES

1. Berkowitz GS, Lapinski RH, Dolgin SE, et al. Prevalence and natural history of cryptorchidism. Pediatrics 1993;92:44.
2. Scorer CG. The descent of the testis. Arch Dis Child 1964;39:605.
3. Thorsson AV, Christiansen P, Ritzen M. Efficacy and safety of hormonal treatment of cryptorchidism: current state of the art. Acta Paediatr 2007;96:628.
4. Sijstermans K, Hack WW, Meijer RW, et al. The frequency of undescended testis from birth to adulthood: a review. Int J Androl 2008;31:1.
5. Chilvers C, Pike MC, Forman D, et al. Apparent doubling of frequency of undescended testis in England and Wales in 1962–81. Lancet 1984;2:330.
6. Simpson AS, Laugesen M, Silva PA, et al. The prevalence of retained testes in Dunedin. N Z Med J 1985;98:758.
7. Boyd HA, Myrup C, Wohlfahrt J, et al. Maternal serum alpha-fetoprotein level during pregnancy and isolated cryptorchidism in male offspring. Am J Epidemiol 2006;164:478.
8. Damgaard IN, Jensen TK, Petersen JH, et al. Risk factors for congenital cryptorchidism in a prospective birth cohort study. PLoS One 2008;3:e3051.
9. Virtanen HE, Toppari J. Epidemiology and pathogenesis of cryptorchidism. Hum Reprod Update 2008;14:49.
10. Forest MG, Sizonenko PC, Cathiard AM, et al. Hypophyso-gonadal function in humans during the first year of life. 1. Evidence for testicular activity in early infancy. J Clin Invest 1974;53:819.
11. Gendrel D, Job JC, Roger M. Reduced post-natal rise of testosterone in plasma of cryptorchid infants. Acta Endocrinol (Copenh) 1978;89:372.
12. Hadziselimovic F, Thommen L, Girard J, et al. The significance of postnatal gonadotropin surge for testicular development in normal and cryptorchid testes. J Urol 1986;136:274.
13. Job JC, Toublanc JE, Chaussain JL, et al. The pituitary-gonadal axis in cryptorchid infants and children. Eur J Pediatr 1987;146(Suppl 2):S2.
14. Pierik FH, Deddens JA, Burdorf A, et al. The hypothalamus-pituitary-testis axis in boys during the first six months of life: a comparison of cryptorchidism and hypospadias cases with controls. Int J Androl 2009;32:453.
15. Barthold JS, Manson J, Regan V, et al. Reproductive hormone levels in infants with cryptorchidism during postnatal activation of the pituitary-testicular axis. J Urol 2004;172:1736.
16. Suomi AM, Main KM, Kaleva M, et al. Hormonal changes in 3-month-old cryptorchid boys. J Clin Endocrinol Metab 2006;91:953.
17. Schnack TH, Zdravkovic S, Myrup C, et al. Familial aggregation of cryptorchidism–a nationwide cohort study. Am J Epidemiol 2008;167:1453.
18. Czeizel A, Erodi E, Toth J. Genetics of undescended testis. J Urol 1981;126:528.
19. Elert A, Jahn K, Heidenreich A, et al. Population-based investigation of familial undescended testis and its association with other urogenital anomalies. J Pediatr Urol 2005;1:403.
20. Jones IR, Young ID. Familial incidence of cryptorchidism. J Urol 1982;127:508.
21. Main KM, Skakkebaek NE, Toppari J. Cryptorchidism as part of the testicular dysgenesis syndrome: the environmental connection. Endocr Dev 2009;14:167.
22. Sharpe RM, Skakkebaek NE. Testicular dysgenesis syndrome: mechanistic insights and potential new downstream effects. Fertil Steril 2008;89:e33.
23. Palmer JR, Herbst AL, Noller KL, et al. Urogenital abnormalities in men exposed to diethylstilbestrol in utero: a cohort study. Environ Health 2009;8:37.
24. Damgaard IN, Skakkebaek NE, Toppari J, et al. Persistent pesticides in human breast milk and cryptorchidism. Environ Health Perspect 2006;114:1133.
25. Fernandez MF, Olmos B, Granada A, et al. Human exposure to endocrine-disrupting chemicals and prenatal risk factors for cryptorchidism and hypospadias: a nested case-control study. Environ Health Perspect 2007;115(Suppl 1):8.
26. Main KM, Mortensen GK, Kaleva MM, et al. Human breast milk contamination with phthalates and alterations of endogenous reproductive hormones in infants three months of age. Environ Health Perspect 2006;114:270.
27. Pierik FH, Burdorf A, Deddens JA, et al. Maternal and paternal risk factors for cryptorchidism and hypospadias: a case-control study in newborn boys. Environ Health Perspect 2004;112:1570.
28. Weidner IS, Moller H, Jensen TK, et al. Cryptorchidism and hypospadias in sons of gardeners and farmers. Environ Health Perspect 1998;106:793.
29. Akre O, Richiardi L. Does a testicular dysgenesis syndrome exist? Hum Reprod 2009;24:2053.
30. van der Schoot P. Towards a rational terminology in the study of the gubernaculum testis: arguments in support of the notion that the cremasteric sac should be considered the gubernaculum in

postnatal rats and other mammals. J Anat 1996; 189(Pt 1):97.

31. Hutson JM, Hasthorpe S. Abnormalities of testicular descent. Cell Tissue Res 2005;322:155.

32. Husmann DA. Testicular descent: a hypothesis and review of current controversies. Pediatr Endocrinol Rev 2009;6:491.

33. Kubota Y, Temelcos C, Bathgate RA, et al. The role of insulin 3, testosterone, Mullerian inhibiting substance and relaxin in rat gubernacular growth. Mol Hum Reprod 2002;8:900.

34. Nef S, Parada LF. Cryptorchidism in mice mutant for Insl3. Nat Genet 1999;22:295.

35. Zimmermann S, Steding G, Emmen JM, et al. Targeted disruption of the Insl3 gene causes bilateral cryptorchidism. Mol Endocrinol 1999; 13:681.

36. Anand-Ivell R, Ivell R, Driscoll D, et al. Insulin-like factor 3 levels in amniotic fluid of human male fetuses. Hum Reprod 2008;23:1180.

37. Bay K, Cohen AS, Jorgensen FS, et al. Insulin-like factor 3 levels in second-trimester amniotic fluid. J Clin Endocrinol Metab 2008;93:4048.

38. Emmen JM, McLuskey A, Adham IM, et al. Hormonal control of gubernaculum development during testis descent: gubernaculum outgrowth in vitro requires both insulin-like factor and androgen. Endocrinology 2000;141:4720.

39. Husmann DA, Boone TB, McPhaul MJ. Flutamide-induced testicular undescent in the rat is associated with alterations in genitofemoral nerve morphology. J Urol 1994;151:509.

40. Hrabovszky Z, Farmer PJ, Hutson JM. Undescended testis is accompanied by calcitonin gene related peptide accumulation within the sensory nucleus of the genitofemoral nerve in trans-scrotal rats. J Urol 2001;165:1015.

41. Barthold JS, McCahan SM, Singh AV, et al. Altered expression of muscle- and cytoskeleton-related genes in a rat strain with inherited cryptorchidism. J Androl 2008;29:352.

42. Barthold JS, Kumasi-Rivers K, Upadhyay J, et al. Testicular position in the androgen insensitivity syndrome: implications for the role of androgens in testicular descent. J Urol 2000;164:497.

43. Aschim EL, Nordenskjold A, Giwercman A, et al. Linkage between cryptorchidism, hypospadias, and GGN repeat length in the androgen receptor gene. J Clin Endocrinol Metab 2004;89:5105.

44. Ferlin A, Garolla A, Bettella A, et al. Androgen receptor gene CAG and GGC repeat lengths in cryptorchidism. Eur J Endocrinol 2005;152:419.

45. Radpour R, Rezaee M, Tavasoly A, et al. Association of long polyglycine tracts (GGN repeats) in exon 1 of the androgen receptor gene with cryptorchidism and penile hypospadias in Iranian patients. J Androl 2007;28:164.

46. Sasagawa I, Suzuki Y, Muroya K, et al. Androgen receptor gene and male genital anomaly. Arch Androl 2002;48:461.

47. Silva-Ramos M, Oliveira JM, Cabeda JM, et al. The CAG repeat within the androgen receptor gene and its relationship to cryptorchidism. Int Braz J Urol 2006;32:330.

48. Wiener JS, Marcelli M, Gonzales ET Jr, et al. Androgen receptor gene alterations are not associated with isolated cryptorchidism. J Urol 1998;160: 863.

49. Kumagai J, Hsu SY, Matsumi H, et al. INSL3/Leydig insulin-like peptide activates the LGR8 receptor important in testis descent. J Biol Chem 2002; 277:31283.

50. Foresta C, Zuccarello D, Garolla A, et al. Role of hormones, genes, and environment in human cryptorchidism. Endocr Rev 2008;29:560.

51. Bogatcheva NV, Ferlin A, Feng S, et al. T222P mutation of the insulin-like 3 hormone receptor LGR8 is associated with testicular maldescent and hinders receptor expression on the cell surface membrane. Am J Physiol Endocrinol Metab 2007;292:E138.

52. El Houate B, Rouba H, Imken L, et al. No association between T222P/LGR8 mutation and cryptorchidism in the Moroccan population. Horm Res 2008; 70:236.

53. Nuti F, Marinari E, Erdei E, et al. The leucine-rich repeat-containing G protein-coupled receptor 8 gene T222P mutation does not cause cryptorchidism. J Clin Endocrinol Metab 2008;93:1072.

54. Bay K, Virtanen HE, Hartung S, et al. Insulin-like factor 3 levels in cord blood and serum from children: effects of age, postnatal hypothalamic-pituitary-gonadal axis activation, and cryptorchidism. J Clin Endocrinol Metab 2007;92:4020.

55. Branford WW, Benson GV, Ma L, et al. Characterization of Hoxa-10/Hoxa-11 transheterozygotes reveals functional redundancy and regulatory interactions. Dev Biol 2000;224:373.

56. Satokata I, Benson G, Maas R. Sexually dimorphic sterility phenotypes in Hoxa10-deficient mice. Nature 1995;374:460.

57. Bertini V, Bertelloni S, Valetto A, et al. Homeobox HOXA10 gene analysis in cryptorchidism. J Pediatr Endocrinol Metab 2004;17:41.

58. Kolon TF, Wiener JS, Lewitton M, et al. Analysis of homeobox gene HOXA10 mutations in cryptorchidism. J Urol 1999;161:275.

59. Wang Y, Barthold J, Kanetsky PA, et al. Allelic variants in HOX genes in cryptorchidism. Birth Defects Res A Clin Mol Teratol 2007;79:269.

60. Galan JJ, Guarducci E, Nuti F, et al. Molecular analysis of estrogen receptor alpha gene AGATA haplotype and SNP12 in European populations: potential protective effect for cryptorchidism and lack of

association with male infertility. Hum Reprod 2007; 22:444.

61. Wang Y, Barthold J, Figueroa E, et al. Analysis of five single nucleotide polymorphisms in the ESR1 gene in cryptorchidism. Birth Defects Res A Clin Mol Teratol 2008;82:482.

62. Watanabe M, Yoshida R, Ueoka K, et al. Haplotype analysis of the estrogen receptor 1 gene in male genital and reproductive abnormalities. Hum Reprod 2007;22:1279.

63. Yoshida R, Fukami M, Sasagawa I, et al. Association of cryptorchidism with a specific haplotype of the estrogen receptor alpha gene: implication for the susceptibility to estrogenic environmental endocrine disruptors. J Clin Endocrinol Metab 2005;90:4716.

64. Barthold JS, Gonzalez R. The epidemiology of congenital cryptorchidism, testicular ascent and orchiopexy. J Urol 2003;170:2396.

65. Rusnack SL, Wu HY, Huff DS, et al. The ascending testis and the testis undescended since birth share the same histopathology. J Urol 2002;168:2590.

66. Acerini CL, Miles HL, Dunger DB, et al. The descriptive epidemiology of congenital and acquired cryptorchidism in a UK infant cohort. Arch Dis Child 2009;94:868.

67. Wohlfahrt-Veje C, Boisen KA, Boas M, et al. Acquired cryptorchidism is frequent in infancy and childhood. Int J Androl 2009;32:423.

68. Agarwal PK, Diaz M, Elder JS. Retractile testis–is it really a normal variant? J Urol 2006;175:1496.

69. La Scala GC, Ein SH. Retractile testes: an outcome analysis on 150 patients. J Pediatr Surg 2004;39:1014.

70. Stec AA, Thomas JC, DeMarco RT, et al. Incidence of testicular ascent in boys with retractile testes. J Urol 2007;178:1722.

71. Wyllie GG. The retractile testis. Med J Aust 1984; 140:403.

72. Cendron M, Huff DS, Keating MA, et al. Anatomical, morphological and volumetric analysis: a review of 759 cases of testicular maldescent. J Urol 1993;149:570.

73. Moul JW, Belman AB. A review of surgical treatment of undescended testes with emphasis on anatomical position. J Urol 1988;140:125.

74. Cisek LJ, Peters CA, Atala A, et al. Current findings in diagnostic laparoscopic evaluation of the non-palpable testis. J Urol 1998;160:1145.

75. Kirsch AJ, Escala J, Duckett JW, et al. Surgical management of the nonpalpable testis: the Children's Hospital of Philadelphia experience. J Urol 1998;159:1340.

76. Patil KK, Green JS, Duffy PG. Laparoscopy for impalpable testes. BJU Int 2005;95:704.

77. Radmayr C, Oswald J, Schwentner C, et al. Long-term outcome of laparoscopically managed non-palpable testes. J Urol 2003;170:2409.

78. Hegarty PK, Mushtaq I, Sebire NJ. Natural history of testicular regression syndrome and consequences for clinical management. J Pediatr Urol 2007;3:206.

79. Mesrobian HG, Chassaignac JM, Laud PW. The presence or absence of an impalpable testis can be predicted from clinical observations alone. BJU Int 2002;90:97.

80. Cox MJ, Coplen DE, Austin PF. The incidence of disorders of sexual differentiation and chromosomal abnormalities of cryptorchidism and hypospadias stratified by meatal location. J Urol 2008; 180:2649.

81. Kaefer M, Diamond D, Hendren WH, et al. The incidence of intersexuality in children with cryptorchidism and hypospadias: stratification based on gonadal palpability and meatal position. J Urol 1999;162:1003.

82. Hrebinko RL, Bellinger MF. The limited role of imaging techniques in managing children with undescended testes. J Urol 1993;150:458.

83. Elder JS. Ultrasonography is unnecessary in evaluating boys with a nonpalpable testis. Pediatrics 2002;110:748.

84. Cain MP, Garra B, Gibbons MD. Scrotal-inguinal ultrasonography: a technique for identifying the nonpalpable inguinal testis without laparoscopy. J Urol 1996;156:791.

85. Nijs SM, Eijsbouts SW, Madern GC, et al. Nonpalpable testes: is there a relationship between ultrasonographic and operative findings? Pediatr Radiol 2007;37:374.

86. Yeung CK, Tam YH, Chan YL, et al. A new management algorithm for impalpable undescended testis with gadolinium enhanced magnetic resonance angiography. J Urol 1999;162:998.

87. Desireddi NV, Liu DB, Maizels M, et al. Magnetic resonance arteriography/venography is not accurate to structure management of the impalpable testis. J Urol 1805;180:2008.

88. De Rosa M, Lupoli G, Mennitti M, et al. Congenital bilateral anorchia: clinical, hormonal and imaging study in 12 cases. Andrologia 1996;28:281.

89. Lustig RH, Conte FA, Kogan BA, et al. Ontogeny of gonadotropin secretion in congenital anorchism: sexual dimorphism versus syndrome of gonadal dysgenesis and diagnostic considerations. J Urol 1987;138:587.

90. Grumbach MM. A window of opportunity: the diagnosis of gonadotropin deficiency in the male infant. J Clin Endocrinol Metab 2005;90:3122.

91. Henna MR, Del Nero RG, Sampaio CZ, et al. Hormonal cryptorchidism therapy: systematic review with metanalysis of randomized clinical trials. Pediatr Surg Int 2004;20:357.

92. Ong C, Hasthorpe S, Hutson JM. Germ cell development in the descended and cryptorchid testis

and the effects of hormonal manipulation. Pediatr Surg Int 2005;21:240.

93. Pyorala S, Huttunen NP, Uhari M. A review and meta-analysis of hormonal treatment of cryptorchidism. J Clin Endocrinol Metab 1995;80:2795.

94. Bica DT, Hadziselimovic F. Buserelin treatment of cryptorchidism: a randomized, double-blind, placebo-controlled study. J Urol 1992;148:617.

95. Hadziselimovic F, Huff D, Duckett J, et al. Long-term effect of luteinizing hormone-releasing hormone analogue (buserelin) on cryptorchid testes. J Urol 1987;138:1043.

96. Barthold JS. Is adjuvant hormonal therapy indicated in cryptorchidism? Nat Clin Pract Urol 2005;2:366.

97. Al-Mandil M, Khoury AE, El-Hout Y, et al. Potential complications with the prescrotal approach for the palpable undescended testis? A comparison of single prescrotal incision to the traditional inguinal approach. J Urol 2008;180:686.

98. Bassel YS, Scherz HC, Kirsch AJ. Scrotal incision orchiopexy for undescended testes with or without a patent processus vaginalis. J Urol 2007;177:1516.

99. Bianchi A, Squire BR. Transscrotal orchidopexy:orchidopexy revised. Pediatr Surg Int 1989;4:189.

100. Dayanc M, Kibar Y, Irkilata HC, et al. Long-term outcome of scrotal incision orchiopexy for undescended testis. Urology 2007;70:786.

101. Rajimwale A, Brant WO, Koyle MA. High scrotal (Bianchi) single-incision orchidopexy: a "tailored" approach to the palpable undescended testis. Pediatr Surg Int 2004;20:618.

102. Russinko PJ, Siddiq FM, Tackett LD, et al. Prescrotal orchiopexy: an alternative surgical approach for the palpable undescended testis. J Urol 2003;170:2436.

103. Takahashi M, Kurokawa Y, Nakanishi R, et al. Low transscrotal orchidopexy is a safe and effective approach for undescended testes distal to the external inguinal ring. Urol Int 2009;82:92.

104. Dessanti A, Falchetti D, Iannuccelli M, et al. Cryptorchidism with short spermatic vessels: staged orchiopexy preserving spermatic vessels. J Urol 2009;182:1163.

105. Belman AB, Rushton HG. Is an empty left hemiscrotum and hypertrophied right descended testis predictive of perinatal torsion? J Urol 2003;170:1674.

106. Snodgrass WT, Yucel S, Ziada A. Scrotal exploration for unilateral nonpalpable testis. J Urol 2007;178:1718.

107. Handa R, Kale R, Harjai MM. Laparoscopic orchiopexy: is closure of the internal ring necessary? J Postgrad Med 2005;51:266.

108. Riquelme M, Aranda A, Rodriguez C, et al. Incidence and management of the inguinal hernia during laparoscopic orchiopexy in palpable cryptoorchidism: preliminary report. Pediatr Surg Int 2007;23:301.

109. Baker LA, Docimo SG, Surer I, et al. A multi-institutional analysis of laparoscopic orchidopexy. BJU Int 2001;87:484.

110. Chang M, Franco I. Laparoscopic Fowler-Stephens orchiopexy: the Westchester Medical Center experience. J Endourol 2008;22:1315.

111. Denes FT, Saito FJ, Silva FA, et al. Laparoscopic diagnosis and treatment of nonpalpable testis. Int Braz J Urol 2008;34:329.

112. Esposito C, Damiano R, Gonzalez Sabin MA, et al. Laparoscopy-assisted orchiopexy: an ideal treatment for children with intra-abdominal testes. J Endourol 2002;16:659.

113. Esposito C, Garipoli V. The value of 2-step laparoscopic Fowler-Stephens orchiopexy for intraabdominal testes. J Urol 1952;158:1997.

114. Jordan GH, Winslow BH. Laparoscopic single stage and staged orchiopexy. J Urol 1994;152:1249.

115. Lotan G, Klin B, Efrati Y, et al. Laparoscopic evaluation and management of nonpalpable testis in children. World J Surg 2001;25:1542.

116. Robertson SA, Munro FD, Mackinlay GA. Two-stage Fowler-Stephens orchiopexy preserving the gubernacular vessels and a purely laparoscopic second stage. J Laparoendosc Adv Surg Tech A 2007;17:101.

117. Samadi AA, Palmer LS, Franco I. Laparoscopic orchiopexy: report of 203 cases with review of diagnosis, operative technique, and lessons learned. J Endourol 2003;17:365.

118. Dym M, Kokkinaki M, He Z. Spermatogonial stem cells: mouse and human comparisons. Birth Defects Res C Embryo Today 2009;87:27.

119. Huff DS, Hadziselimovic F, Snyder HM 3rd, et al. Histologic maldevelopment of unilaterally cryptorchid testes and their descended partners. Eur J Pediatr 1993;152(Suppl 2):S11.

120. Mancini RE, Rosemberg E, Cullen M, et al. Cryptorchid and scrotal human testes. I. Cytological, cytochemical and quantitative studies. J Clin Endocrinol Metab 1965;25:927.

121. Cortes D, Thorup J, Lindenberg S, et al. Infertility despite surgery for cryptorchidism in childhood can be classified by patients with normal or elevated follicle-stimulating hormone and identified at orchidopexy. BJU Int 2003;91:670.

122. Rusnack SL, Wu HY, Huff DS, et al. Testis histopathology in boys with cryptorchidism correlates with future fertility potential. J Urol 2003;169:659.

123. Hadziselimovic F, Hocht B, Herzog B, et al. Infertility in cryptorchidism is linked to the stage of germ cell development at orchidopexy. Horm Res 2007;68:46.

124. Hadziselimovic F, Hoecht B. Testicular histology related to fertility outcome and postpubertal hormone status in cryptorchidism. Klin Padiatr 2008;220:302.

125. Tasian GE, Hittelman AB, Kim GE, et al. Age at orchiopexy and testis palpability predict germ and Leydig cell loss: clinical predictors of adverse histological features of cryptorchidism. J Urol 2009;182:704.

126. Lackgren G, Ploen L. The morphology of the human undescended testis with special reference to the Sertoli cell and puberty. Int J Androl 1984; 7:23.

127. Regadera J, Martinez-Garcia F, Gonzalez-Peramato P, et al. Androgen receptor expression in Sertoli cells as a function of seminiferous tubule maturation in the human cryptorchid testis. J Clin Endocrinol Metab 2001;86:413.

128. Rune GM, Mayr J, Neugebauer H, et al. Pattern of Sertoli cell degeneration in cryptorchid prepubertal testes. Int J Androl 1992;15:19.

129. Zivkovic D, Hadziselimovic F. Development of Sertoli cells during mini-puberty in normal and cryptorchid testes. Urol Int 2009;82:89.

130. Chilvers C, Dudley NE, Gough MH, et al. Undescended testis: the effect of treatment on subsequent risk of subfertility and malignancy. J Pediatr Surg 1986;21:691.

131. Cortes D, Thorup JM, Visfeldt J. Cryptorchidism: aspects of fertility and neoplasms. A study including data of 1,335 consecutive boys who underwent testicular biopsy simultaneously with surgery for cryptorchidism. Horm Res 2001;55:21.

132. Gracia J, Sanchez Zalabardo J, Sanchez Garcia J, et al. Clinical, physical, sperm and hormonal data in 251 adults operated on for cryptorchidism in childhood. BJU Int 2000;85:1100.

133. Okuyama A, Nonomura N, Nakamura M, et al. Surgical management of undescended testis: retrospective study of potential fertility in 274 cases. J Urol 1989;142:749.

134. Lee PA. Fertility after cryptorchidism: epidemiology and other outcome studies. Urology 2005;66:427.

135. Sonne SB, Almstrup K, Dalgaard M, et al. Analysis of gene expression profiles of microdissected cell populations indicates that testicular carcinoma in situ is an arrested gonocyte. Cancer Res 2009; 69:5241.

136. Wood HM, Elder JS. Cryptorchidism and testicular cancer: separating fact from fiction. J Urol 2009; 181:452.

137. Akre O, Pettersson A, Richiardi L. Risk of contralateral testicular cancer among men with unilaterally undescended testis: a meta analysis. Int J Cancer 2009;124:687.

138. Pettersson A, Richiardi L, Nordenskjold A, et al. Age at surgery for undescended testis and risk of testicular cancer. N Engl J Med 2007;356:1835.

139. Walsh TJ, Dall'Era MA, Croughan MS, et al. Prepubertal orchiopexy for cryptorchidism may be associated with lower risk of testicular cancer. J Urol 2007;178:1440.

A Practical Approach to Ambiguous Genitalia in the Newborn Period

Sarah M. Lambert, MD[a], Eric J.N. Vilain, MD, PhD[b],
Thomas F. Kolon, MD[a],*

KEYWORDS

- Ambiguous genitalia • Congenital adrenal hyperplasia
- Disorders of sex development • Neonates

CHAPTER

The evaluation and management of a newborn with ambiguous genitalia must be undertaken with immediacy and great sensitivity. The pediatric urologist, endocrinologist, geneticist, and child psychiatrist or psychologist should work closely with the family in pursuing a dual goal: to establish the correct diagnosis of the abnormality and, with input from the parents, determine gender based on the karyotype, endocrine function, and anatomy of the child. In this section the authors outline a practical approach to the neonate born with a disorder of sex development (DSD).

Nomenclature

Genital ambiguity in the neonate has been described for centuries and evidence for disorders of sexual differentiation exists from many ancient civilizations.[1] The actual incidence of DSD is difficult to accurately determine because of the heterogeneity of the clinical presentation and the varied etiologies. Using birth registries, some authors have attempted to estimate the incidence of ambiguous genitalia at birth; The estimated incidence of clinically detectable ambiguous genitalia at birth in Germany is 2.2 per 10,000 births.[2] Congenital adrenal hyperplasia is estimated to occur in approximately 1 per 16,000 births.[3] Historically, the term intersex was used to characterize DSD and subcategories included male pseudohermaphrodite, female pseudohermaphrodite, and true hermaphrodite. These terms used gender in the nomenclature and were often considered controversial or disparaging. Therefore a revised nomenclature was proposed that incorporated genetic etiology and descriptive terminology while removing gender references.[4] The main categories include sex chromosome DSD, 46,XX DSD, and 46,XY DSD. Some conditions can be placed into more than one category. Additionally, although the majority of infants with 46,XX DSD will be diagnosed with congenital adrenal hyperplasia (CAH), only approximately 50% of children with 46, XY DSD will have a definitive clinical diagnosis.[5]

Diagnosis

Chromosomal sex is established at fertilization and the undifferentiated gonads subsequently develop into either testes or ovaries. A child's phenotypic sex results from the differentiation of internal ducts and external genitalia under the influence of hormones and transcription factors. Any discordance among these processes results in ambiguous genitalia or DSD. Currently, the main categories of DSD are 46,XX DSD, 46,XY DSD, sex chromosome DSD, ovotesticular DSD, and 46,XX testicular DSD.

[a] Children's Hospital of Philadelphia, University of Pennsylvania School of Medicine, 39th Street and Civic Center Boulevard, Philadelphia, PA 19104, USA
[b] David Geffen School of Medicine at UCLA, 695 Charles Young Drive South, Los Angeles, CA 90095, USA
* Corresponding author.
E-mail address: kolon@email.chop.edu

Urol Clin N Am 37 (2010) 195–205
doi:10.1016/j.ucl.2010.03.014
0094-0143/10/$ – see front matter © 2010 Elsevier Inc. All rights reserved.

46,XX disorder of sex development

Girls with 46,XX DSD, the most common DSD, are 46,XX with normal ovaries and Müllerian derivatives. The sexual ambiguity is limited to masculinization of the external genitalia that occurs as a result of exposure to androgens in utero. Congenital adrenal hyperplasia (CAH), which accounts for the majority of patients with 46,XX DSD, describes a group of autosomal recessive disorders that arises from a deficiency in one of five genes required for the synthesis of cortisol (**Fig. 1**). These five genes and the enzymes they encode are include *CYP21*: 21-hydroxylase; *CYP11*: 11β-hydroxylase, 18-hydroxylase and 18-oxidase; *CYP 17*: 17α-hydroxylase and 17,20 lyase; *3β2HSD*: 3β–hydroxysteroid dehydrogenase; and *StAR*: side chain cleavage enzyme. Although these biochemical defects are characterized by impaired cortisol secretion, only deficiencies in *CYP21* and *CYP11* are predominantly masculinizing disorders, and *3β2HSD* to a lesser extent. Although the female fetus is masculinized because of overproduction of adrenal androgens and precursors, the affected boys have no genital abnormalities. In contrast, *3β2HSD*, *CYP17*, and *StAR* deficiencies block cortisol synthesis and gonadal steroid production. Thus, boys have varying degrees of undermasculinization, whereas girls generally have normal external genitalia.[6–8]

CAH resulting in genital ambiguity in boys is discussed in detail later in this article.

The most common cause of CAH is inactivation of *CYP21*, which catalyzes the conversion 17-OH progesterone to 11-deoxycortisol, a precursor of cortisol, and the conversion of progesterone to deoxycorticosterone, a precursor of aldosterone. A spectrum of phenotypes from mild to severe clitoromegaly is possible. Classic 21α-hydroxylase deficiency is comprised of two forms of CAH: a severe, salt-wasting type with a defect in aldosterone biosynthesis and a simple, virilizing type with normal aldosterone synthesis. A mild, nonclassic form also exists that can be asymptomatic or associated with signs of postnatal androgen excess.[9] There are two *CYP11* genes: *CYP11B1* and *CYP11B2*. *CYP11B1* converts 11-deoxycortisol to cortisol.[10,11] Alternatively, *CYP11B2* converts deoxycorticosterone (DOC) to corticosterone, corticosterone to 18-hydroxycorticosterone, and 18-hydroxycorticosterone to aldosterone. Hypertension, which occurs in about two thirds of patients, is presumptively a consequence of excess DOC, with resultant salt and water retention. Excess androgen secretion in utero masculinizes the external genitalia of the female fetus. After birth, untreated male and female neonates progressively virilize and experience rapid somatic growth and skeletal maturation.

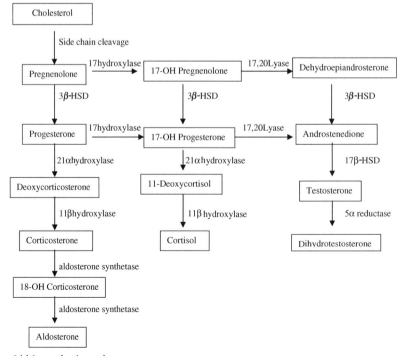

Fig. 1. The steroid biosynthetic pathway.

3β2HSD catalyzes three reactions: pregnenolone to progesterone; 17-OH pregnenolone to 17-OH progesterone; and dehydroepiandrosterone (DHEA) into androstenedione.[6,8] Complete deficiency of *3β2HSD* impairs synthesis of adrenal aldosterone and cortisol, and gonadal testosterone and estradiol. These newborns have severe CAH and exhibit signs of mineralocorticoid and glucocorticoid deficiency in the first week of life. Masculinization occurs as a result of DHEA conversion to testosterone in fetal placenta and peripheral tissues manifesting as mild to moderate clitoromegaly.

CYP17 also catalyzes three reactions: pregnenolone to 17-OH pregnenolone, 17-OH pregnenolone to dehydroepiandrosterone, and progesterone to 17-OH progesterone.[8] Phenotypically, affected girls have normal internal and external genitalia, but demonstrate immature sexual development because of an inability of the ovaries to secrete estrogens at puberty. In mild defects, aldosterone secretion may be normal and hypertension absent.[12]

StAR deficiency, also called lipoid adrenal hyperplasia, is a rare form of CAH and represents the most severe genetic defect in steroidogenesis. *StAR* deficiency is associated with severe glucocorticoid and mineralocorticoid deficiencies because of a failure to transport cholesterol from the outer to the inner mitochondrial membrane, which blocks conversion of cholesterol to pregnenolone.[13] These children are at risk for neonatal demise because of missed adrenal crisis. Neonates suspected to have adrenal insufficiency should be closely monitored for hypoglycemia, hyponatremia, and adrenal insufficiency. Affected girls demonstrate normal internal and external genitalia. Most of these women undergo spontaneous puberty but are at risk for irregular menses, ovarian cysts, and premature menopause.[14]

Ovotesticular disorder of sex development

Ovotesticular DSD requires expression of ovarian and testicular tissue. The most common karyotype in the United States is 46,XX, although 46,XY, mosaicism, or chimerism (46,XX/46,XY) can occur. Although mosaicism may occur from chromosomal nondisjunction, chimerism may result from a double fertilization (an X and a Y sperm) or from fusion of two fertilized eggs. This fairly uncommon condition can be further classified into three groups: lateral ovotesticular DSD has a testis on one side and an ovary on the contralateral (usually left) side; bilateral ovotesticular DSD has an ovotestis on each side; and, most commonly, unilateral ovotesticular DSD has an ovotestis on one side and either a testis or an ovary on the contralateral side. Furthermore, the external genitalia are ambiguous with hypospadias, cryptorchidism, and incomplete fusion of the labioscrotal folds. The genital duct differentiation in these patients generally follows that of the ipsilateral gonad on that side, such as a fallopian tube with an ovary and a vas deferens with a testis.[15]

46,XY disorder of sex development

The 46,XY DSD is a heterogeneous disorder in which testes are present but the internal ducts system or the external genitalia are incompletely masculinized. The phenotype is variable and ranges from completely female external genitalia to the mild male phenotype of isolated hypospadias or cryptorchidism. The 46,XY DSD can be classified into eight basic etiologic categories: (1) Leydig cell failure, (2) testosterone biosynthesis defects, (3) androgen insensitivity syndrome, (4) 5a-Reductase deficiency, (5) persistent Müllerian duct syndrome, (6) primary testicular failure or vanishing testes syndrome, (7) exogenous insults, and (8) gonadal dysgenesis.

Leydig cell failure The presence of testosterone, produced by testicular Leydig cells, induces male differentiation of the wolffian ducts and external genitalia. The 46,XY DSD can result from Leydig cell unresponsiveness to human chorionic gonadotrophin hormone (hCG) and luteinizing hormone (LH). The phenotypes of these patients vary from normal female to hypoplastic external male genitalia.

Testosterone biosynthesis enzyme defects Described earlier in this article for 46,XX DSD, defects in four of the steps of the steroid biosynthetic pathway from cholesterol to testosterone may also produce genital ambiguity in the male.[7,8] These defects include the less common forms of congenital adrenal hyperplasia: *3β2HSD* deficiency, *CYP17* deficiency, *StAR* protein deficiency, and *17bHSD* deficiency. Although DHEA conversion into testosterone results in virilization in females, this same process insufficiently masculinizes affected boys. Thus, male infants exhibit ambiguous genitalia with variable degrees of hypospadias, cryptorchidism, penoscrotal transposition, and a blind vaginal pouch. Boys with *CYP17* deficiency display a developmental spectrum from the normal female phenotype to the ambiguous hypospadiac male phenotype.[12,16] The magnitude of the decreased masculinization in the male infant correlates with the severity of the block in 17α-hydroxylation. Affected boys with *StAR* deficiency have severe testosterone deficiencies and exhibit female external genitalia with a blind vaginal pouch.[17,18] No surviving patients with 46,XY have demonstrated testis function at puberty. The affected 46,XY boys with *17βHSD* deficiency have external female genitalia, inguinal testes, internal male ducts, and a blind vaginal pouch. At puberty, these patients demonstrate an increase in their levels of gonadotropins, androstenedione, estrone and testosterone. Delayed virilization may ensue if some testosterone levels approach the normal range.[19,20]

Androgen insensitivity syndrome The broad spectrum of androgen insensitivity syndrome (AIS) ranges from patients with 46,XY with complete AIS, or testicular feminization, to partial AIS. This syndrome is the result of mutations of the steroid-binding domain of the androgen receptor resulting in receptors unable to bind androgens or receptors that bind to androgens but exhibit qualitative abnormalities and do not function properly. This disorder affects 1 in 20,000 live male births with a maternal inheritance pattern, because the androgen receptor gene is located on the long arm of the X chromosome.[21]

The external genitalia of a child with complete androgen insensitivity resembles normal female genitalia although the karyotype is XY and testes are located internally. These children are raised as girls. Most children are not diagnosed until puberty during an evaluation for primary amenorrhea. Occasionally, it is also discovered that at the time of inguinal hernia repair, or more recently, when the prenatal karyotype does not match the external phenotype of the newborn child.

5α-reductase deficiency 5α-reductase deficiency was first described as pseudovaginal perineal scrotal hypospadias.[22] In this autosomal recessive condition, patients have a defect in the conversion of testosterone to dihydrotestosterone (DHT). These patients have a 46,XY karyotype and ambiguous external genitalia but normally differentiated testes with male internal ducts. However, at puberty, significant virilization occurs as testosterone levels increase into the adult male range while dihydrotestosterone remains disproportionately low. There are three genetic isolates of this disorder that have been described: the Dominican Republic, the New Guinea Samba Tribe, and in Turkey. Many of these patients undergo a change of their gender identity from female to male after puberty.[23,24] Virilization can be secondary to slightly increased plasma DHT levels and to the chronic effect of adult T levels on the androgen receptor.

Persistent Müllerian duct syndrome Antimüllerian hormone (AMH), or Müllerian inhibitory substance

(MIS), is secreted by the Sertoli cells from the time of fetal seminiferous tubule differentiation until puberty. MIS binds to a receptor in the mesenchyme surrounding the Müllerian ducts before 8-weeks gestation causing apoptosis and regression of the Müllerian duct.[25] Because the diagnosis of persistent Müllerian duct syndrome (PMDS) is often made at the time of inguinal hernia repair or orchiopexy, this syndrome is commonly referred to as hernia uteri inguinalis. PMDS can occur from a failure of the testes to synthesize or secrete MIS because of an AMH gene mutation or from a defect in the response of the duct to MIS because of an AMH2 receptor gene mutation. PMDS is inherited in a sex-linked autosomal recessive manner and AMH mutations are most common in Mediterranean or Arab countries with high rates of consanguinity.[26] Most of these familial mutations are homozygous and the patients have low or undetectable levels of serum MIS. In contrast, AMH2 receptor mutations are often heterozygous and are more common in France and Northern Europe. These patients usually have high-normal or elevated MIS concentrations.[27]

Congenital anorchia Congenital anorchia or vanishing testes syndrome encompasses a spectrum of anomalies resulting from cessation of testicular function.[28] A loss of testes before 8-weeks gestation results in patients with 46,XY with female external and internal genitalia and either no gonads or streak gonads. A loss of testes at 8 to 10 weeks in development leads to ambiguous genitalia and variable ductal development. A loss of testis function after the critical male differentiation period, which is at 12- to 14-weeks gestation, results in a normal male phenotype externally along with anorchia internally. Sporadic and familial forms of anorchia exist. The familial cases, including some reports of monozygotic twins, support the presence of an as yet unidentified mutant gene in some patients with the syndrome.

Exogenous source Exogenous insults to normal male development include maternal ingestion of progesterone or estrogen or various environmental hazards. As early as 1942, Courrier and Jost[29] demonstrated an antiandrogen effect on the male fetus induced by a synthetic progestagen, and more recently, Silver and colleagues[30] showed an increased incidence of hypospadias in male offspring conceived by in vitro fertilization. They hypothesized that the increased risk may be secondary to maternal progesterone ingestion. Sharpe and Skakkebaek[31] have further postulated that the increase in reproductive abnormalities in men is related to an increase in the in utero exposure to environmental estrogens.

Gonadal dysgenesis

Dysgenetic 46,XY DSD exhibits ambiguous development of the internal genital ducts, the urogenital sinus and the external genitalia. Dysgenetic testes can result from mutations or deletions of any of the genes involved in the testis determination cascade, namely SRY, DAX, WT1, and SOX9. The SRY gene is a single exon gene located on the short arm of the Y chromosome.[32] SRY gene mutations usually result in complete gonadal dysgenesis and XY sex reversal or Swyer syndrome. The DSS locus (dosage-sensitive sex reversal) has been mapped to the Xp21 region, which contains the DAX1 gene. Duplication of the DSS locus has been associated with dysgenetic 46,XY DSD. The DSS locus has been theorized to contain a wolffian inhibitory factor, which acts as an inhibitory gene of the testis determination pathway.[33] Swain and colleagues[34] have shown that DAX1 antagonizes SRY action in mammalian sex determination. Male patients with Denys-Drash syndrome have ambiguous genitalia with streak or dysgenetic gonads, progressive nephropathy, and Wilms tumor. Analysis of these patients revealed heterozygous mutations of the Wilms tumor suppressor gene (WT1) at 11p13.[35] The WAGR syndrome (Wilms tumor, aniridia, genitourinary abnormalities, mental retardation) is also associated with WT1 alterations.[29] The urogenital anomalies seen in the WAGR syndrome are usually less severe than in Denys-Drash syndrome. The SOX9 gene has been associated with campomelic dysplasia, an often lethal skeletal malformation with dysgenetic 46,XY DSD.[36] Affected 46,XY children have phenotypic variability from normal boys to normal girls, depending on the function of the gonads.

Swyer syndrome represents an uncommon form of pure gonadal dysgenesis. These children have female external genitalia and have a uterus and fallopian tubes, however, the karyotype is 46,XY with a Y chromosome that usually does not work and two dysgenetic gonads in the abdomen.[37]

Partial gonadal dysgenesis refers to disorders with partial testicular development, including mixed gonadal dysgenesis, dysgenetic male pseudohermaphroditism, and some forms of testicular or ovarian regression. Mixed or partial gonadal dysgenesis (45,XX/46,XY or 46,XY) involves a streak gonad on one side and a testis, often dysgenetic, on the other side. Patients with a Y chromosome in the karyotype are at a higher risk than the general population to develop a tumor in the streak or dysgenetic gonad. Gonadoblastoma,

a benign growth, is the most common tumor.[38] Because of the 20% to 25% age-related risk for malignant transformation into a dysgerminoma,[39] surgical removal of the gonad is recommended. Patients with a 45,XX/46,XY karyotype and normal testis biopsy could retain the testis if it is descended or can be placed in the scrotum. These children would then need a close follow-up of the testis by monthly self examinations for tumor formation.

Sex chromosome disorder of sex development

Sex chromosome anomalies comprise another category of DSD. Klinefelter syndrome (47,XXY) usually becomes evident during adolescence as patients develop gynecomastia, variable androgen deficiency, and small atrophic testes with hyalinization of the seminiferous tubules. These patients demonstrate azoospermia and increasing gonadotropin levels. Boys with 47,XXY may develop through nondisjunction of the sex chromosomes during the first or second meiotic division in either parent, or less commonly, through mitotic nondisjunction in the zygote at or after fertilization. These abnormalities almost always occur in parents with normal sex chromosomes. The 46,XY/47,XXY mosaicism is the most common form of the Klinefelter variants. The mosaics, in general, manifest a much milder phenotype than patients with classic Klinefelter. Testes differentiation and a lack of ovarian development in these patients indicates that a single Y chromosome with SRY expression is enough for testis organogenesis and male sex differentiation in the presence of as many as four X chromosomes in some patients with Klinefelter. These testes are not truly normal, however, since they are usually small and azoospermic. Although there are sporadic reports of paternity, most fertile Klinefelter individuals have sex chromosome mosaicism.[40–42] Pure gonadal dysgenesis (PGD) describes a 46,XX or 46,XY child with streak gonads or more commonly, a child with Turner syndrome (45,XO or 45,XO/46,XX).

46,XX testicular disorder of sex development

Categories of 46,XX testicular DSD include boys with classic XX with apparently normal phenotypes, boys with non-classic XX with some degree of sexual ambiguity, and XX ovotesticular DSD.[43] Eighty percent to ninety percent of boys with 46,XX result from an anomalous Y to X translocation involving the SRY gene during meiosis. In general, the greater the amount of Y-DNA present, the more virilized the phenotype. Although 8% to 20% of boys with XX have no detectable Y sequences, including SRY, about 1 in 20,000 phenotypic boys have a 46,XX karyotype. Most of these patients have ambiguous genitalia, but reports of boys with classic XX without the SRY gene do exist.[26,33,38,39,43,44] This phenomenon again raises the possibility of mutation of a downstream wolffian inhibitory factor when cases of normal virilization are seen without the presence of the SRY gene. Some patients with 46,XX testicular DSD have the SRY gene translocated from the Y to the X chromosome. However, for most patients, the genes responsible are not yet identified.[45,46]

History and Physical Examination

Patients with bilaterally impalpable testes or a unilaterally impalpable testis and hypospadias should be regarded as having DSD until proven otherwise, whether or not the genitalia appear ambiguous. Patient history should include the degree of prematurity, ingestion of exogenous maternal hormones used in assisted reproductive techniques, and maternal use of oral contraceptives during pregnancy. A family history should be obtained to document any urologic abnormalities, neonatal deaths, precocious puberty, amenorrhea, infertility, or consanguinity. Any abnormal virilization or cushingoid appearance of the child's mother should also be noted. Abnormalities of the prenatal maternal ultrasound are also helpful, such as discordance of the fetal karyotype with the genitalia by sonogram.

For differential diagnosis and treatment purposes, the most important physical finding is the presence of one or two gonads. If no gonads are palpable, all DSD categories are possible. Of these, 46,XX DSD is most commonly seen followed by 45,X/46,XY. A palpable gonad is highly suggestive of a testis, or rarely, an ovotestis, because ovaries and streak gonads do not descend. If one gonad is palpable, 46,XX DSD is less likely, whereas 45,X/46,XY, ovotesticular DSD, and 46,XY remain possibilities. If two gonads are palpable, 46,XY, and rarely ovotesticular DSD, are the most likely diagnoses (**Fig. 2**).

Patients should be examined in a warm room supine in the frog leg position with both legs free. It is important to determine size, location, and texture of both gonads, if palpable. The undescended testis may be found in the inguinal canal, the superficial inguinal pouch, at the upper scrotum, or rarely in the femoral, perineal, or contralateral scrotal regions. One should also note the development and pigmentation of the labioscrotal folds along with any other congenital anomalies of other body systems. An abnormal phallic size should be documented by width and stretched length measurements. Micropenis is defined as a stretched penile length of less than 2 cm in a term male neonate.[47–50] One should describe the position of the urethral meatus and the amount of penile curvature and note the number of perineal orifices.

Another critical finding on physical examination is the presence of a uterus that is palpable by digital rectal examination as an anterior midline, cord-like structure. Of course, a thorough general physical examination must also be performed. A blood pressure should be taken to rule out hypertension. The presence of hyperpigmentation should also be documented. Dysmorphic features indicating syndromic manifestations (eg, short broad neck, widely spaced nipples, or aniridia) should also be noted.

Patient Evaluation

In the immediate newborn period, all patients require a karyotype and laboratory evaluation by serum electrolytes, 17-OH progesterone, testosterone, luteinizing hormone, follicle stimulation hormone, and urinalysis. The karyotype can be determined from peripheral blood or skin fibroblasts from genital skin. It is important to remember that chromosomal studies from an amniocentesis do not negate the need for a postnatal karyotype. Once the karyotype is determined, serum analysis will assist in narrowing the differential diagnosis. If the 17-OH progesterone level is elevated, a diagnosis of CAH can be made. Determining the 11-deoxycortisol and deoxycorticosterone levels will help differentiate between 21-hydroxylase and 11β-hydroxylase deficiencies. If the levels are elevated, then a diagnosis of 11β-hydroxylase deficiency can be made, whereas low levels confirm 21-hydroxylase deficiency. If the 17-OH progesterone level is normal, a testosterone to DHT ratio along with androgen precursors before and after hCG stimulation will help elucidate the 46,XY DSD etiology. A testosterone to DHT ratio of greater than 20 is suggestive of a 5 alpha reductase deficiency. A failure to respond to hCG in combination with elevated LH and FSH levels is consistent with anorchia. It is important to remember that for the first 60 to 90 days of life, a normal gonadotropic surge occurs with a resultant increase in the testosterone level and its precursors. During this specific time period, hCG stimulation for androgen evaluation can be postponed. Serum levels of AMH and inhibin B can also be measured in the immediate postnatal period to document the existence of normal testicular tissue.

Genetic Tests

The initial genetic testing is the assessment of the chromosomes by karyotype. This testing can be

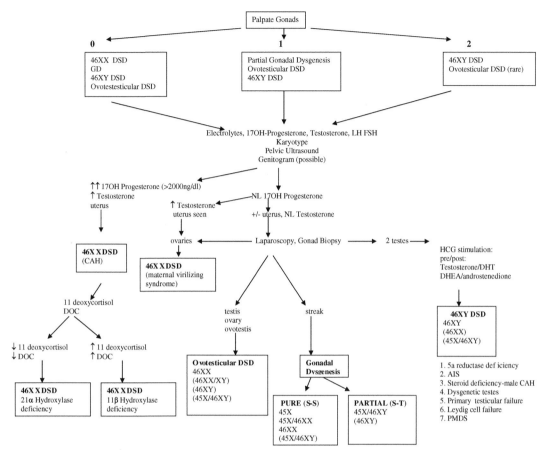

Fig. 2. Anatomic and endocrine approach to DSD evaluation. NL, normal; S, streak gonad; T, testis.

done by regular, meta-phasic, karyotype, but if the question asked is limited to the nature of the sex chromosomes, an interphasic FISH (fluorescent in situ hybridization) should be performed with X- and Y-specific probes, providing the number of and the quality of sex chromosomes in less than 48 hours. If a mosaic is detected or suspected, a large number of interphasic nuclei can be assessed by FISH (typically 200–300) to evaluate the percentage of each clone accurately (**Fig. 3**).

The follow-up genetic tests are diagnostic. They are of two kinds: one is the direct sequencing of a specific gene and the other the evaluation of copy number variants (CNV) by micro-array analysis. If there are enough phenotypic features to orient the physician toward a specific diagnosis, direct sequencing of the causal gene is preferred. This sequencing would typically happen in cases of complete androgen insensitivity, or congenital adrenal hyperplasia, for which the diagnostic indicators are strong. Several genes can be sequenced on a clinical basis by molecular laboratories (eg, AR, CYP21, SRY, SOX9, SF1), and the list is growing.

If the DSD does not have an obvious genetic cause, whether it is syndromic or isolated, a screen for CNVs (micro-deletions or micro-duplications) is recommended. This screen is performed in clinical laboratories using micro-array–based comparative genomic hybridization (CGH) methods. Although the techniques and the sensitivity of the array vary, all methods detect CNVs that can then be confirmed by FISH. For best sensitivity, oligonucleotide-based arrays are preferred, and may detect CNVs as small as 10 to 50 kb. The use of direct molecular sequencing and array-CGH is presented in the diagnostic algorithm shown in **Fig. 1**. The interpretation of genetic testing can be challenging. If the test detects point mutations or CNVs known to cause a DSD, the genetic diagnosis is certain, and the testing of parents as potential carriers will then be performed for the purpose of genetic counseling.

If the test detects unknown point mutations or CNVs, the investigation of parental DNA becomes essential. A de novo (not present in parents) CNV or point mutation in patients with a DSD is likely

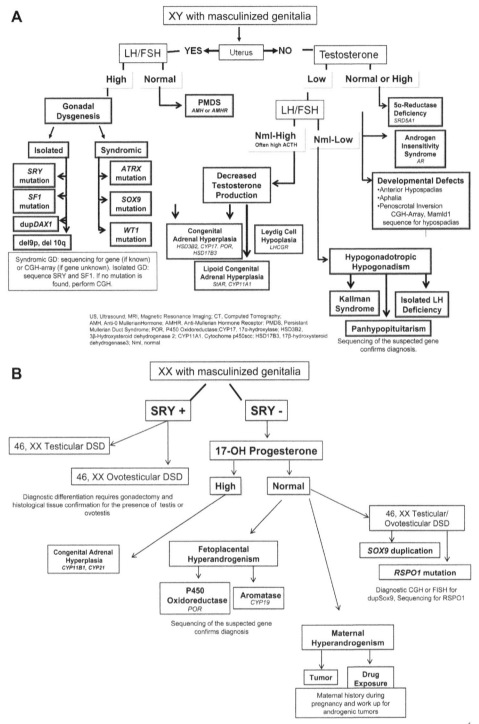

Fig. 3. (A) Genetic evaluation of XY patient with masculinized genitalia. AMHR, Anti-Mullerian Hormone Receptor; CYP11A1, Cytochome p450scc; CYP17, 17α-hydroxylase; HSD3B2, 3β-Hydroxysteroid dehydrogenase 2; HSD17B3, 17β-hydroxysteroid dehydrogenase3; Nml, normal; POR, P450 Oxidoreductase; US, Ultrasound. (B) Genetic evaluation of XX patient with masculinized genitalia. (Data from Fleming A, Vilain E. The endless quest for sex determination genes. Clin Genet 2005;67(1):15–25).

to be causative. An inherited, unknown variant (present in one of the parents) is more difficult to interpret and requires a specialized genetics consultation. In all cases, pre- and post-test genetic counseling is essential to ensure that the family understands the interpretation of the test and the risk for recurrence in future pregnancies.

Radiographic Tests

Examination of the internal genital can be achieved using many modalities, including abdominal and pelvic ultrasound, MRI, fluoroscopy, endoscopy, or laparoscopy. Noninvasive, quick, and inexpensive, an ultrasound should be the first radiologic examination obtained. Although only 50% accurate in detecting intra-abdominal testes,[51] ultrasound can detect gonads in the inguinal region and can assess Müllerian structures. For example, the presence of Müllerian structures visible on a pelvic ultrasound can often differentiate between pure gonadal dysgenesis and complete AIS in an adolescent with primary amenorrhea.[52] Although more expensive, MRI scan can further delineate the anatomy. Ectopic gonads, testes, and immature ovaries have an intermediate signal intensity on T-1 weighted images and a high signal intensity with an intermediate signal intensity surrounding rim on T-2 weighted images.[53] A genitogram should be performed to evaluate a urogenital sinus, including the entry of the urethra in the vagina and the presence of a cervical impression.[51] Infants with intra-abdominal or non-palpable testes in whom ovotesticular DSD; 45,X/46,XY DSD; or 46,XY DSD is considered will require an open or laparoscopic exploration with bilateral deep longitudinal gonadal biopsies for histologic evaluation, which will determine the presence of ovotestes, streak gonads, or dysgenetic testes thereby confirming the diagnosis. This procedure is a diagnostic maneuver; therefore, removal of gonads or reproductive organs should be deferred until the final pathology report is available, a diagnosis achieved, a discussion has occurred between the family and all consultants, and a gender decision reached.[54]

Multidisciplinary Team

Most children with DSD are evaluated at tertiary centers with familiarity in all aspects of management throughout childhood and into adulthood. At these centers, children with DSD should be managed with a well-established multidisciplinary team, including genetics, neonatology, endocrinology, urology, and psychology/psychiatry. In addition to the genetic, endocrine, and radiographic evaluation, the clinical data must be thoughtfully and carefully construed to the family. A team approach that includes family discussions should begin immediately. The importance of a clinical psychologist or psychiatrist who is familiar with DSD cannot be underestimated. In addition to support from the medical team, many families find support groups useful.[55]

Although the preferred gender assignment is not always clear, a thorough examination of endocrine function, karyotype, and potential for fertility should guide the determination. Current DSD guidelines recommend that all individuals receive a gender assignment in infancy and family participation in that decision-making process is essential.[4] A single-institution survey of parents of girls with CAH reported that 52% of respondents were completely satisfied with the information they were given during the neonatal period, whereas 43% were only partially satisfied.[56] This study reinforces the need for open and direct communication between the family and medical team as a core component of satisfactory patient care. This sentiment is confirmed by a survey of fellows in the urology section of the American Academy of Pediatrics that documented that the overwhelming majority of pediatric urologists believe a team approach and parental involvement are recommended and important in the care of patients with DSD.[57] The decision of whether or not to pursue surgical intervention should be based upon anatomy, functional status, and a consensus of opinion between the family and medical team; this decision must be individualized for each patient with DSD.

REFERENCES

1. Rogers BO. History of external genital surgery. In: Horton CE, editor. Plastic and reconstructive surgery of the external genitalia. Boston: Little Brown and Company; 1973. p. 3–50.
2. Thyen U, Lanz K, Holterus PM, et al. Epidemiology and initial management of ambiguous genitalia at birth in Germany. Horm Res 2006;66:195.
3. Speiser PW, White PC. Congenital adrenal hyperplasia. N Engl J Med 2003;349:776.
4. Hughes IA, Houk C, Ahmed SF, et al. Consensus statement on management of intersex disorders. Arch Dis Child 2006;91(7):554.
5. Morel Y, Rey R, Teinturier C, et al. Aetiological diagnosis of male sex ambiguity: a collaborative study. Eur J Pediatr 2002;161:49.
6. New MI. Congenital adrenal hyperplasia. In: De Groot L, editor. Endocrinology. 3rd edition. Philadelphia: WB Saunders; 1995. p. 1813–35.
7. Donohue PA, Parker K, Migeon CJ. Congenital adrenal hyperplasia. In: Scriver CR, Beaudet AL,

Sly WS, et al, editors. The metabolic and molecular basis of inherited disease. 7th edition. New York: McGraw-Hill; 1995. p. 2929–66.

8. Miller WL, Tyrell JB. The adrenal cortex. In: Felig P, Baxter JD, Frohmer LA, editors. Endocrinology and metabolism. 3rd edition. New York: McGraw-Hill; 1995. p. 555–711.

9. White PC, Speiser PW. Congenital adrenal hyperplasia due to 21-hydroxylase deficiency. Endocr Rev 2000;21:245–91.

10. Simard J, Rheaume E, Mebarki F, et al. Molecular basis of human 3β-hydroxysteroid dehydrogenase deficiency. J Steroid Biochem Mol Biol 1995;53: 127–38.

11. Rheaume E, Simard J, Morel Y, et al. Congenital adrenal hyperplasia due to point mutations in the type II 3β-hydroxysteroid dehydrogenase gene. Nat Genet 1992;1:239–45.

12. Miura K, Yasuda K, Yanase K, et al. Mutation of cytochrome P-45017α gene (CYP17) in a Japanese patient previously reported as having glucocorticoid-responsive hyperaldosteronism: with a review of Japanese patients with mutations of CYP17. J Clin Endocrinol Metab 1996;81:3797–801.

13. Saenger P. New developments in congenital lipoid adrenal hyperplasia and steroidogenic acute regulatory protein. Pediatr Clin North Am 1997;44(2): 397–421.

14. Bhangoo A, Buyuk E, Oktay K, et al. Phenotypic features of 46, XX females with StAR protein mutations. Pediatr Endocrinol Rev 2007;5(2):633.

15. Hadjiathanasion CG, Brauner R, Lortat-Jacob S, et al. True hermaphroditism: genetic variants and clinical management. J Pediatr 1994;125:738–43.

16. Geller DH, Auchus RJ, Mendonca BB, et al. The genetic and functional basis of isolated 17,20-lyase deficiency. Nat Genet 1997;17:201–5.

17. Bose HS, Sugawara T, Strauss JF III, et al. The pathophysiology and genetics of congenital lipoid adrenal hyperplasia. N Engl J Med 1996;335: 1870–8.

18. Matsuo N, Tsuzaki S, Anzo M, et al. The phenotypic definition of congenital lipoid adrenal hyperplasia: analysis of the 67 Japanese patients [abstract 200]. Horm Res 1994;41:106 33rd Annual European Society of Pediatric Endocrinology Meeting.

19. Geissler WM, Davis DL, Wu I, et al. Male pseudohermaphroditism caused by mutations of testicular 17β-hydroxysteroid dehydrogenase 3. Nat Genet 1994; 7:34–9.

20. Saez JM, de Peretti E, Morera AM, et al. Familial male pseudohermaphroditism with gynecomastia due to a testicular 17-ketosteroid reductase defect. I. In vivo studies. J Clin Endocrinol Metab 1971;32: 604–10.

21. Bangsboll S, Qvist I, Lebech PE, et al. Testicular feminization syndrome and associated gonadal tumors in Denmark. Acta Obstet Gynecol Scand 1992;71:63–6.

22. Nowakowski H, Lenz W. Genetic aspects in male hypogonadism. Recent Prog Horm Res 1961;17: 53–95.

23. Imperato-McGinley JL, Guerrero L, Gautier T, et al. Steroid 5α-reductase deficiency in man: an inherited form of male pseudohermaphroditism. Science 1974;186:1213–5.

24. Boudon C, Lobaccaro JM, Lumbroso S, et al. A new deletion of 5α-reductase type 2 gene in a Turkish family with 5α-reductase deficiency. Clin Endocrinol 1995;43:183–8.

25. Baarends WM, van Helmond MJ, Post M, et al. A novel member of the transmembrane serine/threonine kinase receptor family is specifically expressed in the gonads and in mesenchymal cells adjacent to the mullerian duct. Development 1994;120:189–97.

26. Imbeaud S, Carre-Eusebe D, Rey R, et al. Molecular genetics of the persistent mullerian duct syndrome: a study of 19 families. Hum Mol Genet 1994;3:125–31.

27. Hook EB, Warburton D. The distribution of chromosome genotypes associated with Turner's syndrome: livebirth prevalence rates and evidence for diminished fetal mortality and severity in genotypes associated with structural X abnormalities or mosaicism. Hum Genet 1983;64:24–7.

28. Grumbach MM, Barr ML. Cytological tests of chromosomal sex in relation to sexual anomalies in man. Recent Prog Horm Res 1958;14:255–334.

29. Courrier R, Jost A. Intersexualite totale provoque par la pregnenilone au cours de la grossesse. CR Soc Biol 1942;136:395–6.

30. Silver RI, Rodriguez R, Chang TS, et al. In vitro fertilization is associated with an increased risk of hypospadias. J Urol 1999;161:1954–7.

31. Sharpe RM, Skakkebaek NE. Are oestrogens involved in falling sperm counts and disorders of the male reproductive tract? Lancet 1993;341: 1392–5.

32. Goodfellow PA, Lovell-Badge R. SRY and sex determination in mammals. Annu Rev Genet 1993;27:71–92.

33. Kolon TF, Ferrer FA, McKenna PH. Clinical and molecular analysis of XX sex reversed patients. J Urol 1998;160:1169–72.

34. Swain A, Narvaez V, Burgoyne P, et al. DAX1 antagonizes SRY action in mammalian sex determination. Nature 1998;391:761–7.

35. Pelletier J, Bruening W, Kashtan CE, et al. Germline mutations in the Wilms tumor suppressor gene are associated with abnormal urogenital development in Denys-Drash syndrome. Cell 1991;67:437–47.

36. Foster JW, Dominguez-Steglich MA, Guioli S, et al. Campomelic dysplasia and autosomal sex reversal

caused by mutations in an SRY-related gene. Nature 1994;372:525–30.

37. Hsu LYF. Phenotype/karyotype correlations of Y chromosome aneuploidy with emphasis on structural aberrations in postnatally diagnosed cases. Am J Med Genet 1994;53:108–40.

38. Jorgenson N, Muller J, Jaubert F, et al. Heterogeneity of gonadoblastoma germ cells: similarities with immature germ cells, spermatogonia, and testicular carcinoma in situ cells. Histopathology 1997;30:177–86.

39. Casey AC, Bhodauria S, Shapter A, et al. Dysgerminoma: the role of conservative surgery. Gynecol Oncol 1996;63:352–7.

40. Cozzi J, Chevret S, Rousseaux S, et al. Achievement of meiosis in XXY-germ cells: study of 543 sperm karyotypes from an XY/XXY mosaic patient. Hum Genet 1994;93:32–4.

41. Jacobs PA, Hassold TJ, Whittington E, et al. Klinefelter's syndrome: an analysis of the origin of the additional sex chromosome using molecular probes. Ann Hum Genet 1988;52:147–51.

42. Ferguson-Smith MA, Mack WS, Ellis PM, et al. Parental age and the source of the X chromosomes in XXY Klinefelter's syndrome. Lancet 1964;1:46.

43. Boucekkine C, Toublanc JE, Abbas N, et al. Clinical and anatomical spectrum in XX sex-reversed patients: relationship to the presence of Y-specific DNA sequences. Clin Endocrinol 1994;40:733–42.

44. Palmer MS, Sinclair AH, Berta P, et al. Genetic evidence that ZFY is not the testis-determining factor. Nature 1989;342:937–9.

45. Fechner PY, Rosenberg C, Stetten G, et al. Nonrandom inactivation of the Y-bearing X chromosome in a 46, XX individual: evidence for the etiology of 46, XX true hermaphroditism. Cytogenet Cell Genet 1994;66:22–6.

46. Braun A, Kammerer S, Cleve A, et al. True hermaphroditism in a 46 XY individual caused by a postzygotic somatic point mutation in the male gonadal sex-determining locus (SRY): molecular genetics and histological findings in a sporadic case. Am J Hum Genet 1993;52:578–85.

47. Feldman KW, Smith DW. Fetal phallic growth and penile standards for newborn male infants. J Pediatr 1975;86:395.

48. Parisi MA, Ramsdell LA, Burns MW, et al. A gender assessment team: experience with 250 patients over a period of 25 years. Genet Med 2007;9(6):348.

49. Garry LW, Jeffrey DZ. Evaluation of a child with ambiguous genitalia: a practical guide to diagnosis and management. In: Meena PD, Vijayalaxmi B, Menon PSN, editors. Pediatric endocrine disorders. Andhra Pradesh (India): Orient Longman Ltd; 2001. p. 257–76.

50. Bergada I, Milani C, Bedecarras P, et al. Time course of the serum gonadotropin surge, inhibins, and anti-Mullerian hormone in normal newborn males during the first month of life. J Clin Endocrinol Metab 2006; 91(10):4092.

51. Kolon TF. Intersex. In: Schwartz MW, editor. The 5-minute pediatric consult. New York: Lippincott, Williams & Wilkins; 2003. p. 480–1.

52. Chavhan GB, Parra DA, Oudjhane K, et al. Imaging of ambiguous genitalia: classification and diagnostic approach. Radiographics 2008;28:1891.

53. Gambino J, Caldwell B, Dietrich R, et al. Congenital disorders of sexual differentiation: MR findings. AJR Am J Roentgenol 1992;158:363.

54. Diamond DA. Sexual differentiation: normal and abnormal. In: Walsh PC, Retik AB, Vaughan, Jr. ED, et al, editors. Campbell's urology. 8th edition. New York: Saunders; 2002. Chapter 68.

55. Warne G. Support groups for CAH and AIS. Endocrinologist 2003;13:175.

56. Dayner JE, Lee PA, Houk CP. Medical treatment of intersex: parental perspectives. J Urol 2004;172:1762.

57. Diamond DA, Burns JP, Mitchell C, et al. Sex assignment for newborns with ambiguous genitalia and exposure to fetal testosterone: attitudes and practices of pediatric urologists. J Pediatr 2006; 148:445.

Urologic Care of the Neurogenic Bladder in Children

Warren T. Snodgrass, MD*, Patricio C. Gargollo, MD

KEYWORDS

- Neurogenic bladder • Spina bifida
- Urodynamic evaluation • Incontinence

INITIAL MANAGEMENT

In a prior article,[1] the authors reviewed controversies regarding the urologic care of infants diagnosed with neurogenic bladder, primarily caused by spina bifida. Briefly summarized, initial management options include (1) universal institution of anticholinergics and intermittent catheterization (CIC), (2) observation using periodic radiologic imaging, reserving anticholinergics and CIC for infants developing bladder trabeculation, reflux, and/or hydronephrosis, or (3) urodynamic-based management using preemptive anticholinergics and CIC for infants with adverse findings.

Proposed advantages of urodynamic-based management include avoidance of therapy in infants with low intravesical pressures, and prevention of bladder and upper tract damage in those with high pressures. Risk assessment according to bladder pressures is based on the observation by McGuire and colleagues[2] that 80% of patients with intravesical pressures greater than 40 cm H_2O at urinary leakage (detrusor leak point pressure [DLPP]) had reflux and/or hydronephrosis. Accordingly, infants with DLPP greater than 40 cm H_2O, and/or detrusor sphincter dyssynergia believed to be an additional risk factor,[3] have been prescribed anticholinergics and CIC prophylactically rather than at observation of secondary radiologic deterioration.

Although McGuire found a DLPP greater than 40 cm H_2O predictive for upper tract risk, others subsequently suggested that sustained intravesical pressures as low as 20 cm H_2O increase likelihood for bladder damage.[4] Furthermore, how many infants with initially low intravesical pressures will subsequently manifest increased pressures with risk for bladder and upper tract deterioration is unclear, although two reports suggest it occurs in up to 40% of patients,[5,6] usually within the first 6 months of life. Together, these observations have led to early treatment of more infants.

However, determining DLPP in infants has potential pitfalls, because intravesical pressures vary according to infusion rate[7] and catheter size.[8] Similarly, ability to diagnose detrusor sphincter dyssynergia with commonly used perineal patch electrodes rather than concentric needles has been questioned.[6]

CURRENT TEXAS SCOTTISH RITE HOSPITAL PROTOCOL

The authors perform initial evaluation using renal ultrasound and fluoroscopic urodynamic evaluation at approximately 6 weeks of age, when spinal shock from newborn back closure appears resolved. A 5-French transurethral urodynamic catheter and a rectal balloon are used to measure detrusor and intra-abdominal pressures, respectively. Contrast medium is infused through a pump with a filling rate based on 10% of estimated bladder capacity (approximately 5 mL/min). Infants with areflexic detrusor pressures exceeding 40 cm H_2O start oxybutynin (0.2 mg/kg twice daily) and CIC (every 3 hours), with repeat

Department of Urology, University of Texas Southwestern Medical Center and Children's Medical Center, 2350 Stemmons Freeway, Suite F4300, Mail Stop F4.04, Dallas, TX 75207, USA
* Corresponding author.
E-mail address: warren.snodgrass@childrens.com

Urol Clin N Am 37 (2010) 207–214
doi:10.1016/j.ucl.2010.03.004
0094-0143/10/$ – see front matter © 2010 Elsevier Inc. All rights reserved.

testing within 12 weeks to confirm lower pressures.

The authors do not treat uninhibited contractions (UBC), which can be seen in normal infants, unless baseline pressures before contraction exceed 40 cm H_2O, nor do they diagnose detrusor sphincter dyssynergia. All others with pressures less than 40 cm H_2O are observed without active bladder management.

Urodynamic evaluation is repeated at 12 months and approximately 36 months of age. Renal ultrasonography provides surveillance for hydronephrosis every 6 months. Development of hydronephrosis, or new onset of febrile urinary tracts infections, prompts additional fluoroscopic urodynamic evaluation. Data from this protocol are being collected prospectively to document the number of infants diagnosed with high pressures through initial urodynamics at 6 weeks, and the number of patients initially believed to be at low risk who develop high pressures, reflux, or hydronephrosis over time.

Assuming fewer than 10% of children with congenital neurogenic bladder will develop satisfactory bladder control without need for CIC, all parents are initially counseled and reminded at periodic follow-ups to expect this intervention by the age of toilet training if urodynamic evaluation does not indicate earlier management.

MANAGEMENT AT TOILET TRAINING AGE

Classifying the neurogenic bladder into high and low pressures also helps predict continence at toilet training (**Fig. 1**). Those with baseline pressures greater than 40 cm H_2O often become dry with anticholinergics (oxybutynin 0.2 mg/kg three to four times daily) and CIC (every 3 hours) alone. Most patients with high pressures have already been diagnosed and started on this medical regimen as a result of earlier urodynamic study.

Those with persistent incontinence undergo repeat testing to determine adequacy of oxybutynin for reducing pressures to less than 40 cm H_2O and abolishing UBC. Persistent high pressure or UBC is treated by increasing oral oxybutynin to tolerance and/or adding intravesical instillation of 5 mg twice to three times daily as needed. In unusual cases with continued UBC, Botox injection is recommended. The indication for augmentation is persistent high pressure or UBC despite these medical treatments.

Sphincteric Insufficiency

Children who are incontinent on CIC and/or have a history of stress urinary incontinence and found to have detrusor areflexia and pressures less than 40 cm H_2O are diagnosed with sphincteric insufficiency.[9,10] Treatment requires surgical enhancement of outlet resistance using one of several bladder neck (BN) options: injection, reconstruction, sling, artificial sphincter, or closure.

In a series of patients with mixed causes of incontinence and mean follow-up of 28 months, BN injection using dextranomer/hyaluronic acid polymer resulted in a dry interval of 4 hours in 48% of 27 children with neuropathic bladders, 4 of whom underwent failed treatment with slings.[11] Similarly, polydimethylsiloxane injection ended pad use in 34% of 44 children with neurogenic bladders, 24 of whom underwent prior bladder neck procedures, at median follow-up of 28 months.[12] No difference in outcomes was seen between those who underwent prior interventions and those who did not. Both series used a mean volume per injection of approximately 3.5 mL, found that more than 2 additional injections were unlikely to succeed, and noted that the number of patients considered continent declined during the first 12 months and then seemed to stabilize.

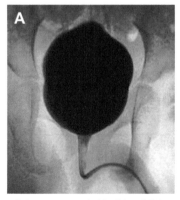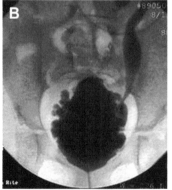

Fig. 1. Classification of the neurogenic bladder: (A) low pressure; (B) high pressure.

BN procedures designed to achieve continence through urethral lengthening for neuropathic outlet incompetency include those described by Kropp and Angwafo[13] and Salle.[14] Each uses the anterior bladder wall to extend the urethra beyond the bladder neck into the bladder, through tubularization versus an onlay-type flap, respectively. Reported outcomes for these reconstructions and various modifications are summarized in **Table 1**.

Fascial sling for neurogenic incontinence was first reported by McGuire and colleagues,[9] and is currently the most commonly used procedure in the United States for this condition in children. Technical aspects in published series vary; for example, McGuire and colleagues[9] described a pubovaginal fascial sling elevated until the bladder neck was observed cystoscopically to close. Others have placed the sling around the bladder neck/proximal urethra in a U or X configuration[15] or 360° wrap,[16] adjusting tension "loosely,"[17] "snug,"[18] or "tight"[16] without cystoscopy. Increase in DLPP averaged approximately 10 to 15 cm H_2O, regardless of technique.[9,16,19] Outcomes are listed in **Table 2**.

The artificial sphincter compresses the bladder outlet circumferentially. Continence rates greater than 80% are reported[20,21] for functioning devices, but concerns for mechanical failure and/or erosion have limited the use of the artificial urinary sphincter (AUS) in children. Long-term follow-up indicates most failures occur within the initial 3 to 5 years of placement,[21,22] with a mean device survival time of 12 years.[22]

BN closure is not generally considered first-line therapy for neurogenic incontinence in the United States, although historically Paul Mitrofanoff developed appendicovesicostomy in the mid-1970s to facilitate CIC after closing the outlet. He reviewed his outcomes in 22 patients with a mean follow-up of 20 years.[23] Of these, 5 (23%) had persistent incontinence requiring reclosure, 4 of whom were said to have developed high detrusor pressures, but no mention was made of urodynamic findings or anticholinergic use in this series. Others reported BN closure, with simultaneous augmentation in most, achieving continence in more than 80% of patients at a mean of 20 months follow-up.[24] Some children had urinary leakage from the stoma, whereas others experienced difficulty with catheterization because of stomal stenosis, a potentially serious complication after closing the bladder outlet.

Changes in Bladder Pressure After Outlet Procedures

These bladder outlet procedures have been associated with increased detrusor pressures, resulting in trabeculation, vesicoureteral reflux, and/or hydronephrosis. However, risk for adverse changes is unknown and factors, including preoperative urodynamic parameters, that might predict likelihood for their development have not been well defined. Further complicating evaluation is lack of universal criteria to diagnose outlet insufficiency in neurogenic bladders, for pre- and postoperative anticholinergic use and CIC intervals, to define postoperative continence, and to determine need for simultaneous or subsequent augmentation.

Table 1
Bladder neck reconstruction for neurogenic incontinence

Authors	Number of Patient (Male/Female)	Mean Follow-up	Number of "Dry" (%)	New Vesicoureteral Reflux (%)	Augmentation Prior/ Simultaneous	Subsequent	Total (%)
Nill et al[37]	24 (10/14)	1.5–7 y	20 (83)	10 (42)			"all"
Belman, Kaplan[34]	18 (10/8)	ns	14 (78)	4 (22)	16	1	17 (94)
Mollard et al[36]	16 (0/16)	12–36 mo	13 (81)	ns[a]	7		7 (44)
Snodgrass[38]	22 (13/9)	ns	20 (91)	9 (50)[b]	19		19 (86)
Salle et al[14]	17 (7/10)	26 mo	12 (70)	2 (12)[c]	12	1	13 (76)
Hayes et al[35]	28 (12/16)	28 mo	18 (64)	ns	23		23 (82)

Abbreviation: ns, not stated.
[a] Reimplant for refluxing or insufficient intraureteric distance for tube in 12 patients.
[b] Six underwent simultaneous reimplant.
[c] One of ten despite reimplant; one of seven without reimplant.

Table 2
Sling for neurogenic incontinence

Authors	Number of Patients (Male/Female)	Mean Follow-up (mo)	Number of "Dry" (%)	Augmentation Prior/ Simultaneous	Subsequent	Total (%)
Gormley et al[31]	10 (0/10)	49	10 (100)	3	0	3 (30)
Bauer et al[18]	11 (0/11)	12	8 (73)	4		4 (36)
Elder[43]	14 (4/10)	12	13 (93)	13		13 (93)
Decter[42]	10 (4/6)	26	5 (50)	6	3	9 (90)
Walker et al[45]	17 (8/9)	16	16 (94)	11		11 (65)
Perez et al[15]	36 (13/23)	17	22 (61)	35		35 (90)[a]
Kurzrock et al[44]	24 (15/9)	9–14	19 (79)	24		24 (100)
Barthold et al[39]	27 (7/20)	≥12	10 (37)	20	2	22 (81)
Austin et al[17]	18 (8/10)	21	14 (78)	6		6 (33)
Bugg, Joseph[40]	15 (1/14)	10–36	9 (60)	15		15 (100)
Castellan et al[19]	58 (15/43)	50	51 (88)	58		58 (100)
Snodgrass et al[16]	30 (18/12)	22	17 (57)	0	1	1 (3)
Chrzan et al[41]	89 (46/43)	72	42 (47)	11	9	20 (22)[b]

[a] Series comprised of 39 patients; 36 with neurogenic bladder. Diagnosis unclear in 4 patients without augmentation.
[b] Simultaneous detrusorrhapy was present in 59 patients; only 19 patients had sling alone.

Accordingly, variation most likely exists in not only surgical procedures but also patient selection for outlet enhancement as well as their postoperative management.

Lessons from Artificial Urinary Sphincter

The AUS was introduced in 1972 and used to treat incontinence from various causes. Although continence rates exceeded those achieved by other available means, mechanical failures, erosion, and upper tract changes were noted complications. A report by Roth and colleagues[25] in 1986 highlighted the development of hydronephrosis in a series of children implanted with AUS for neurogenic incontinence, occurring in 11 (25%) of 44 with a functioning device (excluding 1 with female epispadias). In 4 patients, 3 who had prior augmentation, dilation was attributed to urinary retention from noncompliance with CIC, and resolved with resumed catheterization and "neuropharmacology," although 1 patient was recognized later to have decreased bladder compliance. Another patient with a known "hypertonic bladder" preoperatively awaited augmentation. The remaining 6 were believed to have new onset of decreased bladder compliance based on either cystometry or voiding cystourethrogram showing trabeculation. Of these, 3 had no preoperative urodynamic evaluation and 3 relied on combined valsalva voiding and CIC. No mention was made of anticholinergic use or changes in

medical regimen in response to hydronephrosis, but augmentation was recommended for each. This report also failed to disclose medical therapy and prior or simultaneous augmentation in the other 33 children without hydronephrosis, and did not report on overall follow-up for their patients.

That same year, another report[26] found new loss of bladder compliance or UBC developed in 6 of 35 children treated with AUS for neurogenic incontinence. However, 3 of these were also noted to have spinal cord tethering with new leg spasticity, 2 of whom had detethering with resolution of bladder changes, whereas the other 3 were treated with a trial of anticholinergics before augmentation. Similar to the report by Roth and colleagues,[25] medical management for the entire group, prior or simultaneous augmentation, and postoperative follow-up were not described.

Light and Prieto[27] evaluated 15 patients with myelodysplastic syndromes who had detrusor hyperreflexia or areflexia with decreased compliance after AUS, selected from a nonspecified population of patients at Baylor, where the device was developed. Anticholinergics improved findings in 11 patients, and it should be emphasized CIC was not used in these patients. Of the 13 patients with decreased compliance postoperatively, "almost all" showed changes "immediately postoperatively," with 10 experiencing response to anticholinergics, indicating functional rather than structural bladder changes. Only 2 of these patients with adverse pressures that did not respond to anticholinergics underwent augmentation.

These articles raised concern that urinary continence achieved through outlet procedures may be associated with decreased bladder compliance. However, the risk for change cannot be determined from this earlier era in which the AUS was implanted without preoperative urodynamic evaluation, sometimes in already trabeculated bladders, in patients who often had no systematic follow-up while asymptomatic and were often not being treated with anticholinergics or CIC. Furthermore, the question arose as to whether diminished bladder capacity was masked by the incompetent outlet or was caused by a change in bladder dynamics after outlet surgery. For example, McGuire and colleagues[9] noted that urodynamic evaluation with BN occlusion in five patients leaking at 50 mL showed decreased compliance in three and a flat filling curve in the other two. However, despite subsequent statements that preoperative urodynamic evaluation with the BN occluded by a Foley balloon is therefore "mandatory,"[28] no publication seems to report urodynamics with versus without BN occlusion in children experiencing sphincteric insufficiency.

Instead, two centers used preoperative urodynamics with BN occlusion in their decision making before AUS placement and evaluated postoperative results. de Badiola and colleagues[29] found preoperative compliance of less than 2 mL/cm H_2O predicted need for postoperative augmentation, performed a mean of 14 months after AUS implantation. From a population of 23 children with neurogenic outlet incompetency, augmentation occurred in 7 (30%), whereas another 5 (22%) had increased postoperative capacity and the other 11 were only described as continent without hydronephrosis or reflux postoperatively. Preoperative anticholinergic responsiveness in those with poor compliance was not discussed.

In contrast, in a report focused on AUS device survival, Levesque and colleagues[22] also performed preoperative urodynamics with BN occlusion. Criteria for augmentation included pressure greater than 20 cm H_2O at 50% or less predicted or functional capacity for age, and were met by 15 (37%) of 41 patients, 13 of whom did not have UBC or decreased compliance detected with preoperative urodynamics.

Preoperative UD findings did not reliably correlate with postoperative need for augmentation, which is not surprising given the variations in performing cystometry, which included not only whether the outlet was occluded but also use of slow vs rapid "provocative" filling rates, and even gas-versus-fluid infusions. Additionally, variations in postoperative bladder-emptying routines

(valsalva vs CIC), anticholinergics, and UD and radiologic testing further influenced impressions of bladder changes. Another confounding factor was the lack of definition for what constituted need for augmentation.

After reviewing experience reported by de Badiola and colleagues[29] and Levesque and colleagues,[22] Kronner and colleagues[30] declared that determining which patients need augmentation during or after AUS is "challenging," admitting that decision making in their center was based on surgeon judgment without relying on formal urodynamic criteria. This approach resulted in 35 (44%) of 80 children with neurogenic incontinence undergoing simultaneous augmentation, and subsequent augmentation in another 15 because of decreased compliance and/or upper tract changes, for a total rate of 63%. As in other studies from this era, technical aspects of urodynamics varied among patients, some having gas-versus-liquid cystometry performed with or without BN occlusion. Postoperative intervals for radiologic imaging, and CIC and anticholinergic regimens were not specified. Nevertheless, a trend toward increasing augmentation was seen compared with prior reports.

SLINGS AND AUGMENTS

Kryger and colleagues[20] reviewed publications regarding AUS, finding reported overall augmentation rates between 33% and 58%. Slings gained popularity as an alternative to the AUS and bladder neck reconstructions and, although they do not compress the outlet to the same extent as AUS,[31] simultaneous augmentation rates increased.

In a review of published series, Perez and colleagues[15] stated that 70% of patients undergoing slings for neurogenic incontinence were augmented. Their own enterocystoplasty rate was 90%, partly because continence seemed improved, and also because of concern that preoperative urodynamics may not detect adverse bladder characteristics in the presence of outlet incompetency.

This article's authors attempted urodynamics using a Foley balloon adjacent to a urodynamic catheter and found that the outlet was often poorly occluded. After the death of two patients from bladder rupture after enterocystoplasty performed for continence, and realizing that indications for cystoplasty were not clearly defined, the authors decided to perform slings without augmentation in all patients diagnosed with neurogenic outlet incompetency.[16] Sphincteric insufficiency was defined as DLPP less than 50 cm H_2O in patients with areflexia (with and/or without anticholinergics) and a nontrabeculated bladder, and/or stress incontinence. Postoperative continence was categorized as "dry" when there was no, or rare, pad use; "improved" when 1 to 2 pads per 24 hours were used; or "wet" when more than 2 pads per 24 hours were used. In an initial series of 30 consecutive children, with data prospectively maintained in a database, 83% were dry (57%) or improved (27%), which reflect similar results to those in the literature.

One boy was augmented 15 months later. He originally was dry with CIC and only underwent appendicovesicostomy. Immediately postoperatively he became incontinent, with repeat urodynamics showing decreased capacity and sphincter insufficiency. A sling was performed, but he remained incontinent and capacity continued to decrease despite anticholinergics. MRI showed no apparent cord tethering, and upper tracts remained normal. BN closure with augmentation was performed. Another boy with a failed sling had BN closure and augmentation by another surgeon, whereas a girl complaining of pain in the pubic region 4 years after sling placement underwent augmentation by another surgeon despite being continent with stable findings of a smooth bladder with end filling pressures of 15 cm H_2O.

Subsequently, the authors[32] used standardized questionnaires to assess patient-reported continence, anticholinergic use, CIC interval, and health-related quality of life (HRQOL) in two cohorts: one after sling placement plus augment and the other after sling alone. Medication requirements were significantly greater in those without augmentation, and mean CIC interval was 3 hours without augment versus 3.5 hours after augment. However, continence and HRQOL were the same in both groups.

The authors[33] recently reviewed urodynamic results after sling without augmentation, comparing preoperative, initial postoperative (within 12 months after surgery), and most recent studies (at least 18 months postoperatively), with mean follow-up 39 months. Of 26 patients, 73% had DLPP less than 25 cm H_2O before sling. Postoperative urodynamics within 12 months showed increased pressures and/or UBC in 8 patients (31%). After adjustments in anticholinergics, 6 of these had decreased end-filling pressures on their latest urodynamic evaluation, whereas the other 2 remained stable. All other patients similarly remained stable or had decreased pressures on their latest urodynamic evaluation after sling placement. No trend toward loss of bladder compliance was seen, and no patient developed trabeculation, hydronephrosis, or reflux. The authors concluded that early adverse changes after surgery should prompt adjustments in medical therapy rather than augmentation.

The authors' 360° tight fascial sling achieved "dryness" in only 57% of patients, prompting consideration of means to improve continence. Evaluation of those still using pads showed continued outlet incompetency, rather than UBC or decreased compliance, as the cause for persistent incontinence. Consequently, they added Leadbetter/Mitchell proximal urethra/BN reconstruction to reduce diameter by 50%, theoretically increasing efficiency of the sling to provide compression.[16]

Early results compared with initial results after sling alone showed a significant increase in continence rates from 57% to 93%. Postoperative urodynamics within 12 months showed an increase in pressures to greater than 40 cm H_2O in 22% of patients with sling placement, versus 18% of those who underwent leadbetter mitchell sling (LMS). However, after LMS, 1 boy developed pressures to 100 cm H_2O and four bladder cellules with transient unilateral grade 2 reflux before increased anticholinergics and overnight continuous catheter drainage reduced the pressures to 45 cm H_2O. No patient had hydronephrosis or persistent reflux. All patients continue with annual urodynamic evaluation and renal sonography.

The authors' experience agrees with the impression of Light and Prieto[27] that adverse bladder changes occur in a minority of patients early after surgery, and are most often responsive to anticholinergics and CIC, sometimes with overnight catheter drainage. The anticholinergic regimen they use consists of oral oxybutynin, 0.2 mg/kg, three to four times daily (or extended-release oxybutynin twice daily). When used, intravesical oxybutynin, 5 to 10 mg, is instilled twice daily in preteens and teens, respectively. Children with pressures greater than 40 cm H_2O may require augmentation, a finding at last urodynamic evaluation in less than 10% our patients.

SUMMARY

Initial care of newborns with spina bifida centers on preventing bladder and upper tract damage from DLPP of greater than 40 cm H_2O. The authors recommend using urodynamic-based management to select patients with elevated pressures for anticholinergic therapy and CIC, using diapers and observation with biannual renal sonography for the remainder.

At the age of toilet training, children who have urodynamic evidence of UBC and/or rising pressure during filling are started on anticholinergics and CIC, or have their dosage increased until pressures less than 40 cm H_2O and areflexia are achieved.

Sphincter incompetency is diagnosed in incontinent children with pressures less than 40 cm H_2O

and areflexia and/or stress incontinence. The authors currently use Leadbetter/Mitchell bladder neck revision and a 360° tight rectus fascial sling with appendicovesicostomy to provide continence and facilitate CIC.

Augmentation is indicated in patients with hydronephrosis and/or reflux and end-filling pressures or DLPP greater than 40 cm H_2O despite medical management to the point of patient tolerance. A minority of patients, not yet well-defined, will also need augmentation after bladder outlet surgery for similar postoperative indications.

REFERENCES

1. Snodgrass W, Keefover-Hicks A, Prieto J, et al. Comparing outcomes of slings with versus without enterocystoplasty for neurogenic urinary incontinence. J Urol 2009;181:2709.
2. McGuire EJ, Woodside JR, Borden TA, et al. Prognostic value of urodynamic testing in myelodysplastic patients. J Urol 1981;126:205.
3. Edelstein RA, Bauer SB, Kelly MD, et al. The long-term urological response of neonates with myelodysplasia treated proactively with intermittent catheterization and anticholinergic therapy. J Urol 1995;154:1500.
4. Backhaus BO, Kaefer M, Haberstroh KM, et al. Alterations in the molecular determinants of bladder compliance at hydrostatic pressures less than 40 cm. H2O. J Urol 2002;168:2600.
5. Roach MB, Switters DM, Stone AR. The changing urodynamic pattern in infants with myelomeningocele. J Urol 1993;150:944.
6. Sillen U, Hansson E, Hermansson G, et al. Development of the urodynamic pattern in infants with myelomeningocele. Br J Urol 1996;78:596.
7. Joseph DB. The effect of medium-fill and slow-fill saline cystometry on detrusor pressure in infants and children with myelodysplasia. J Urol 1992;147:444.
8. Decter RM, Harpster L. Pitfalls in determination of leak point pressure. J Urol 1992;148:588.
9. McGuire EJ, Wang CC, Usitalo H, et al. Modified pubovaginal sling in girls with myelodysplasia. J Urol 1986;135:94.
10. Wang SC, McGuire EJ, Bloom DA. A bladder pressure management system for myelodysplasia–clinical outcome. J Urol 1988;140:1499.
11. Lottmann H, Traxer O, Aigrain Y, et al. [Posterior approach to the bladder for implantation of the 800 AMS artificial sphincter in children and adolescents: techniques and results in eight patients]. Ann Urol (Paris) 1999;33:357 [in French].
12. Guys JM, Breaud J, Hery G, et al. Endoscopic injection with polydimethylsiloxane for the treatment of pediatric urinary incontinence in the neurogenic bladder: long-term results. J Urol 2006;175:1106.
13. Kropp KA, Angwafo FF. Urethral lengthening and reimplantation for neurogenic incontinence in children. J Urol 1986;135:533.
14. Salle JL, McLorie GA, Bagli DJ, et al. Urethral lengthening with anterior bladder wall flap (Pippi Salle procedure): modifications and extended indications of the technique. J Urol 1997;158:585.
15. Perez LM, Smith EA, Broecker BH, et al. Outcome of sling cystourethropexy in the pediatric population: a critical review. J Urol 1996;156:642.
16. Snodgrass WT, Elmore J, Adams R. Bladder neck sling and appendicovesicostomy without augmentation for neurogenic incontinence in children. J Urol 2007;177:1510.
17. Austin PF, Westney OL, Leng WW, et al. Advantages of rectus fascial slings for urinary incontinence in children with neuropathic bladders. J Urol 2001;165:2369.
18. Bauer SB, Peters CA, Colodny AH, et al. The use of rectus fascia to manage urinary incontinence. J Urol 1989;142:516.
19. Castellan M, Gosalbez R, Labbie A, et al. Bladder neck sling for treatment of neurogenic incontinence in children with augmentation cystoplasty: long-term follow-up. J Urol 2005;173:2128.
20. Kryger JV, Gonzalez R, Barthold JS. Surgical management of urinary incontinence in children with neurogenic sphincteric incompetence. J Urol 2000;163:256.
21. Hafez AT, McLorie G, Bagli D, et al. A single-centre long-term outcome analysis of artificial urinary sphincter placement in children. BJU Int 2002;89:82.
22. Levesque PE, Bauer SB, Atala A, et al. Ten-year experience with the artificial urinary sphincter in children. J Urol 1996;156:625.
23. Liard A, Seguier-Lipszyc E, Mathiot A, et al. The Mitrofanoff procedure: 20 years later. J Urol 2001;165:2394.
24. Bergman J, Lerman SE, Kristo B, et al. Outcomes of bladder neck closure for intractable urinary incontinence in patients with neurogenic bladders. J Pediatr Urol 2006;2:528.
25. Roth DR, Vyas PR, Kroovand RL, et al. Urinary tract deterioration associated with the artificial urinary sphincter. J Urol 1986;135:528.
26. Bauer SB, Reda EF, Colodny AH, et al. Detrusor instability: a delayed complication in association with the artificial sphincter. J Urol 1986;135:1212.
27. Light JK, Pietro T. Alteration in detrusor behavior and the effect on renal function following insertion of the artificial urinary sphincter. J Urol 1986;136:632.
28. Bosco PJ, Bauer SB, Colodny AH, et al. The long-term results of artificial sphincters in children. J Urol 1991;146:396.
29. de Badiola FI, Castro-Diaz D, Hart-Austin C, et al. Influence of preoperative bladder capacity and compliance on the outcome of artificial sphincter

implantation in patients with neurogenic sphincter incompetence. J Urol 1992;148:1493.

30. Kronner KM, Rink RC, Simmons G, et al. Artificial urinary sphincter in the treatment of urinary incontinence: preoperative urodynamics do not predict the need for future bladder augmentation. J Urol 1998; 160:1093.

31. Gormley EA, Bloom DA, McGuire EJ, et al. Pubovaginal slings for the management of urinary incontinence in female adolescents. J Urol 1994;152:822.

32. Snodgrass W, Keefover-Hicks A, Prieto J, et al. Comparing outcomes of slings with versus without enterocystoplasty for neurogenic urinary incontinence. J Urol 2009;181:2709.

33. Snodgrass W, Barber T, Cost N. Detrusor compliance changes after bladder neck sling without augmentation in children with neurogenic urinary incontinence. J Urol 2010, in press.

34. Belman AB, Kaplan GW. Experience with the Kropp anti-incontinence procedure. J Urol 1989;141:1160.

35. Hayes MC, Bulusu A, Terry T, et al. The Pippi Salle urethral lengthening procedure; experience and outcome from three United Kingdom centres. BJU Int 1999;84:701.

36. Mollard P, Mouriquand P, Joubert P. Urethral lengthening for neurogenic urinary incontinence (Kropp's procedure) results of 16 cases. J Urol 1990;143:95.

37. Nill TG, Peller PA, Kropp KA. Management of urinary incontinence by bladder tube urethral lengthening and submucosal reimplantation. J Urol 1990;144:559.

38. Snodgrass W. A simplified Kropp procedure for incontinence. J Urol 1997;158:1049.

39. Barthold JS, Rodriguez E, Freedman AL, et al. Results of the rectus fascial sling and wrap procedures for the treatment of neurogenic sphincteric incontinence. J Urol 1999;161:272.

40. Bugg CE Jr, Joseph DB. Bladder neck cinch for pediatric neurogenic outlet deficiency. J Urol 2003; 170:1501.

41. Chrzan R, Dik P, Klijn AJ, et al. Sling suspension of the bladder neck for pediatric urinary incontinence. J Pediatr Urol 2009;5:82.

42. Decter RM. Use of the fascial sling for neurogenic incontinence: lessons learned. J Urol 1993;150:683.

43. Elder JS. Periurethral and puboprostatic sling repair for incontinence in patients with myelodysplasia. J Urol 1990;144:434.

44. Kurzrock EA, Lowe P, Hardy BE. Bladder wall pedicle wraparound sling for neurogenic urinary incontinence in children. J Urol 1996;155:305.

45. Walker RD 3rd, Flack CE, Hawkins-Lee B, et al. Rectus fascial wrap: early results of a modification of the rectus fascial sling. J Urol 1995;154:771.

Lower Urinary Tract Dysfunction in Childhood

Nathaniel K. Ballek, MD, Patrick H. McKenna, MD*

KEYWORDS

- Pediatric • Incontinence • Dysfunctional voiding
- Constipation • Biofeedback

Identification and treatment of lower urinary tract dysfunction (LUTD) of childhood is a common problem facing pediatric urologists. Children with LUTD may present with incontinence, urinary tract infection (UTI), vesicoureteral reflux (VUR), and constipation alone or in combination. About 20% to 30% of children are estimated to experience symptoms related to dysfunctional voiding (DV).[1,2] Epidemiologic studies have found that the rates of incontinence and enuresis is as high as 20% in school-aged children.[3] These problems alone may account for 30% to 40% of visits to the pediatric urologist.[4,5]

Proper management of LUTD has evolved with the understanding of the pathophysiological mechanism of DV and the overactive bladder of childhood. Focus has moved from primarily pharmacologic treatment, consisting mainly of anticholinergic and antibiotic prophylaxes, to programs of education, hydration, treatment of constipation, and computer-assisted pelvic floor muscle retraining (PFMR). Current recommendations emphasize conservative management and a less invasive approach. This article discusses the proper evaluation, diagnosis, and management of the neurologically normal child presenting with symptoms of incontinence, based on the current understanding of this common yet under-recognized pediatric problem.

DEFINITIONS

The International Continence in Children Society (ICCS) recently updated the standard definitions of commonly used terms to describe abnormalities of lower urinary tract function. "Frequency" can be either increased or decreased. Increased frequency refers to 8 or more voids daily whereas decreased frequency refers to 3 or fewer voids daily in a child older than 5 years. "Incontinence" is uncontrolled leakage of urine and may be categorized as "continuous" or "intermittent". Continuous refers to constant urine leakage that is seen nearly exclusively in congenital abnormalities whereas intermittent refers to discrete urine leakage in children older than 5 years. "Enuresis" describes intermittent incontinence at night and refers to any discrete leakage of urine at night. The term "Diurnal enuresis" is no longer used and instead "diurnal incontinence" or "daytime incontinence" is used to describe incontinence during wakeful hours. "Nocturia" refers to waking to void separate from waking secondary to enuresis. "Urgency" refers to sudden and unexpected experience of an immediate need to void. "Voiding dysfunction" has been used as a broad term to describe LUTD and is no longer an acceptable term. "Dysfunctional voiding" describes habitual contraction of the urethral sphincter and has been used if a uroflow pattern of staccato voiding is seen or confirmed with urodynamics. Recently, the ICCS published terms describing DV that broaden the definition to include cases of urodynamically proven muscle dysfunction associated with low flow.[6]

DEVELOPMENT OF BLADDER CONTROL AND ETIOLOGY OF LUTD

Mechanism of urinary control in infants is not fully understood; however, it is postulated that micturition is controlled largely by the pontine mesencephalic

Department of Surgery, Division of Urology Southern Illinois University School of Medicine, St John's Pavilion, 301 North Eighth Street, PO Box 19665, Springfield, IL 62794, USA
* Corresponding author.
E-mail address: pmckenna@siumed.edu

Urol Clin N Am 37 (2010) 215–228
doi:10.1016/j.ucl.2010.03.001

micturition center.[7] Volitional control starts in children aged around 1 year, when the cortical pathways begin to develop that inhibit the brainstem. This development allows children to achieve full continence at around age 3 to 4 years.[8]

Frequency is considerably different in children when compared with adults due to the latter's maturation of the bladder and continence mechanism. As children age, the bladder capacity and voluntary control of the external sphincter increases. This change results in a decrease in frequency of voiding from up to 24 times a day in infants to around 4 to 6 times in normal adults. The change to adult voiding patterns occurs around the age of 4.[9] Normal increase in bladder capacity is calculated by the formulas[10]:

$2 \times$ age (in years) $+ 2 =$ capacity (in ounces) for children less than 2 years old

Age in years/2 $+ 6 =$ capacity (in ounces) for those 2 years old or older

Disturbances to normal bladder function in a child without neurologic lesions have been theorized to be largely behavioral in origin. The ability of the central nervous system (CNS) to cause a functional obstruction by volitional contraction of the external sphincter has been well recognized since Hinman and Baumann[11] first described the functional discoordination between detrusor contraction and the external sphincter. Evidence that stressors during or after toilet training can lead to LUTD that may perpetuate infantile voiding patterns supports this theory.[12] Sexual abuse, especially in female patients, has been linked to new onset of DV.[13] In addition, children with attention-deficit/hyperactivity disorder (ADHD) have higher rates of DV.[14,15]

As a result of studies of DV diagnosed in infancy, a congenital or genetic component to the disorder has been postulated recently. Small series of infants with signs and symptoms consistent with nonneurogenic neurogenic bladder (NNNB) syndromes have been reported.[16,17] Furthermore, DV has been linked to the Ochoa syndrome, a genetic disorder with an autosomal recessive inheritance pattern. The gene locus at chromosome 10q23-q24 is identified as the defective gene in Ochoa syndrome. It is postulated to be the possible gene locus of the NNNB described by Hinman and Allan.[18] This information casts doubt on the commonly held belief that disturbance of behavior is the sole cause of NNNB because these findings are present at or near the time of birth.

Animal and human studies have supported the evidence of a multifactorial cause of DV that involves complex interplay of the nervous systems and end organs. This has been referred to the neuroplastic model of DV in which adverse neural remodeling of the bowel and bladder occurs due to an unidentified trophic factor released in response to pelvic floor activity.[19] Steers and De Groat[20] demonstrated in a rodent model that obstruction of the urethra leads to an exaggerated spinal reflex contributing to bladder instability and hypertrophy. Yamanishi and colleagues[21] have shown that the modulation of the CNS influences overactive bladder symptoms. Their work on intractable overactive bladder symptoms with biofeedback has shown that the CNS can modulate bladder activity once thought to be largely reflexive in nature. The hypothalamus has been shown to have feedback of neurons from the pelvic nerve that has stimulatory and inhibitory activity on the bladder.[22] Electrostimulation of the anterior hypothalamus stimulates bladder contraction, and electrostimulation of the posterior hypothalamus has been shown to be inhibitory.[23] Modification of the peripheral nervous system through selective dorsal root rhizotomy has led to improvement of urodynamic parameters in patients with spastic cerebral palsy.[24] In addition, stimulation of peripheral afferent neurons leads to an inhibitory effect of detrusor through inhibition of the dorsal horn.[25] Finally, visceral afferent input to the detrusor muscle can be modified through cervical and rectal stimulation.[26,27] Together, these findings support the theory that LUTD may not be fully explained by disturbances of behavior alone. The complex interplay of pelvic floor dysfunction (PFD) that leads to end-organ changes through abnormalities in neural networks is yet to be fully elucidated.

CLASSIFICATION OF LUTD

Disturbances of the lower urinary tract function in neurologically normal children can be categorized by the bladder cycle. Problems related to the filling phase include overactive bladder syndrome, functional urinary incontinence, and giggle incontinence. Disturbances of the emptying phase include DV, lazy bladder syndrome, Hinman syndrome, and post-void dribbling.[9] Confusion can occur in identifying these syndromes as they may exist as a single entity or in combination and can be progressive.

Overactive bladder (OAB) syndrome includes involuntary detrusor contractions and urethral instability. OAB has replaced "unstable bladder of childhood" in the ICCS definitions.[6] This syndrome is found to coincide in a third of children with VUR and recurrent UTIs.[7–28] In children, OAB is the result of sudden and overwhelming urge to void that requires immediate urethral compression by the pelvic floor or by external maneuvers such as the Vincent curtsy. This syndrome may also result in constipation from chronic pelvic musculature contraction. The diagnosis of OAB syndrome can be made on examining the history of incontinence related to urgency, and does not require urodynamic evidence of uninhibited detrusor activity.

Functional urinary incontinence is the failure of the sphincteric mechanism to maintain continence in anatomically normal children. True stress urinary incontinence in which there is an anatomic insufficiency of the sphincteric mechanism to hold urine in transmission of abdominal pressures to the bladder is rare in children.

Giggle incontinence is a rare disorder seen almost exclusively in female patients in which large-volume incontinence occurs with laughter. This disorder may represent a type of cataplexy, as methylphenidate has been shown to alleviate some of the symptoms in this disorder.[29] Recently, PFMR has been shown to be a possible treatment method.[30]

Dysfunctional voiding is an abnormal contraction of the voluntary sphincter mechanism during voiding that is thought to be an acquired disorder that may progress to complete loss of bladder function. Staccato and fractionated voiding are seen in these children in uroflow studies. Due to the abnormal contraction of the pelvic floor, constipation is common in these children. Dysfunctional elimination syndrome (DES) is often used to describe this disorder because this term accounts for the link between the difficulty in voiding and defecation caused by the abnormal contraction of the pelvic floor.[31]

Lazy bladder syndrome is the loss of detrusor activity that requires the Valsalva maneuver to fully empty the bladder. Long-term fractionated voiding is thought to be the cause of this syndrome in which long voiding times result in loss of the normal detrusor function. Children often present with a history of infrequent large voids, and urodynamics may reveal large bladder capacity with low detrusor pressures and high abdominal pressures during voiding.

Hinman syndrome is often interchanged with *occult neuropathic bladder* and represents full decompensation of the voiding mechanism. Children will present with day and nighttime incontinence, chronic UTIs, and chronic constipation.[32] Urodynamic studies will often show uninhibited detrusor activity during filling, high filling pressures, large post-void residual (PVR) volumes,

and abnormal activity of the pelvic floor musculature during voiding.[9] Imaging studies results are frequently abnormal with hydroureteronephrosis secondary to VUR being common.

Post-void dribbling is a disorder in which incontinence of urine occurs immediately after micturition. This syndrome is more common in female patients and is thought to be secondary to retained urine in the vagina that leaks after standing. This syndrome is generally thought to be harmless and resolves with age. It is best treated by having the patient sit backward on the toilet, causing the legs to spread widely apart. Once the child is able to void with a clear stream in this position, voiding can occur in a normal position.

VESICOURETERAL REFLUX AND UTI IN LUTD

VUR in LUTD is theorized to be not the result of a short mucosal tunnel, but of high filling and voiding pressures.[33] Whereas VUR in boys is typically detected prenatally by ultrasonography, VUR in girls is often detected at an older age with UTIs and DV symptoms.[34–36] Children with PFD are more likely to have recurrent UTIs, have mild bilateral reflux with less spontaneous resolution, and are less likely to have success with surgical management.[33]

VUR and UTI are not independent of DV, as found by Chen and colleagues.[37] Surprisingly, DES was found more often in children with VUR and UTI, but presence of DES was not predictive of VUR. This is in line with the neuroplastic theory that postulates that hypertrophy of the bladder and bowel musculature is caused by trophic factors released during pelvic floor hyperactivity secondary to central nervous disturbances.[33] Hypertrophy can lead to an increase in risk factors that predispose the urinary tract to more UTIs and more severe VUR including anatomic bladder abnormalities, constipation, increased residual urine, higher voiding pressures, and increased urethral bacteria colonization secondary to turbulent flow.[38,39] Turbulent flow is of particular importance as eddy currents formed by nonlaminar flow leads to reflux of periurethral bacterial to the proximal urethra and bladder, causing recurrent infections.

The pelvic floor musculature is closely related to bowel and bladder. Isolated contraction of the pelvic floor musculature was found to lead to spontaneous contraction of the bladder.[33] The cycle of PFD contributing to recurrent UTIs and VUR can cause worsening bladder and bowel symptoms, and increased PFD with functional obstruction. Eventually this can lead to a hypertrophied, small-capacity bladder with high-pressure voiding that will lead to renal damage. The integral relationship between the pelvic floor activity with UTIs and VUR can be used as a model for developing treatment strategies in affected children to address the cognitive and behavioral aspects of DV and prevent irreversible damage to the upper urinary tract.

CONSTIPATION AND LUTD

According to the North American Society for Pediatric Gastroenterology and Nutrition (NASPGN), constipation is defined as "a delay or difficulty in defecation, present for 2 weeks or more, and sufficient to cause significant distress to the patient."[40] Constipation is a cofactor in PFD that contributes to voiding symptomatology, and should be factored into management programs.[33,38] The close link between bladder and bowel function is evident in embryologic development with the formation of the pelvic floor where both organs empty to, and shared innervations of sacral spinal nerves. This link may be under-recognized by clinicians and parents who have children with wetting problems. In one study of children with enuresis, more than one-third of patients had constipation despite only 14% of parents reporting any difficulties with stooling.[41]

Children with constipation may present with DV and suffer from high residual volumes and reflux due to distention of the bowel that inhibits normal contraction. Resolution of constipation has been identified as an independent risk factor in the management of VUR.[42] Upadhyay and colleagues[43] also showed that improvement in bowel-function scores on the Dysfunctional Voiding Symptom Score (DVSS) correlated directly with improvements in VUR. Treatment of constipation also decreases UTIs, most likely through modification of the bowel flora.[44] Constipation and distention of the rectal vault can lead to obstruction of the urethra, which may be one reason why treatment of constipation reduces residual volumes of urine.[45]

EVALUATION

Children with DV typically present symptoms that start soon after toilet training. Children will often continue to have daytime or nighttime incontinence, or both. Initial examination of patient history should focus on relevant questions pertaining to frequency, daily patterns of voids, volume of voids, and symptoms of urgency. Fluid intake data including caffeine consumption can be elicited. Developmental history should focus on birth history, developmental milestones, age of toilet training, any troubles with toilet training, and behavioral or mental deficiencies. History of UTI and vesicoureteral reflux is also relevant. Social history should be assessed for any new stressors including recent move, interruption of home life, recent separation from loved ones, or school performance. Relevant questions pertaining to constipation, soiling, and encopresis should be assessed. Parents are often unaware of their child's bowel habits, including abdominal pain or anxiety associated with defecation. Voiding diaries are useful to accurately record fluid intake, frequency, urgency symptoms, incontinence episodes, voiding patterns, and voiding volumes.

Physical examination should be focused and rule out any signs of neurologic deficits. Inspection of the back should focus on signs of spinal dysraphism or sacral agenesis. A neurologic examination to assess strength and reflexes of the extremities, gait, perineal sensation, rectal tone, and bulbocavernosal reflex is useful to reveal any neurologic deficit. Abdominal examination may reveal impacted stool in the colon. A genitourinary examination should focus on the urethral meatus to ensure patency. Perineal soiling or excoriation of the skin may be present as well as fecal staining of undergarments.

Laboratory assessment should occur at the initial visit and include a urinalysis with cultures and sensitivities. For children presenting with LUTD and recurrent febrile UTIs, ultrasonography of the kidneys and bladder with pre- or post-void volumes should be performed. The ultrasonographic scan can be assessed for thickened bladder wall, obstructive uropathy, or ureterocele. Voiding cystourethrogram (VCUG) is indicated in patients with documented UTIs. Significant findings include spinning top deformity in girls with DV, keyhole sign in boys with posterior urethral valves, VUR, ureterocele, and bladder trabeculation.

Full urodynamic studies are considered invasive and should be reserved for children with neurogenic bladder dysfunction, severe DV, or symptoms that do not improve with therapy. Less invasive uroflowmetry, perineal electromyography, and PVR comprise the preferred modality at the authors' institution for screening and monitoring response to treatment. Before flow study, bladder ultrasonography is used to ensure adequate volume and exclude patients with overdistention of the bladder. Overdistention of the bladder can obscure results, causing an artificial increase in PVR volumes in normal children.[46] A typical uroflow pattern in children with DV is a staccato pattern with a low prolonged flow rate. Children with detrusor underactivity will demonstrate low interrupted flows, abdominal straining, and large voided volumes (**Fig. 1**).

In the evaluation of boys with OAB symptoms, anatomic abnormalities must be considered before the initiation of therapy. In flow studies, male patients may present with symptoms of frequency, urgency, or dysuria, and a flattened curve without pelvic floor activity. In a recent series from the authors' institution, nearly 50% of these patients will have correctable surgical abnormalities including posterior urethral valves, strictures, or anterior urethral valves.[47] Although the CNS is a major factor in OAB syndrome, these findings discount the theory that a CNS is the sole cause of OAB.

For assessment of constipation abdominal examination may used, but rectal examinations are generally not performed due to emotional distress of the child. Abdominal ultrasonography can be performed to diagnose and quantify constipation.[48] An increased rectal diameter may indicate the diagnosis of impaction in some cases.

This method may be useful in the management because a decrease in rectal diameter correlates with successful treatment.[49] Bowel diaries and Bristol stool scales are also used to evaluate and monitor treatment in LUTD and constipation.

Recently, there has been an effort to standardize a scoring system in the evaluation of children with DV.[4,50,51] This scoring system would be beneficial in classifying the type and severity of DV to determine necessary treatment modalities. A small prospective cohort was analyzed by Upadhyay and colleagues[43] to determine the validity of the DVSS in children with reflux. A positive correlation between symptom score improvement and resolution of VUR was found. The validity of these scoring systems has not yet been evaluated in large prospective trials.

TREATMENT OF LUTD

The most successful treatment programs use an escalating treatment program that institutes

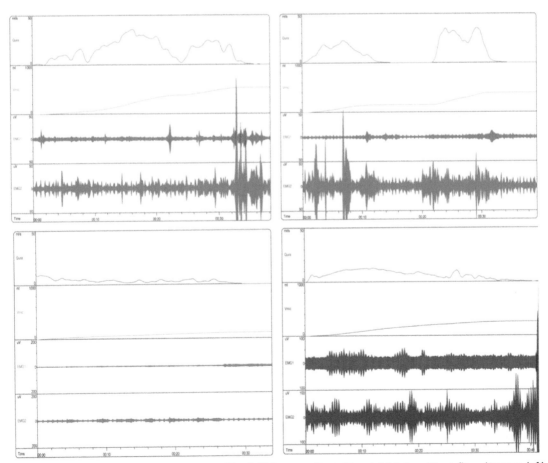

Fig. 1. Examples of uroflow studies in LUTD. (*Top left*) Staccato flow. (*Top right*) Intermittent flow. (*Bottom left*) Low flow with low electromyographic (EMG) activity. (*Bottom right*) Low flow with high EMG activity.

education and modification of lifestyle at an early stage, followed by PFMR and pharmacologic therapy (**Fig. 2**).[52,53] Conservative management is the initial treatment strategy for children presenting with the primary complaint of incontinence or UTI without anatomic abnormality. Focus should be on modification of the child's urinary and bowel habits in an attempt to ameliorate the incontinence and prevent UTI prior to more invasive testing or treatment strategies (**Fig. 3**). Bowel function management in the treatment of LUTD is one of the main goals in managing voiding symptoms, VUR, and UTIs. Many conservative treatment programs implement bowel management as a treatment strategy to manage LUTD. Programs differ in exact protocol; however, most emphasize education, increased hydration, timed voiding, correction of constipation, and proper hygiene.

Education is a key component of the initial management for LUTD for voiding habits and hygiene. In one prospective study, education emphasizing timed voiding, fluid management, and pelvic floor exercises had a large impact of daytime incontinence, with nearly 60% of patients having improvement at the end of 5 years of treatment.[54] In addition, education concerning proper posture during voiding should be emphasized to minimize abdominal musculature straining. Research has shown the link between abdominal musculature contraction and concomitant pelvic floor contraction.[55,56] Proper sitting technique with buttock and foot support and comfortable hip position is necessary to enable voiding without recruitment of the abdominal muscles.[57] Hygiene education is also important to limit local skin inflammation that may contribute to holding maneuvers and DV. In this way, coordinated voiding with a relaxed pelvic floor can be facilitated at the initiation of management.

Constipation has been identified as an integral component in the conservative management approach of DV.[38,42,43] Treatment of constipation alone has been shown to resolve lower urinary tract abnormalities (**Table 1**). In one study by Loening-Baucke,[58] enuresis resolved in 63% and daytime incontinence in 89% of patients presenting with constipation and incontinence. In the same study, resolution of constipation also resolved recurrent UTIs. Initial treatment with aggressive use of laxatives, stool softeners, and enemas is recommended by the NASPGN if fecal

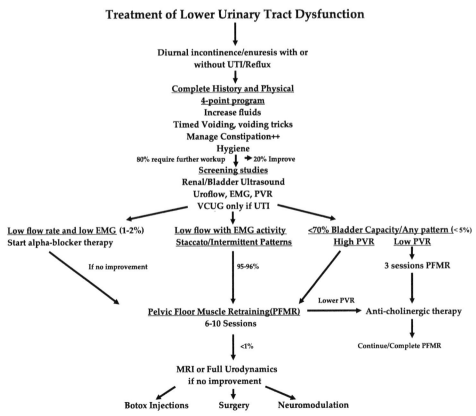

Fig. 2. An escalating management strategy for LUTD.

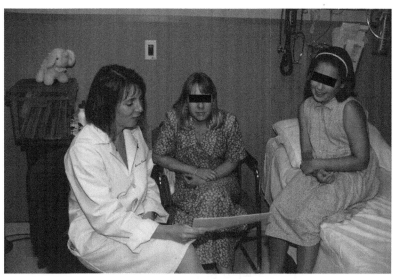

Fig. 3. Treatment strategies focusing on education begins with teaching by a nurse educator with parents and patients.

impaction is present. Oral medications such as mineral oil or polyethylene glycol are effective. Phosphate soda, saline, or mineral oil enemas are recommended because they do not have the potential risk of toxicity that soap suds, tap water, or magnesium enemas carry. Oral and invasive rectal treatments are equally effective, although enemas have a faster resolution of impaction.[40] Fecal impaction must be managed prior to maintenance therapy to be successful. Maintenance with balanced diet, fiber supplementation, and laxatives are recommended to maintain a goal of one bulky bowel movement a day.

PFMR using biofeedback therapy is the next line of treatment after conservative approaches have been initiated. Goals of biofeedback therapy differ for the type of LUTD, but in each case the awareness of the pelvic floor to alter the patient's voiding habits is the main objective. In children with hyperactive pelvic floor, biofeedback therapy focuses on the relaxation and a return of normal flow. For children with overactive bladder and incontinence, use of the guarding reflex of the pelvic floor musculature can maintain continence during uninhibited contractions. In addition, biofeedback can teach these children to void optimally and ensure that there is no decompensation of the detrusor muscle that occurs with the lazy bladder syndrome.[59]

There is no standard protocol for the correct teaching of biofeedback, but in general there are 2 methods. The first uses real-time flow rates viewed by the patient with pelvic floor exercises to modify flow. This method is recommended in children with pelvic floor hyperactivity and no OAB symptoms. The method requires a sophisticated flowmeter with immediate feedback. In selected patients, this type of biofeedback may provide resolution of symptoms in fewer sessions.[52,60] The second method uses pelvic and abdominal surface electromyography (EMG) to record activity and provide input back to the patient regarding the use of these muscle groups. The advantage in using this method lies in its ability to teach a guarding reflex in addition to the relaxation of the pelvic floor during voiding.[59] Children with mixed DV may benefit more from this type of biofeedback therapy.

At the authors' institution, PFMR is administered by a urotherapist in 6 to 10 individual 1-hour sessions (**Fig. 4**). The first session concentrates on isolation of the pelvic floor musculature through Kegel exercises in patients while being monitored on EMG. Surface EMG leads are placed at the 4- and 10-o'clock positions on the perineum, and an abdominal lead is placed on the rectus abdominis muscle. If Kegel exercises are difficult to achieve, then the pelvic floor is actively contracted by rolling the knees and feet in and out with each leg held straight and heel in place. This exercise forces the patient to use the pelvic floor and become aware of its contraction, necessary for the subsequent Kegel exercises. Each following session begins with a discussion on the patient's progress regarding UTIs, incontinence, constipation, and doing Kegel exercises at home. The session then moves to relaxation exercises followed by short repetitions of quick flicks monitored on EMG to ensure isolation of the pelvic floor with relaxation of the abdomen. The session

Table 1
Effect of constipation treatment alone on urinary tract abnormalities

Study	Number of Patients	UTI	Reflux	High Residual	Incontinence/Enuresis
Dohil et al[45]	29	Not evaluated	64% of patients with reflux had resolution	68% of patients resolved or decreased	Not evaluated
Loening-Baucke[58]	234	100% resolution if no anatomic abnormalities	Not evaluated	Not evaluated	89% incontinence resolved; 63% enuresis resolved
Neumann et al[77]	63	88% vs 9% recurrence rate of untreated vs treated constipation	Not evaluated	Not evaluated	Not evaluated
Hagstroem et al[78]	45	Not evaluated	Not evaluated	Not evaluated	17% had wetting resolve

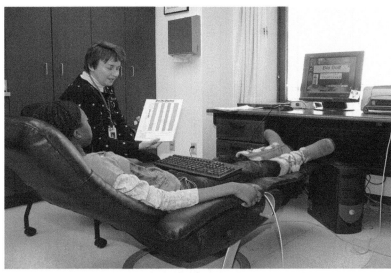

Fig. 4. Biofeedback sessions begin with review of voiding habits by the urotherapist and warm-up exercises.

advances to cycles of contraction, relaxation, and quick flick exercises while being monitored with EMG. The contraction and relaxation of the pelvic floor is used in video games to achieve goals in video games such as golf, growing flowers, or spaceships (see **Fig. 4; Fig. 5**). Use of this type of biofeedback has been successful, with 87% of patients reporting subjective improvement.[19]

Improvement in incontinence, UTIs, VUR, and constipation with biofeedback therapy is well documented in the literature (**Table 2**). Factors that have been found to improve efficacy of biofeedback include compliance, normal bladder capacity, number of sessions, and use of animation. Independent risk factors to predict failure identified by Herndon and colleagues[19] are small bladder capacity and compliance to therapy. In this study, children with small bladder capacity and low residual were found more likely to respond to therapy if anticholinergics were given. Recently, Drzewiecki and colleagues[61] demonstrated that 3 sessions were required to have improvement in most ideal patients using biofeedback with animation. Children with neurologic and other issues that would limit compliance were excluded in this study. Although this study shows the minimum amount of sessions using a specific methodology, it is significant in that it showed a dose-dependent effect based on several sessions. In one study, use of animation was found to lower the number of minimum sessions by more than half.[62] Use of animations enforces behavior with biofeedback through the use of rewards for obtaining objectives.

PHARMACOLOGIC THERAPY IN THE TREATMENT OF LUTD

The use of pharmacologic therapy in the treatment of LUTD is used as an adjunct to standard urotherapy. Pharmacotherapy may be used generally in 2

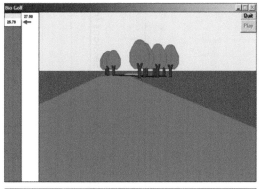

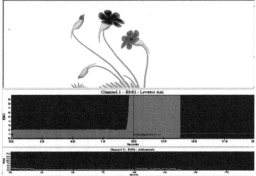

Fig. 5. Examples of video games that are used for PFMR.

Table 2
Results of pelvic floor retraining with biofeedback in LUTD

Study	Number of Patients	Number of Sessions (mean)	Follow-up	Outcome
Herndon et al[19]	168	5	24 mo	87% improved incontinence
Yamanishi et al[21]	33	–	6 mo	Refractory overactive bladder resolved in 30% and improved in 54%
Shei Dei Yang and Wang[60]	20	2.2	18.9 mo	Short course of uroflowmetry and electromyographic biofeedback improved in 90% of patients
Schulman et al[53]	102	1–3	1.8 y	100% had improvement with nurse coaching during flow studies, 91% improved with animated biofeedback
Drzewiecki et al[61]	77	3 (median)	–	64.5% improved incontinence
Kaye and Palmer[62]	120	3.6 vs 7.6	5.4	Animated required fewer sessions than nonanimated. 90% of both groups had improvement
Herndon et al[33]	51	–	24 mo	90% reduction in need for surgical intervention for reflux
Porena et al[79]	43	11	4 y	80% cured of incontinence
Chin-Peukert et al[80]	87	5	6 mo	61% improvement in urinary symptoms
Pfister et al[81]	15	12	3–4 mo	100% clinical improvement
Combs et al[82]	21	4	34 mo	81% urodynamic improvement

ways: to enhance bladder emptying and bladder filling. α-Adrenergic blockade of receptors at the bladder neck and urethra results in relaxation of smooth muscle and theoretically enables more complete bladder emptying. Several studies have shown efficacy in reducing subjective symptoms and improving objective urinary parameters in children with DV and increased PVR.[63–66] α-Blockers that have low flow rate, low EMG activity, and delayed initiation of voiding are used early in the treatment course of male patients without anatomic abnormality. Dramatic improvement in flow, initiation of voiding, and PVR was documented in one study by Donohoe and colleagues.[65] All children that met the criteria of primary bladder neck dysfunction improved with α-blocker therapy and those that discontinued therapy returned to baseline symptoms. In one prospective randomized trial, α-blockers were given to a group of children with DV. In most patients, there was little change in objective parameter except in 2 patients that had significant improvement.[66] This study supports the practice of using alpha blockers in select cases of patients with aforementioned findings on uroflow and EMG.

Botulinum toxin A has also been proposed as a possible treatment regimen to improve bladder emptying for children with DV who have failed standard therapy. Several small studies have demonstrated improvement.[67–71] The limitations of the studies advocating the use of botulinum toxin are small sample size, lack of standard dosing, and nonrandomization.

Anticholinergic therapy is used to facilitate bladder filling by inhibiting detrusor contractions. The place of anticholinergics has moved from being a primary intervention in the treatment of overactive bladder syndrome to a more ancillary role with biofeedback. For patients with small bladder capacity and low PVR in which LUTD did not improve with 3 sessions of biofeedback, oxybutynin is effective. For children with small-capacity bladders and high PVR, a full biofeedback session is often necessary to isolate pelvic floor muscles and lower PVR before initiation of anticholinergics. About 87% of these patients with small-capacity bladders who do not improve with biofeedback will improve with the addition of anticholinergics.[19] Solifenacin has also been demonstrated to treat incontinence in refractory OAB, with an 85% response rate and only a 6.5% side effect rate.[72]

Anticholinergic therapy as a primary treatment modality has been documented to have an 84% efficacy in children without UTIs, but efficacy dropped to 40% in the presence of UTI.[28] More recently, Bolduc and colleagues[73] demonstrated

that double anticholinergic therapy could be used to treat OAB syndrome that is not responsive to single-agent anticholinergic therapy, with little increase in side effects. Double-dose treatment led to a 100% continence rate in 52% of patients and 90% continence rate in 42% of patients. Despite proven efficacy, indiscriminate use of anticholinergic therapy as a primary management strategy in OAB syndrome in children is not advocated by most investigators, because of the side effect profile and similar rates of success with biofeedback.

OTHER TREATMENT MODALITIES IN LUTD

Clean intermittent catheterization (CIC) has been shown to be useful in children with high PVR volumes that do not improve with standard therapy. CIC as the primary therapy has demonstrated improvement in continence and a lower rate of UTIs in neurologically normal children with high PVR.[74] Its use may also be implemented to temporize symptoms while standard therapy has time to take effect in the OAB syndrome.[59]

Neuromodulation has been successful in children with refractory OAB syndromes, but the invasiveness of permanent sacral modulation has limited its use in children without neurologic deficits. Less invasive neuromodulatory devices such as tibial nerve stimulation and transcutaneous electrical nerve stimulation (TENS) have been proposed as treatment modalities. Tibial nerve stimulation has been successful in improving symptoms related to DV and OAB syndrome at rates of up to 100% in one series.[75] TENS has had success in the treatment of OAB syndrome when compared with placebo in one prospective trial.[76] The use of neuromodulation as treatment modality in refractory LUTD is promising, but larger prospective trials will be necessary to solidify its role as a treatment modality.

SUMMARY

LUTD is a common disorder that may be under-reported by parents and clinicians. Although the prognosis is favorable in most cases, serious long-term complications can occur, including renal failure. Thorough history, physical, and stepwise evaluation will determine appropriate treatment strategies. Advances in the understanding of the underlying pathology of this common disorder have led to a revolution in management, from expensive and potentially harmful medications and surgeries to noninvasive, effective behavioral modifications.

REFERENCES

1. Whelan CM, McKenna PH. Urologic applications of biofeedback therapy. Contemp Urol 2004;58:23–34.
2. Hellstrom AL, Hanson E, Hansson S, et al. Micturition habits and incontinence in 7-year-old Swedish school entrants. Eur J Pediatr 1990;149:434–7.
3. Lee SD, Sohn DW, Lee JZ, et al. An epidemiological study of enuresis in Korean children. BJU Int 2000; 85(7):869–73.
4. Farhat W, Bagli D, Capolicchio G, et al. The dysfunctional voiding scoring system: quantitative standardization of dysfunctional voiding symptoms in children. J Urol 2000;164:1011.
5. Rushton HG. Wetting and functional voiding disorders. Urol Clin North Am 1995;22:75–93.
6. Nevéus T, von Gontard A, Hoebeke P, et al. The standardization of terminology of lower urinary tract function in children and adolescents: report from the Standardization Committee of the International Children's Continence Society. J Urol 2006;176:314–24.
7. Bauer SB. Special considerations of the overactive bladder in children. Urology 2002;60(Suppl 5A):43–8.
8. Yeung CK, Godley ML, Ho CKW, et al. Some new insights into bladder function in infancy. Br J Urol 1995;76:235–40.
9. Bauer SB, Yeung CK, Sihoe JD. Voiding dysfunction in children: neurogenic and non-neurogenic. In: Kavoussi LR, Novick AC, Partin AW, et al, editors. Campbell's urology. 9th edition. Philadelphia: WB Saunders Co; 2007. p. 3604–55.
10. Kaefer M, Zurakowski D, Bauer SB, et al. Estimating normal bladder capacity in children. J Urol 1997; 158:2261–4.
11. Hinman F, Baumann FW. Vesical and ureteral damage from voiding dysfunction in boys without neurologic or obstructive disease. J Urol 1973;109: 727–32.
12. Feldman AS, Bauer SB. Diagnosis and management of dysfunctional voiding. Curr Opin Pediatr 2006;18: 139–47.
13. Ellsworth PI, Merguerian PA, Copening ME. Sexual abuse: another causative factor in dysfunctional voiding. J Urol 1995;153:773–6.
14. Duel BP, Steinberg-Epstein R, Hill M, et al. A survey of voiding dysfunction in children with attention deficit-hyperactivity disorder. J Urol 2003;170: 1521–3.
15. Bhatia MS, Nigam VR, Bohra N, et al. Attention deficit disorder with hyperactivity among paediatric outpatients. J Child Psychol Psychiatry 1991;32: 297–306.
16. Jayanthi VR, Khoury AE, McLorie GA, et al. The non-neurogenic neurogenic bladder of early infancy. J Urol 1997;158(3 Pt 2):1281–5.
17. Al Mosawi AJ. Identification of nonneurogenic neurogenic bladder in infants. Urology 2007;70(2):355–6.
18. Ochoa B. Can a congenital dysfunctional bladder be diagnosed from a smile? The Ochoa syndrome updated. Pediatr Nephrol 2004;19(1):6–12.
19. Herndon CD, Decambre M, McKenna PH. Interactive computer games for treatment of pelvic floor dysfunction. J Urol 2001;166:1893–8.
20. Steers WD, De Groat WC. Effect of bladder outlet obstruction on micturition reflex pathways in the rat. J Urol 1988;140:864–71.
21. Yamanishi T, Yasuda K, Murayama N, et al. Biofeedback training for detrusor overactivity in children. J Urol 2000;164:1686–90.
22. Marson L. Identification of central nervous system neurons that innervate the bladder body, bladder base, or external urethral sphincter of female rats: a transneuronal tracing study using pseudorabies virus. J Comp Neurol 1997;389:584–602.
23. Morrison JF. Bladder control: role of higher levels of the central nervous system. In: Torrens M, Morrison JF, editors. The physiology of the lower urinary tract. New York: Springer-Verlag; 1987. p. 238–74.
24. Houle AM, Vernet O, Jednak VR, et al. Bladder function before and after selective dorsal rhizotomy in children with cerebral palsy. J Urol 1998;160: 1088–91.
25. Steers WD. New strategies in the diagnosis and management of voiding dysfunction. J Urol 2000; 163:1234–5.
26. De Groat WC. Inhibition and excitation of sacral parasympathetic neurons by visceral and cutaneous stimuli in the cat. Brain Res 1971;33:499–503.
27. Sato A, Schmidt RF. The modulation of visceral function by somatic afferent activity. Jpn J Physiol 1987;37:1.
28. Bauer SB, Retic AB, Colodny AH, et al. The unstable bladder of childhood. Urol Clin North Am 1980;7:321–36.
29. Berry AK, Zderic S, Carr M. Methylphenidate in giggle incontinence. J Urol 2009;182(4):2028–32.
30. Richardson I, Palmer LS. Successful treatment for giggle incontinence with biofeedback. J Urol 2009; 182:2062–6.
31. Koff SA, Wagner TT, Jayanthi VR. The relationship among dysfunctional elimination syndromes, primary vesicoureteral reflux and urinary tract infections in children. J Urol 1998;160:1019–22.
32. Hinman F. Nonneurogenic neurogenic bladder (the Hinman syndrome)—15 years later. J Urol 1986; 136:769–77.
33. Herndon CDA, Decambre M, McKenna PH. Changing concepts concerning the management of vesicoureteral reflux. J Urol 2001;166:1439–43.
34. Kokoua A, Homsy Y, Lavigne JF, et al. Maturation of the bladder external urinary sphincter: a comparative histotopographic study in humans. J Urol 1993;150: 617–22.

35. Snodgrass W. The impact of treated dysfunctional voiding on the nonsurgical management of vesicoureteral reflux. J Urol 1998;160:1823–5.

36. Soygur T, Arikan N, Yesillin C, et al. Relationship among pediatric voiding dysfunction and vesicoureteral reflux and renal scars. Urology 1999;54:905–8.

37. Chen JJ, Mao W, Homayoon K, et al. A multivariate analysis of dysfunctional elimination syndrome and its relationships with gender, urinary tract infection and vesicoureteral reflux in children. J Urol 2004; 171:1907–10.

38. Whelan CM, McKenna PH. Dysfunctional voiding as a co-factor of recurrent UTI. Contemp Urol 2004;16: 58–73.

39. Hinman F. Mechanisms for the entry of bacteria and the establishment of urinary infection in female children. J Urol 1966;96(4):546–50.

40. Baker SS, Liptak GS, Colletti RB, et al. Constipation in infants and children: evaluation and treatment. J Pediatr Gastroenterol Nutr 1999;29:612–26.

41. Mcgrath KH, Caldwell PH, Jones MP. The frequency of constipation in children with nocturnal enuresis: a comparison with parental reporting. J Paediatr Child Health 2008;44:19–27.

42. Silva JMP, Diniz JSS, Lima EM, et al. Predictive factors of resolution of primary vesico-ureteric reflux: a multivariate analysis. BJU Int 2006;97(5):1063–8.

43. Upadhyay J, Bolduc S, Bagli DJ, et al. Use of the dysfunctional voiding symptom score to predict resolution of vesicouretereal reflux in children with voiding dysfunction. J Urol 2003;169:1842–6.

44. Zoppi G, Cinquetti M, Luciano A, et al. The intestinal ecosystem in chronic functional constipation. Acta Paediatr 1998;87(8):152–4.

45. Dohil R, Roberts E, Jones KV, et al. Constipation and reversible urinary tract abnormalities. Arch Dis Child 1994;70:56–7.

46. Chang S, Yang S. Variability, related factors, and normal reference value of post-void residual urine in healthy kindergarteners. J Urol 2009;182:1933–8.

47. Miller J, McKenna PH. Uroflowmetric parameters and symptomatologic outcomes in boy with overactive bladders. In: Programs and abstracts of the 83rd Annual Meeting North Central Section of the AUA. Arizona; 2009.

48. Bijos AM, Czerwionka-Szaflarska M, Mazur A, et al. The usefulness of ultrasound examination of the bowel as a method of assessment of functional chronic constipation in children. Pediatr Radiol 2007;37:1247–52.

49. Joensson IM, Siggard C, Rittig S, et al. Transabdominal ultrasound of the rectum as a diagnostic tool in childhood constipation. J Urol 2008;179:1997–2002.

50. Akbal C, Genc Y, Burgu B, et al. Dysfunctional voiding and incontinence scoring system: Quantitative evaluation of incontinence symptoms in pediatric population. J Urol 2005;173:969–73.

51. Afshar K, Mirbagheri A, MacNeily A, et al. Development of a symptom score for dysfunctional elimination syndrome. J Urol 2009;182:1939–43.

52. Herndon CD, Connery S, McKenna PH, et al. Pelvic floor muscle retraining for pediatric voiding dysfunction using interactive computer games. J Urol 1999; 162(3):1056–62.

53. Schulman SL, Von Zuben FC, Plachter N, et al. Biofeedback methodology: does it matter how we teach children how to relax the pelvic floor during voiding? J Urol 2001;166:2423–6.

54. Wiener JS, Scales MT, Hampton J, et al. Long term efficacy of simple behavioral therapy for daytime wetting in children. J Urol 2000;164:786–90.

55. Neumann P, Gill V. Pelvic floor and abdominal muscle interaction: EMG activity and intra-abdominal pressure. Int Urogynecol J Pelvic Floor Dysfunct 2002;13:125–32.

56. Sapsford R, Hodges PW, Richardson CA, et al. Co-activation of the abdominal and pelvic floor muscles during voluntary exercises. Neurourol Urodyn 2001;20:31–42.

57. Wennergren H, Oberg B, Sandstedt P. The importance of leg support for relaxation of the pelvic floor muscles: a surface electromyography study in healthy girls. Scand J Urol Nephrol 1991;25:205–13.

58. Loening-Baucke V. Urinary incontinence and urinary tract infection and their resolution with treatment of chronic constipation of childhood. Pediatrics 1997; 100:228.

59. van Gool JD, de Jonge GA. Urge syndrome and urge incontinence. Arch Dis Child 1989;64:1629–34.

60. Shei Dei Yang SS, Wang CC. Outpatient biofeedback relaxation of the pelvic floor in treating pediatric dysfunctional voiding: a short-course program is effective. Urol Int 2005;74:118–22.

61. Drzewiecki BA, Kelly PR, Marinaccio B, et al. Biofeedback training for lower urinary tract symptoms: factors affecting efficacy. J Urol 2009;182: 2050–5.

62. Kaye JD, Palmer LS. Animated biofeedback yields more rapid results than nonanimated biofeedback in the treatment of dysfunctional voiding in girls. J Urol 2008;180(1):300–5.

63. Austin PF, Homsy YL, Masel JL, et al. Alpha-Adrenergic blockade in children with neuropathic and nonneuropathic voiding dysfunction. J Urol 1999; 162(3 Pt 2):1064–7.

64. Cain MP, Wu SD, Austin PF, et al. Alpha blocker therapy for children with dysfunctional voiding and urinary retention. J Urol 2003;170:1514–5.

65. Donohoe JM, Combs AJ, Glassberg KI. Primary bladder neck dysfunction in children and adolescents II: results of treatment with alpha-adrenergic antagonists. J Urol 2005;173(1):212–6.

66. Kramer SA, Rathbun SR, Elkins D, et al. Double-blind placebo controlled study of alpha-adrenergic

receptor antagonists (doxazosin) for treatment of voiding dysfunction in the pediatric population. J Urol 2005;173:2121.

67. Grazko MA, Polo KB, Jabbari B. Botulinum toxin A for spasticity, muscle spasms, and rigidity. Neurology 1995;45:712–7.

68. Mokhless I, Gaafar S, Fouda K, et al. Botulinum A toxin urethral sphincter injection in children with non-neurogenic neurogenic bladder. J Urol 2006;176: 1767–70.

69. Petronijevic V, Lazovic M, Vlajkovic M, et al. Botulinum toxin type A in combination with standard urotherapy for children with dysfunctional voiding. J Urol 2007;178:2599–602.

70. Steinhardt F, Naseer S, Cruz OA. Botulinum toxin: Novel treatment for dramatic urethral dilatation associated with dysfunctional voiding. J Urol 1997;158: 190–1.

71. Franco I, Landau-Dyer L, Isom-Batz G, et al. The use of botulinum toxin A injection for the management of external sphincter dyssynergia in neurologically normal children. J Urol 2007;178:1775–9.

72. Hoebeke P, De Pooter J, De Caestecker K, et al. Solifenacin for therapy resistant overactive bladder. J Urol 2009;182:2040–4.

73. Bolduc S, Moore K, Lebel S, et al. Double anticholinergic therapy for refractory overactive bladder. J Urol 2009;182:2033–9.

74. Pohl HG, Bauer SB, Borer JG, et al. The outcome of voiding dysfunction managed with clean intermittent catheterization in neurologically and anatomically normal children. BJU Int 2002;89(9):923–7.

75. Capitanucci ML, Camanni D, Demelas F, et al. Long-term efficacy of percutaneous tibial nerve stimulation for different types of lower urinary tract dysfunction in children. J Urol 2009;182:2056–61.

76. Hagstroem S, Mahler B, Madsen B, et al. Transcutaneous electrical nerve stimulation for refractory daytime urinary urge incontinence. J Urol 2009; 182:2072–8.

77. Neumann PZ, deDomenico IJ, Nogrady MB. Constipation and urinary tract infection. Pediatrics 1973; 52(2):241–5.

78. Hagstroem S, Rittig N, Kamperis K, et al. Treatment outcome of day-time urinary incontinence in children. Scand J Urol Nephrol 2008;42:528–33.

79. Porena M, Costantini E, Rociola W, et al. Biofeedback successfully cures detrusor-sphincter dyssynergia in pediatric patients. J Urol 2000;163(6): 1927–31.

80. Chin-Peukert L, Salle JL. A modified biofeedback program for children with detrusor-sphincter dyssynergia: 5 year experience. J Urol 2001;166(4):1470–5.

81. Pfister C, Dacher JN, Gaucher S, et al. The usefulness of a minimal urodynamic evaluation and pelvic floor biofeedback in children with chronic voiding dysfunction. BJU Int 1999;84(9):1054–7.

82. Combs AJ, Glassberg AD, Gerdes D, et al. Biofeedback therapy for children with dysfunctional voiding. Urology 1998;52:312–5.

Urinary Tract Infection in Children: When to Worry

Curtis J. Clark, MD[a], William A. Kennedy II MD[a,b],
Linda D. Shortliffe, MD[a,b],*

KEYWORDS

- Urinary tract infection • Pediatric • Cystitis
- Pyelonephritis • Treatment

Urinary tract infection (UTI) is a significant concern for parents as well as for children who acquire them. While primary care physicians and pediatricians are the front line, dealing with the initial management of UTI, they turn to urologists when faced with more complicated infections. This article reviews the diagnosis and management of UTI, and examines scenarios in which the clinician should have a heightened level of concern when dealing with UTI in the pediatric population.

The comprehensive epidemiology of UTI has been well described.[1] The overall incidence of UTI in the prepubertal pediatric population is 3% in girls and 1% in boys. The incidence of UTI varies with age and sex. Infant girls have an incidence of 0.4% to 0.1%, which increases to 0.9% to 1.4% between the ages 1 and 5 years, and peaks with an incidence of 0.7% to 2.3% in school-aged girls. In contrast, infant boys have an incidence of UTI of 0.188% (circumcised) and 0.702% (uncircumcised), which decreases to 0.1% to 0.2% between ages 1 and 5 years, followed by 0.04% to 0.2% in school-aged boys.[2] In febrile children presenting to the emergency department, UTI is more common than in healthy children, with an incidence between 3% and 5% in most studies.[3] Racial differences also exist, including a low incidence in African American children and higher incidence in Caucasian girls relative to other races.[1]

Other risk factors associated with UTI include anomalies of the urinary tract (anatomic, functional, or neurologic) and systemic abnormalities (diabetes mellitus, compromised immune system, and so forth).

The pathogenesis of UTI is based both on the bacteria that cause infection and on patient-specific factors. Bacteria common in UTI are predominantly of enteric origin. *Escherichia coli* is the most frequent cause of all types of UTI, while group B streptococcal infection is relatively more common in neonates. Bacteria tend to colonize the periurethral area, migrating in a retrograde fashion to reach the urinary tract. Bacteria may also be introduced into the urinary tract via instrumentation. Systemic infections may also result in UTI through seeding of the urinary system. Once present within the urinary tract, bacteria can be cleared by the emptying of urine or can adhere to the urothelial lining, resulting in infection. After colonization of the urinary tract, virulence factors such as fimbriae may assist bacteria in causing an infection.

Diagnosis of UTI is based on clinical symptoms and the results of a urine culture. Classic symptoms of UTI in adults are dysuria, frequency, hesitancy, and flank pain. Unfortunately, young children often lack the ability to identify and describe these symptoms. Symptoms in children

Disclosures: L.D.S. is on the Board of directors of Vivus, Inc.
[a] Department of Urology, Lucile Packard Children's Hospital, Stanford University Medical Center, Stanford University School of Medicine, S-287, 300 Pasteur Drive, Stanford, CA 94305-5118, USA
[b] Department of Pediatric Urology, Lucile Packard Children's Hospital, Stanford University School of Medicine, S-287, 300 Pasteur Drive, Stanford, CA 94305-5118, USA
* Corresponding author. Department of Urology, Lucile Packard Children's Hospital, Stanford University Medical Center, Stanford University School of Medicine, S-287, 300 Pasteur Drive, Stanford, CA 94305-5118.
E-mail address: lindashortliffe@stanford.edu

Urol Clin N Am 37 (2010) 229–241
doi:10.1016/j.ucl.2010.03.009

tend to be less specific in nature and parents commonly report their symptoms as fever, irritability, lethargy, poor feeding, incontinence, and pungent urine odor. Children presenting with these symptoms, or with unexplained fever, should have UTI eliminated as a diagnosis. On performing a genitourinary examination, no specific abnormalities are consistently present. Definitive diagnosis of a UTI requires a properly obtained urine culture. Perineally "bagged" urine is useful only for excluding UTI, as there is a high chance that any growth is the result of skin colonization. Clean catch urine specimens also have a higher false-positive rate in young children, likely due to periurethral colonization. This collection technique can be more useful in older children.

The 2 most reliable sources of urine for culture are a catheterized urine specimen or a suprapubic aspirate. The drawbacks of catheterized urine include the potential for (a) introduction of bacteria, which may lead to an iatrogenic infection, and (b) psychological trauma to the patient. Suprapubic aspirates avoid introduction of pathogens into the urinary tract and give a reliable specimen; however, the use of this technique is limited by physician comfort. A suprapubic aspirate is obtained by blind passage of a small-gauge (21F or 22F) needle through the abdominal wall approximately 1 to 2 cm cephalad to the pubic symphysis into a bladder that is palpably full.[4] The use of bedside ultrasonography enhances the ability to safely perform this technique by ensuring an adequately full bladder and allowing assessment of structures between the abdominal wall and bladder, while topical anesthesia can decrease patient discomfort.

Imaging for UTI is a subject of ongoing debate beyond the scope of this article. Prior teaching deferred imaging for a nonfebrile UTI, while recommending renal/bladder ultrasonography and voiding cystourethrography (VCUG) for a febrile UTI. More recently, the top-down approach has been advocated as a method of avoiding VCUG and concentrating effort on those at greatest risk of renal scarring.[5] This approach, which will be discussed in detail elsewhere in this issue, focuses on using a dimercaptosuccinic acid (DMSA) scan to document pyelonephritis and/or renal scarring. Additional lower tract imaging with a VCUG is performed on patients with documented renal involvement. DMSA scans are considered the gold standard for detection of acute pyelonephritis and renal scarring (**Fig. 1**), with 92% sensitivity when compared with histology in an animal model.[6] As always, limitation of radiation exposure is a goal in pediatrics, and use of imaging modalities that limit radiation exposure while providing

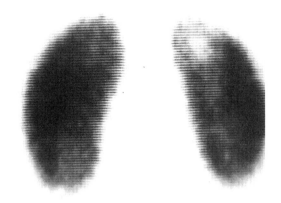

Fig. 1. Renal scarring. In this DMSA scan, note the normal left kidney, while the right kidney shows a photopenic area and loss of renal contour consistent with scarring at the right upper pole.

the necessary details will continue to increase as techniques improve. Magnetic resonance imaging (MRI), including MR urography, has increasingly been used to image the urinary tract and to identify renal scarring, with some literature questioning whether MRI is superior to DMSA.[7] While these studies avoid radiation exposure, they often require sedation or general anesthesia when performed in children. Renal/bladder ultrasonography (RBUS) is less sensitive for detecting pyelonephritis than DMSA scan, with one study noting only 22% detection of DMSA-confirmed scarring using RBUS.[8] Ultrasound, however, does allow for assessment of renal abnormalities, such as hydronephrosis and duplication anomalies, as well as monitoring of renal growth and the presence of parenchymal thinning; it does so without the need for sedation or anesthesia, and without ionizing radiation exposure.

Classification of UTI has been complicated by the number of prior systems that have been used. Classification by site of infection prompts designation as cystitis (bladder infection) or pyelonephritis (kidney infection). Unfortunately, clinical symptoms alone do not always accurately differentiate upper from lower tract UTI. Previous work using ureteral catheterization to localize the site of infection demonstrated upper tract bacteria in less than 50% of those with fever and flank pain, but in 20% of asymptomatic patients.[9] Infections can also be designated as uncomplicated versus complicated, or initial versus recurrent.

Recurrent UTI may be further categorized as unresolved bacteriuria, bacterial persistence, or reinfection. *Unresolved bacteriuria* results from inadequate treatment of a known pathogen. *Persistence* implies appropriate treatment of the UTI, but persistence of the infecting organism within a nidus of infection or within an area that is isolated from treatment. On immediate posttreatment urine culture the same bacterial pathogen will quickly return. *Reinfection* requires repeated UTI with different bacteria, which may include different bacterial serotypes and clones. The importance of differentiating between persistence and reinfection is that persistence may be surgically correctable.

TREATMENT OF UTI

Treatment of UTI focuses on the site of infection, presence of fever, and the pathogen causing the infection. Ampicillin and gentamicin continue to be the mainstay of empirical treatment of pyelonephritis. The use of a third-generation cephalosporin may be considered with the knowledge that its coverage will not include *Enterococcus* and that there is emerging extended-spectrum β-lactam resistance. When a patient has recently been on antibiotics, it is worthwhile to consider using alternative choices due to the possibility of resistant bacteria. Once afebrile for 24 to 48 hours, consideration can be given to transitioning to oral (PO) antibiotics. Improvement in serum markers such as the white blood cell count or C-reactive protein is also encouraging when considering transition to oral antibiotics. The use of longer duration of intravenous (IV) antibiotics has not been shown to be superior to an early transition to PO therapy in preventing scarring based on DMSA scans at 9 months.[10] In all cases, the combination of IV and oral therapy should include 10 to 14 days of appropriate antibiotics, with neonates and more severe infections favoring the longer duration.

Although traditional teaching has been that febrile UTI should be treated promptly with IV antibiotics in an inpatient setting to avoid renal scarring, recent data have brought this teaching into question. In a study by Hewitt and colleagues[11] from Italy, the frequency of renal scarring on DMSA scan at 1 year was similar (approximately 30%) in those treated early in a comparison with treatment by a delayed fashion. Nonetheless, treatment should be started as soon as possible to relieve symptoms and with the hope of avoiding renal scarring. Even with upper tract involvement, outpatient treatment of UTI has been shown to be safe and effective, particularly in older children who are tolerating oral intake and are clinically stable.[12,13] In these cases, outpatient treatment with trimethoprim/sulfamethoxazole (TMP/SMX), cephalosporins, or fluoroquinolones are viable options. Nitrofurantoin is inadequate when renal involvement is suspected as a result of poor tissue levels. In addition, daily intramuscular (IM) injection of a once-a-day broad-spectrum antibiotic (such as ceftriaxone) is an option. This treatment should be continued either until identification/sensitivities can direct oral therapy, or for the entire outpatient course when more convenient than parenteral antibiotics using a peripherally inserted central catheter. A conservative approach of hospital admission for IV antibiotics is justified when the clinical picture, social scenario, or patient age (particularly neonates) dictates. In these cases, IV rehydration and broad-spectrum antibiotics are administered.

Cystitis in children can safely be treated using nitrofurantoin, sulfonamides, TMP/SMX, trimethoprim alone, and cephalosporins. In addition, ciprofloxacin is also used in children, for whom it is approved as a second-line therapy in complicated UTI.[14] Use of ciprofloxacin in children is reserved for more serious cases due to concerns over potential cartilage damage. Fortunately, in studies of children who received ciprofloxacin, complications have been reversible after discontinuation.[15] Most often, TMP/SMX or nitrofurantoin is a good initial therapy for uncomplicated cystitis until final urine culture and sensitivities have returned. Regional resistance to TMP/SMX is known, and this should be taken into account in the decision to use TMP/SMX as initial therapy. Once final sensitivities are reported, treatment should be adjusted to ensure appropriate antibiotic coverage of the infecting organism. The addition of an IM antibiotic dosage has not been shown to be of significant benefit in febrile UTI[16] and its usage in cystitis is likely not warranted. Duration of treatment is largely age based in this population. A 3-day course is adequate in the clinically stable child with uncomplicated cystitis,[17] while longer treatment courses (7–10 days) are likely appropriate for children younger than 2 years. Although a recent study from Canada has shown feasibility of outpatient ambulatory treatment with parenteral antibiotics in 1- to 3-month old children with febrile UTI,[18] the very young and those who are dehydrated, unable to tolerate oral medications, or toxic appearing warrant a conservative approach with admission for parenteral antibiotics and hydration.

WHEN TO WORRY LESS

It is important for clinicians to be familiar with situations in which there is a relatively low risk for patients. These scenarios can be perplexing for parents and primary care physicians who do not encounter such urologic scenarios on a consistent basis. For example, urine cultures growing *Lactobacillus* species, coagulase-negative staphylococci, and *Corynebacterium* species are not considered pathogens in otherwise healthy children of 2 months to 2 years old, and treatment is unnecessary.[19]

During the period of toilet-training, children are at an increased risk of lower UTI because of changes in voiding and stooling habits. Less than optimal hygiene, in combination with the newly developed ability to hold one's urine, can lead to UTIs. While still warranting treatment, these infections may be more related to functional changes. In the case of an isolated UTI during toilet-training, establishing good voiding and stooling habits is the primary goal after initial treatment of the UTI.

The presence of a UTI in the setting of corrected or spontaneously resolved reflux can cause significant anxiety for parents and primary care physicians, while not posing as great a risk as perceived. After the initial diagnosis of vesicoureteral reflux (VUR), parents often become conditioned to associate UTI and the risk of damage to the kidneys. The correction of VUR does not decrease the risk of a child developing a lower UTI but only eliminates the reflux of infected urine into the kidney, thereby preventing or delaying the development of upper UTI. It is important to ensure that parents understand the purpose of VUR correction, are informed that VUR correction does not alter host susceptibility to UTI, and are counseled to seek appropriate treatment for UTI.

Finally, a clinical scenario that is challenging to understand is asymptomatic bacteriuria. Clinical situations exist in which colonization of the urinary tract is inevitable. In these situations, the presence of bacteria is normal and does not require treatment despite a positive urine culture. Examples of scenarios in which the urinary tract can be expected to be colonized are patients with long-term indwelling tubes, patients performing clean intermittent catheterization (CIC), patients with intestinal neobladders or augmented bladders, and patients in whom the urinary tract is opened to the skin (vesicostomy, ureterostomy, and so forth). In these cases, routine bacteria cultured from the urinary tract and not causing significant clinical symptoms (dysuria, incontinence, fever, and so forth) should not be treated. One should also favor observation for bacteria noted on a screening urinalysis performed in an asymptomatic patient without complicating factors. Treatment of these asymptomatic bacteria will only allow recolonization with different, potentially more pathogenic bacteria and increase the risk of antibiotic resistance. Fever in a setting of asymptomatic bacteriuria should be worked up as a fever of unknown origin, including urine culture and blood cultures, with treatment as a UTI reserved for cases in which another source is not identified. Pyuria on a concurrent urine analysis can aid in confirming the diagnosis of clinical UTI. While the aforementioned situations are examples of times when excessive concern is not warranted, one should always use common sense when approaching these issues. When additional symptoms, repeated infections, or a confusing clinical scenario presents, further investigation and an increased clinical index of suspicion for the presence of more serious urologic issues is always reasonable.

WHEN TO WORRY

The authors now focus attention on situations in which UTI is more complicated, often requiring a high index of clinical suspicion and a low threshold to proceed to admission, broad-spectrum antibiotics, further investigation, and pediatric urology consultation. Attempts have been made to sort these infrequent scenarios into more generalized groups; however, many pathologic processes could be placed under multiple headings. The rare nature of very complicated UTI makes research comparing different approaches to treatment difficult. Prospective placebo-controlled studies do not exist. In these complex cases, there are undoubtedly multiple effective ways to approach treatment. When the literature does not provide clear evidence supporting one approach, information is provided on the clinical pathway followed by the authors for managing these difficult situations.

Some general principles apply in these complex clinical scenarios. The presence of abnormal anatomy, particularly abnormal drainage, should always prompt additional workup in the presence of UTI. The presence of prior renal scarring should also prompt additional concern, as these patients are starting with fewer functioning nephrons and have established they are susceptible to renal injury. Failure of a patient to respond to conventional treatment of a UTI should also prompt concern. Additional workup should be performed to confirm that culture-specific antibiotics are being used, that adequate drainage exists, and that the antibiotics reach all sites of bacterial infection.

Bad Pathology

While a single febrile UTI is a cause for concern, the presence of repeated febrile infections should alert all physicians to the need for a more extensive evaluation. One must be concerned about the presence of a physiologic or anatomic patient factor as the origin. While most renal scarring is felt to occur with the first episode of pyelonephritis, the "big bang theory,"[1] recurrent pyelonephritis can cause increased renal scarring. A comprehensive workup, with special focus on voiding and bowel habits, family history of recurrent UTI, and activities preceding the infections, should be undertaken. Urine culture results should be reviewed to assess for evidence of bacterial persistence. If true persistence exists, further imaging should be performed to evaluate for a source of the bacteria. Renal bladder ultrasonography and voiding cystourethrography will allow one to quickly assess the upper and lower tract anatomy while minimizing radiation exposure. Additional imaging may be required based on the clinical situation. In a toilet-trained child, a urinary flow rate and postvoid residual should be obtained to assess bladder emptying. Consideration should be given to antibiotic prophylaxis.

Pyonephrosis and emphysematous pyelonephritis are 2 severe infections of the kidney. Pyonephrosis is the presence of purulence and sediment within the renal collecting system. Presenting with a picture similar to pyelonephritis, these patients may not have resolution with antibiotics alone because of the presence of obstruction. In children most pyonephrotic kidneys are nonfunctional or have very poor function.[20] Treatment always involves broad-spectrum antibiotics and frequently drainage of the collecting system, either via retrograde stent or nephrostomy tube placement. Emphysematous pyelonephritis is an infection with air seen in the collecting system on imaging. This entity is extremely rare in children. Percutaneous drainage and antibiotics should be considered first-line therapy. Nephrectomy, which was previously considered the treatment of choice, should be reserved for those who do not respond to conservative management.

Renal abscesses (**Fig. 2**) have become relatively rare in the pediatric population since the advent of modern antimicrobial drugs. These infections may develop via ascending infection, in which case the offending organism will be those seen in UTI (*E coli* and so forth) or via hematogenous spread, in which case staphylococcal infection is more common. Focal bacterial nephritis (acute lobar nephronia) is an acute form of bacterial nephritis affecting 1 or more renal lobules, with some series demonstrating up to 25% progression to abscess.[21] Symptoms associated with abscesses are often those of severe pyelonephritis. Abscesses of 3 cm or less respond well to conservative management with antibiotics and observation in patients with normal urinary tracts and immune systems.[22] Surgical drainage of the kidney was historically the gold standard of care; however, more recently percutaneous drainage using computed tomography (CT) or ultrasound guidance has been found to be effective. In either situation sampling of the abscess fluid with aerobic, anaerobic, and fungal cultures should be performed to assist in care. A single percutaneous drainage procedure may be adequate with smaller abscesses, whereas very large abscesses may warrant placement of a drain to both avoid reaccumulation and facilitate antibiotic penetration. Broad-spectrum antibiotics should be employed, initially guided by urine or blood culture results, then by culture of the abscess fluid. When a urinary tract source is suspected, ampicillin and gentamicin remain good first options, whereas an extended spectrum penicillin or cephalosporin is a good first choice when a hematogenous source is suspected. Follow-up imaging to confirm resolution of the abscess should be obtained.

Xanthogranulomatous pyelonephritis (XGP) is a grave renal infection resulting from chronic

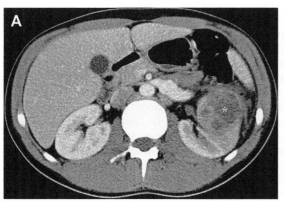 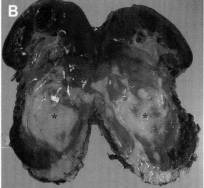

Fig. 2. Renal abscess. (*A*) Note heterogeneous appearing abscess (*asterisk*) in the left kidney on this CT scan with contrast. (*B*) Gross pathology of the left kidney, including the necrotic area of kidney as a result of the abscess (*asterisk*).

bacterial pyelonephritis and obstruction. XGP is named after the xanthoma cell, a foamy lipid-laden histiocyte that is seen on histology in this infection. Although primarily a condition that affects adults, XGP is occasionally seen in children, most often males younger than 8 years. It is most often unilateral, causing significant destruction to a kidney. XGP may lead to a total loss of renal function on the affected side, although it is often focal within the kidney in children.[23] The most common causative organisms are *Proteus mirabilis* and *E coli*. Radiographic imaging is notable for the presence of obstruction, most often due to a calculus. The XGP kidney classically has been described as having an appearance on CT scan similar to a "bear paw" as a result of dilated calyces and abscesses. Pediatric patients with XGP have clinical symptoms ranging from vague complaints to hemodynamic instability and sepsis. In a stable patient with evidence of XGP, drainage of the collecting system, via stent or nephrostomy tube, may allow for true assessment of residual renal function. Placement of additional drains may be needed if nonoperative management is considered safe and desirable. Unfortunately, surgical intervention is required in the majority of cases, often with the need for total nephrectomy. In rare circumstances a partial nephrectomy may be effective.

Bad Anatomy

The presence of anatomically or functionally abnormal segments of the urinary tract can lead to rapid clinical deterioration when a patient develops a UTI. Renal insufficiency is one example of a functional issue. Impairment in renal function, as indicated by an elevated serum creatinine, limits the bioavailability of the antibiotics, making careful monitoring of serum levels necessary. For example, the potentially nephrotoxic antibiotics gentamicin and vancomycin require close management to minimize the risk of renal injury. Imaging options in patients with compromised renal function may also be impacted. IV contrast for CT scans and fluoroscopic examinations can be nephrotoxic, particularly for those with renal insufficiency. Gadolinium, which is used as contrast for MRI, may cause nephrogenic systemic fibrosis when used in patients with an estimated glomerular filtration rate less than 30 mL/min/1.73 m^2.[24] These limitations may cause difficulties in diagnosing more complicated urinary pathology in this patient population. Another situation in which renal function should prompt heightened concern is the solitary kidney. When a patient with a known solitary kidney presents with a febrile

UTI, their clinical condition should be carefully evaluated to ensure appropriate antibiotics and adequate renal drainage.

The presence of poorly functioning and nonfunctional renal segments should prompt additional concern when treating pyelonephritis, as these areas can pose problems caused by poor antibiotic penetration. Examples of UTI in such segments include infection of a dysplastic upper pole moiety in a duplicated system or infection of a devascularized segment of kidney after renal trauma. In these cases, antibiotic administration may be ineffective and facilitating drainage, via ureteral stenting or percutaneous decompression, should be considered. Surgical excision of such segments may also be necessary.

The topic of vesicoureteral reflux (VUR) will be thoroughly addressed elsewhere in this issue. UTI in the setting of VUR can be a cause of significant concern. Previous studies have established that VUR without infection poses little risk for renal scarring or damage.[1] When accompanied by infection, however, VUR can lead to pyelonephritis and subsequent renal scarring, with the potential for reflux nephropathy in severe cases. Primary management of VUR is a subject of much debate, particularly the role of antibiotic prophylaxis. In a patient on antibiotic prophylaxis, development of one or more breakthrough infections is concerning. Assessment of compliance with antibiotic prophylaxis and confirmation of appropriate antibiotic dosing should be performed. Recent studies have shown compliance with continual antibiotic prophylaxis to be only 40%.[25] The patient's social situation should be assessed to ensure that medical care is sought in a timely fashion when UTI symptoms are present. Renal imaging for assessment of renal growth and new scarring should be undertaken. In these situations it may be necessary to consider the options for surgical correction of reflux.

Neuropathic bladder is another scenario in which anatomic and functional concerns can lead to serious consequences in the case of UTI. Inadequate bladder emptying, high-pressure storing of urine, and high-pressure voiding can complicate the management of UTI. When accompanying neurologic issues exist (such as myelomeningocele or spina bifida) or in patients who have undergone bladder reconstruction, the clinical symptoms may be masked. Symptoms may not be present until an infection is severe or septic shock imminent. A high degree of suspicion is necessary in these patients, with a low threshold for imaging of the upper tracts and evaluation of the bladder. High-pressure storage can lead to a trabeculated bladder and secondary VUR with resultant risk to the kidneys if UTI occurs. High-pressure voiding or detrusor-sphincter dyssyner-gia might lead to bladder diverticula and chemical or infectious epididymitis. Inadequate emptying places these patients at risk for bladder stones. Stones may be infectious or noninfectious in origin. Infectious stones are often a source of bacterial persistence that will not resolve until stone extraction is complete.

Patients in whom there is difficulty catheterizing the urethra provide another challenge in the setting of a UTI. Difficulty catheterizing can be due to the size of the patient or the patient's urethra (particu-larly in very premature, very low birth weight babies) or due to variations in urethral anatomy. When urethral issues occur that make routine catheterization difficult, options are more limited in the pediatric population than in adults. Pediatric coudé catheters of small sizes are often not readily available. Frequently these coudé catheters are made of latex. Caution should be observed in using these products in a population with a higher risk of latex allergy. Congenital anomalies such as an enlarged utricle (**Fig. 3**), urogenital sinus abnor-malities, and urethral valves might also make catheterization difficult. A history of complex hypospadias repair can make catheterization diffi-cult for even the most experienced pediatric urol-ogist. Flexible cystoscopy, which would normally be performed at the bedside in adults, is not as convenient or immediate an option in pediatric patients because of the need for general anes-thesia. When there is concern for UTI, a suprapubic aspirate may be necessary to obtain a urine sample. While providing a very reliable urine sample when correctly performed, repeated taps can be of a concern to parents and increase risks of complication. If continuous bladder drainage is required as part of therapy, consideration of a suprapubic tube or vesicostomy may be war-ranted. Prune belly syndrome (PBS) is another potential complicating factor in the treatment of a UTI. PBS is a congenital defect of the anterior abdominal wall musculature (**Fig. 4**A) associated with undescended testes and megacystis/mega-ureters (see **Fig. 4**B). In this case the urinary system, though not obstructed, has a degree of stagnation and impaired flow. Treatment of UTIs in these cases may be compromised by this poor drainage. Less commonly, PBS can be associated with urethral anomalies that include prostatic hypoplasia, urethral atresia, and other obstructive lesions.[26] These urethral anomalies may compli-cate catheterization. The decision to catheterize these patients requires expert care and sterile technique, as the possibility exists of seeding the stagnant urinary system with bacteria if not already infected. Once seeded, clearing infection can be more difficult in these cases.

Bad Drainage

Those patients in whom segmental urine drainage is persistently compromised are also at risk for increased severity of infection. Causes of obstruc-tion can be similar to those seen frequently in adults (stones, strictures, ureteropelvic junction [UPJ] obstruction, and mass effect) or those diagnosed infrequently in adults (ectopic ureter, ureterovesical junction obstruction, megaureter, ureterocele). Symptoms may be difficult to discern in younger children. Fever is often the first sign. Failure to defervesce or improve with appropriate antibiotics should prompt further investigation. This evaluation may lead to the initial diagnosis of segmental obstruction. In children with known

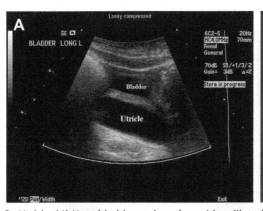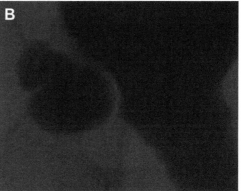

Fig. 3. Utricle. (*A*) Note bladder and urethra with a dilated, fluid-filled structure posteriorly on this bladder ultra-sonograph. Cystoscopy at the time of hypospadias repair confirmed the presence of a large utricle, which compli-cated catheterization. (*B*) Note the presence of a utricle during VCUG in a patient who is extremely difficult to catheterize.

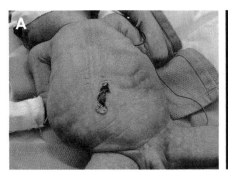
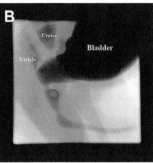

Fig. 4. Prune belly syndrome (PBS). (*A*) Note the lax abdominal wall musculature on physical examination in this patient with PBS. (*B*) VCUG displaying anterior displacement of the bladder and presence of small utricle, which may combine to make catheterization difficult. Also note vesicoureteral reflux with dilated, tortuous ureters.

impaired drainage, the presence of UTI should prompt early evaluation of the affected side(s) with appropriate imaging studies. In all cases of impaired urine drainage, partial or complete, the principles of management follow those in adults (drainage, cultures, and broad-spectrum antibiotics).

Renal stones are less common in children than adults, but may be increasing in frequency.[27] A single infection in the presence of nonobstructing stones requires only standard treatment of the UTI. Imaging to monitor for movement of the stone and careful instruction of the patient/parents regarding the signs and risks of obstruction should be part of the care plan. When obstructing stones (**Fig. 5**A) are present with infection, the principles of treatment parallel those in adults. Drainage is essential, with ureteral stenting (size and length appropriate for the pediatric patient) or percutaneous nephrostomy tube as options. Ureteral stenting will allow passive dilatation of the pediatric ureter and facilitate subsequent stone extraction via ureteroscopy (see **Fig. 5**B). Percutaneous nephrostomy tube placement will provide access to the kidney, and will be helpful if percutaneous nephrolithotomy is planned. The stability of the

patient, availability of staff, and coordination of scheduling are all factors that influence the choice of drainage modality.

UPJ obstruction (UPJO) is the impaired drainage of urine from the renal pelvis into the ureter. The most common causes of UPJO in children are a congenital aperistaltic segment of ureter and compression from a lower pole crossing blood vessel. UPJO is frequently seen in young children, a group particularly vulnerable because of their inability to communicate early signs of infection. Most UPJO are in the spectrum of partial obstruction, and therefore conservative management with careful IV hydration and antibiotics can be the first-line approach. In this situation, close clinical follow-up is essential. Monitoring temperature curves, white blood cell counts, C-reactive protein, and serial ultrasonography (**Fig. 6**) provides guidance in therapeutic decision making. When there is evidence of a deterioration of the patient's clinical condition, drainage via ureteral stent or nephrostomy tube should be performed. Placement of a ureteral stent can often be very challenging due to the small size of the patient, tortuosity of the ureter, and caliber of the ureteral lumen. Severe infections provide additional

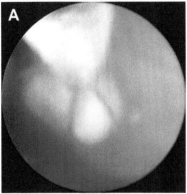
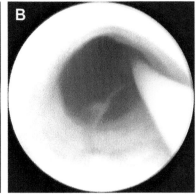

Fig. 5. Ureteral stone. (*A*) Note the impacted ureteral stone obstructing the entire lumen of the ureter as seen during ureteroscopy. (*B*) The stone has been removed endoscopically and the ureter is now patent.

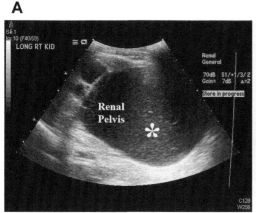
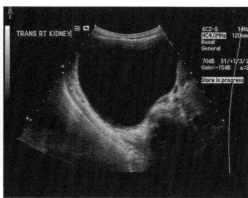

Fig. 6. UPJ obstruction. (*A*) Note the presence of a massively dilated renal pelvis in this patient with UPJ obstruction. This patient presented with a febrile UTI and was found to have significant sediment (*asterisk*) within the kidney. (*B*) When free of infection, the massively dilated pelvis shows no evidence of sediment on ultrasonograph.

evidence to support pyeloplasty once the patient is recovered from the infection. The presence of either a nephrostomy tube or indwelling ureteral stent is likely to cause reactive inflammation in the renal pelvis; however, their presence can be incorporated into the postoperative management strategy. Mid-ureteral obstruction, although rare, may also occur. Common causes are external compression due to mass, congenital strictures, and iatrogenic strictures in the setting of prior instrumentation. Management of infection in these clinical situations proceeds based on the principles described immediately above.

Ureterovesical junction obstruction, ectopic ureters, and ureteroceles are 3 common sources of distal ureteral obstruction that can pose a challenge when treating UTI. If drainage is needed in any of these situations, placement of a ureteral stent can be complicated or near impossible due to difficulty passing guide wires or stents in a retrograde fashion. The length and tortuosity of the obstructed ureter can also be a challenge to retrograde stent placement (**Fig. 7**). In these cases, drainage options include antegrade placement of a ureteral stent, simple nephrostomy tube placement, or placement of a nephroureteral stent. Ectopic ureters can provide an additional challenge for retrograde stenting, as the ureteral orifice often enters at or near the bladder neck, making cystoscopic identification difficult. When ectopic ureters do not insert into the bladder or urethra, locating the distal ureter for stent placement may not be possible. Percutaneous nephrostomy tube placement is preferred, to allow drainage as well as provide an option for subsequent antegrade imaging. Ureteroceles (**Fig. 8**) pose unique opportunities, as internal drainage

to the bladder may be accomplished by creation of a healthy cystoscopic incision into the ureterocele. The possibility of causing future reflux into the moiety associated with the ureterocele is likely in this situation.

Another special challenge of drainage occurs in situations in which urinary tract reconstruction has been performed. Whether through ureteral reimplantation or subtrigonal injection of implant material for VUR, ureterocalycostomy for UPJO,

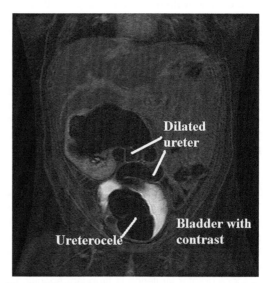

Fig. 7. Dilated, tortuous ureter due to ureterocele. Note the significant tortuosity and dilatation of the ureter to the upper pole of the right kidney in this MRI. The upper pole ureter of this duplicated system is also associated with a large ureterocele, which can be seen filling a large portion of the contrast-filled bladder.

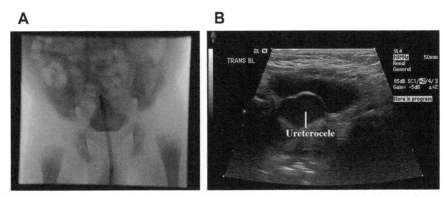

Fig. 8. (*A*) Note the appearance of a ureterocele on VCUG (*arrow*), seen early as the bladder was being filled with contrast. (*B*) Note the appearance of another ureterocele as seen on ultrasonograph of the bladder.

transverse ureteroureterostomy, or ureteropyelostomy for strictures, reconfiguration of the ureters can complicate attempts to drain the affected kidney(s) if obstruction occurs. Cross-trigonal reimplantation in the correction of VUR may cause difficulty in catheterizing the ureteral orifices. Use of flexible cystoscopes, angle-tipped wires, and percutaneous bladder access to provide the appropriate angle for intubating the ureteral orifice are techniques that may aid in stent placement. The presence of extensive bladder trabeculation in the setting of reconfigured ureters can further complicate attempts at internal stenting. This condition may be seen in patients with neuropathic bladders or severe dysfunctional elimination syndrome in whom ureteral reimplantation has been performed. The addition of intravenous indigo carmine or methylene blue may help in locating these ureteral orifices. Subtrigonal injection of dextranomer/hyaluronic acid (Deflux, Oceana Therapeutics, Inc, Edison, NJ, USA) may cause anxiety in the face of UTI by mimicking distal ureteral stones on CT scan.[28] In rare situations, subtrigonal injections have caused obstruction (<0.7%), but ureteral stenting can be accomplished in these settings.[29]

Bad/Rare Bugs

The infecting organism in any UTI plays a large role in how severe an infection becomes, through possession of virulence factors, resistance to antibiotics, and other mechanisms. The classic example of a mechanism through which bacteria possess greater virulence is fimbriae, specifically P-fimbriae. Fimbriae (or pili) are surface structures involved in adherence. P-piliated *E coli* possess fimbriae that bind the human red cell P-group antigen, leading to an increased risk of pyelonephritis. Another factor favoring more virulent bacteria is the presence of mannose-resistant

hemagglutination, which is found in most *E coli* that cause pyelonephritis.[30] Previous work has established that most bacteria causing pyelonephritis in children are associated with P-pili or mannose-resistant hemagglutination.[31] Additional mechanisms used by bacteria include hydrophobic properties and iron-binding capabilities. Additional proteins have been associated with *E coli* causing pyelonephritis; however, none are currently clinically relevant.

Development and usage of new antibiotics has brought about antibiotic resistance in bacteria. While resistance to penicillin remains the highest, in recent years resistance to TMP/SMX has been increasing.[32] In addition, frequent use of fluoroquinolones for a variety of infections has led to increased resistance to these antibiotics, which have high utility and good coverage in the urinary tract. Within pediatrics the issue of antibiotic resistance takes on greater importance because of the limited number of antibiotic options approved for use in children. The most common oral antibiotics used in pediatric urology remain amoxicillin, cephalexin, TMP/SMX, and nitrofurantoin. Antibiotic resistance to nitrofurantoin remains low, leading some to recommend it as first-line treatment for the uncomplicated afebrile UTI.[33] Unfortunately, its lack of tissue levels limits utility in more serious infection.

Examples of bacteria affecting the urinary tract with significant issues related to resistance include: methicillin-resistant *Staphylococcus aureus*, vancomycin-resistant *Enterococcus*, and extended-spectrum β-lactamase (ESBL) bacteria, particularly *E coli*. Increasingly found within hospitals and the community, ESBL bacteria pose significant problems due to the limitations in antibiotics that may be used to treat them. Extended-spectrum β-lactamase–producing enterobacteriae are able to inactivate β-lactam antibiotics via hydrolysis.[34] One study from Taiwan noted an increased risk of ESBL bacteria causing UTI in children on cephalexin prophylaxis.[35] Surveys from multiple countries have demonstrated coresistance to other antibiotics appearing within these bacteria, which has prompted the use of carbapenems as the first-line antibiotics in treating these infections.[34]

Atypical infecting organisms in the urinary tract can also cause infection. A complete discussion of these organisms is beyond the scope of this article. However, these atypical organisms may be more difficult to diagnose due to their slow growth and endemic regions, which may differ greatly from the area of diagnosis. In addition, these atypical organisms may possess antibiotic resistance, causing significant difficulty in treatment. One of the more common atypical causes of UTI is fungal infection. Fungal UTI is most often caused by *Candida albicans* and presents as a nosocomial infection affecting patients on antibiotics with indwelling catheters. In these situations, any indwelling catheter should be changed. Consideration should be given to urine alkalinization and starting antifungal therapy, with the knowledge that resistance to standard antifungals may be present.[36] Bladder irrigation with amphotericin B may be necessary in resistant cases. Upper tract fungal balls may require percutaneous removal followed by antifungal irrigation. *Aspergillosis* is a fungal infection most commonly seen in immunocompromised individuals, which may require amphotericin B irrigation. Other examples of atypical pathogens include tuberculosis, which can occur in the urinary tract leading to strictures; schistosomiasis, which is a parasite frequently leading to bladder fibrosis and an increased risk of bladder cancer; and enterobiasis, which has been implicated in chronic UTI.

Bad Genes/Immune System

Antibiotic use has led to a host of strong pathogens with variable patterns of resistance. Despite exposure to potent pathogens, the majority of people do not develop UTI, pointing to the importance of patient factors in the development of UTI. Unfortunately, this remains an area in which research has not seen significant advances with applicability in the clinical environment. The discovery of P-fimbriae as a virulence factor led to additional research on the P blood group and its role as a receptor. Studies have shown a high prevalence of P1 blood group in both refluxing and nonrefluxing girls with recurrent pyelonephritis. Other blood groups, such as ABO and Lewis, as well as secretor phenotypes may also influence UTI. Certain Lewis blood types (a−b−,

a+b−) have been found to have a 3-times greater risk of recurrent UTI than those with a−b+.[37] While providing a basis for recurrent UTI in some patients, these patient factors are not modifiable nor are they of significant utility in current clinical practice.

A variety of disease states and treatments can impair the immune system and can lead to an increased risk of infection and increased severity of infections that do occur. Examples include the very young (neonates), the immunosuppressed (due to transplants or chemotherapy), human immunodeficiency virus (HIV) patients, and diabetics. Neonates have a higher risk of infection because of an incompletely developed immune system and deficiency of IgA. This risk of infection can be minimized through breastfeeding, which is protective against infection, likely through maternal IgA.[38] These patients require a conservative approach, with a low threshold for admission for febrile UTI.

The prevalence of febrile UTI in transplant patients has ranged from 15% to 33% in studies.[39] Although *E coli* remains the most common bacteria, published series have demonstrated increased frequencies of other bacteria, including those with greater antibiotic resistance. Any infection in these patients causes concern due to immunosuppression and the risks to the transplant kidney. After treatment of the acute infection, consideration should be given to a complete evaluation of anatomic, functional, and social factors that might be contributing to infection. Patients on chemotherapy also represent an at-risk population due to their lowered immunity, frequent inpatient status, and increased likelihood of procedures. UTI in patients on chemotherapy should be treated aggressively with broad-spectrum antibiotics, keeping in mind the potential nephrotoxicity of chemotherapeutic and antibiotic agents. Upper tract imaging to rule out anatomic abnormalities or obstruction should be considered in these patients. Viral UTI is rare in immunocompetent individuals, but not uncommon in the immunocompromised patient. While potentially causing significant symptoms, such as hemorrhagic cystitis, these infections are self-limited and treatment is generally supportive in nature.

Patients with HIV are at increased risk of UTI from routine bacterial pathogens, particularly when CD4 counts fall below 500/mm[3].[40] HIV also increases the risk of UTI due to atypical pathogens such as fungi, parasites, mycobacteria, and viruses. Diabetes is known to increase the risk of UTI in adults and children, with more serious infections being more common in diabetics as well.[41] Because the prevalence of diabetes in children is increasing, the complications of this disease, including UTI, can be expected to increase as well.

Bad Social Situation

How severely a UTI affects a child can be significantly influenced by the social and family situation. Economic, language, racial, and cultural issues may prevent or delay families from seeking care. In these cases, once a patient has presented, careful consideration should be given to the potential risks and benefits of outpatient versus inpatient treatment. Whether a family can afford a prescribed medication, whether they will remember to administer the medication, and whether one considers them reliable should the patient's condition worsen are just 3 of the many factors that must be taken into account. When these questions are posed and uncertainty remains, it may be the safest course to admit the sick child for observation, in the hope of avoiding progression of the infection or loss of renal mass related to medical noncompliance.

Teenage pregnancy is rapidly becoming a social situation in which treatment of UTI can be very challenging. In these patients there can be significant risks due to UTI for both baby and mother. Although asymptomatic bacteriuria would normally not be treated, in pregnant women it increases the risk of symptomatic infection, preterm labor, and low birth weight.[42] As such, in pregnant women all bacteriuria should be treated. Women who have previously displayed an increased risk of infection or who have predisposing factors should be counseled regarding risks as they relate to pregnancy.

Nosocomial Infection

A final situation that warrants brief discussion is nosocomial infections. Nosocomial UTI is an infection acquired while in a hospital. A whole article could be written about the epidemiology, pathology, treatment, and implications of nosocomial UTI. These infections can be significant because they occur in a population that is already ill and often involve resistant bacteria. Financial challenges also exist, as Medicare has eliminated payment for nosocomial UTI treatment and any additional care that occurs as a result of these infections.[43] Basic principles underlie prevention of nosocomial UTI: appropriate hand washing and cleaning, appropriate care for indwelling tubes (including removal at the earliest medically appropriate time), and antibiotics when deemed necessary.

SUMMARY

UTI in children is a frequent cause of worry for parents and physicians. While many infections will not be severe in nature, one should always consider potential complicating factors that may exist in the pediatric population. When a UTI does not resolve routinely or when more complicated scenarios present, knowledge of these complicating factors can allow accurate diagnosis. Consideration should be given to the many approaches to treatment in developing a treatment plan for each individual patient.

REFERENCES

1. Shortliffe LD. Infection and inflammation of the pediatric genitourinary tract. In: Wein A, Kavoussi L, Novick A, et al, editors. Campbell-Walsh urology. 9th edition. Philadelphia: Saunders Elsevier; 2007. p. 3232–68.
2. Foxman B. Epidemiology of urinary tract infections: incidence, morbidity, and economic costs. Am J Med 2002;113(1A):5S–13S.
3. Shaw KN, Gorelick M. Prevalence of urinary tract infection in febrile young children in the emergency department. Pediatrics 1998;102(2):E16.
4. Barkemeyer B. Suprapubic aspiration of urine in very low birth weight infants. Pediatrics 1994;92: 457–9.
5. Hansson S, Dhamey M, Sigström O, et al. Dimercapto-succinic acid scintigraphy instead of voiding cystourethrography for infants with urinary tract infection. J Urol 2004;172:1071–4.
6. Majd M, Nussbaum Blask AR, Markle BM, et al. Acute pyelonephritis: comparison of diagnosis with 99mTc-DMSA, SPECT, spiral CT, MR imaging in an experimental pig model. Radiology 2001;218:101–8.
7. Kavanagh E, Ryan S, Awan A, et al. Can MRI replace DMSA in the detection of renal parenchymal defects in children with urinary tract infections? Pediatr Radiol 2005;35:275–81.
8. Sinha M, Gibson P, Kane T, et al. Accuracy of ultrasonic detection of renal scarring in different centres using DMSA as the gold standard. Nephrol Dial Transplant 2007;22:2213–6.
9. Busch R, Huland H. Correlation of symptoms and results of direct bacterial localization in patients with urinary tract infections. J Urol 1984;132:282–5.
10. Bouissou F, Munzer C, Decramer S, et al. Prospective, randomized trial comparing short and long term intravenous antibiotic treatment of acute pyelonephritis in children: dimercaptosuccinic acid scintigraphic evaluation at 9 months. Pediatrics 2009;121: e553–60.
11. Hewitt I, Zuccheta P, Rigon L, et al. Early treatment of acute pyelonephritis in children fails to reduce

renal scarring: data from the Italian renal infection study trials. Pediatrics 2008;122:486–90.

12. Hoberman A, Wald ER, Hickey RW, et al. Oral versus initial intravenous therapy for urinary tract infections in young febrile children. Pediatrics 1999;104: 79–86.

13. Montini G, Toffolo A, Zucchetta P, et al. Antibiotic treatment for pyelonephritis in children: multicentre randomised controlled non-inferiority trial. BMJ 2007;335:386–92.

14. American Academy of Pediatrics: Committee on Infectious Diseases. The use of systemic fluoroquinolones. Pediatrics 2006;118:1287–92.

15. Grady R. Safety profile of quinolone antibiotics in the pediatric population. Pediatr Infect Dis J 2003; 22(12):1128–32.

16. Baker PC, Nelson DS, Schunk JE. The addition of ceftriaxone to oral therapy does not improve outcomes in febrile children with urinary tract infections. Arch Pediatr Adolesc Med 2001;155(2):135–9.

17. Michael M, Hodson EM, Craig JC, et al. Short versus standard duration oral antibiotic therapy for acute UTI in children. Cochrane Database Syst Rev 2003;(1):CD003966.

18. Doré-Bergeron MJ, Gauthier M, Chevalier I, et al. Urinary tract infections in 1- to 3-month-old infants: ambulatory treatment with intravenous antibiotics. Pediatrics 2009;124:16–22.

19. American Academy of Pediatrics: Committee on Quality Improvement. The diagnosis, treatment, and evaluation of the initial urinary tract infection in febrile infants and young children. Pediatrics 1999; 103(4 Pt 1):843–52.

20. Coleman BG, Arger PH, Mulhern CB. Pyonephrosis: sonography in the diagnosis and management. Am J Roentgenol 1987;137:939–43.

21. Klar A, Hurvitz H, Berkun Y. Focal bacterial nephritis in children. J Pediatr 1996;128(6):850–3.

22. Schaeffer A, Schaeffer E. Infections of the urinary tract. In: Wein A, Kavoussi L, Novick A, et al, editors. Campbell-Walsh urology. 9th edition. Philadelphia: Saunders Elsevier; 2007. p. 223–303.

23. Brown P, Dodson M, Weintrub P. Xanthogranulomatous pyelonephritis: report of nonsurgical management of a case and review of the literature. Clin Infect Dis 1996;22(2):308–14.

24. Prince M, Zhang H, Prowda J, et al. Nephrogenic systemic fibrosis and its impact on abdominal imaging. RadioGraphics 2009;29:1565–74.

25. Copp H, Nelson CP, Shortliffe LD, et al. Compliance with antibiotic prophylaxis in children with vesicoureteral reflux: results from a national pharmacy claims database. J Urol. [Epub ahead of print].

26. Caldamone A, Woodard J. Prune belly syndrome. In: Wein A, Kavoussi L, Novick A, et al, editors. Campbell-Walsh urology. 9th edition. Philadelphia: Saunders Elsevier; 2007. p. 3482–96.

27. VanDervoort K, Wiesen J, Frank R, et al. Urolithiasis in pediatric patients: a single center study of incidence, clinical presentation and outcome. J Urol 2007;177(6):2300–5.

28. Nelson CP, Chow JS. Dextranomer/hyaluronic acid copolymer (Deflux) implants mimicking distal ureteral calculi on CT. Pediatr Radiol 2008;38(1):104–6.

29. Vandersteen DR, Routh JC, Kirsch AJ, et al. Postoperative ureteral obstruction after subureteral injection of dextranomer/hyaluronic acid copolymer. J Urol 2006;176(4):1593–5.

30. Källenius G, Möllby R, Svenson SB, et al. Occurrence of P-fimbriated Escherichia coli in urinary tract infections. Lancet 1981;2:1369–72.

31. Väisänen V, Elo J, Tallgren LG, et al. Mannose-resistant haemagglutination and P antigen recognition are characteristic of Escherichia coli causing primary pyelonephritis. Lancet 1981;2:1366–9.

32. Gupta K, Scholes D, Stamm WE, et al. Increasing prevalence of antimicrobial resistance among uropathogens causing acute uncomplicated cystitis in women. JAMA 1999;281(8):736–8.

33. Kashanian J, Hakimian P, Blute M Jr, et al. Nitrofurantoin: the return of an old friend in the wake of growing resistance. BJU Int 2008;103(7):994–5.

34. Pitout J, Laupland K. Extended spectrum β-lactamase-producing Enterobacteriaceae: an emerging public-health concern. Lancet Infect Dis 2008;8: 159–66.

35. Cheng CH, Tsai MH, Huang YC, et al. Antibiotic resistance patterns of community-acquired urinary tract infections in children with vesicoureteral reflux receiving prophylactic antibiotic therapy. Pediatrics 2008;122:1212–7.

36. Kauffman CA, Vazquez JA, Sobel JD, et al. Prospective multicenter surveillance study of funguria in hospitalized patients. Clin Infect Dis 2000;30(1):14–8.

37. Sheinfeld J, Cordon-Cardo C, Fair WR, et al. Association of type 1 blood group antigens (BGA) with urinary tract infections in children with genitourinary structural abnormalities. J Urol 1990;143:189A.

38. Pisacane A, Graziano L, Mazzarella G, et al. Breast-feeding and urinary tract infection. J Pediatr 1992; 120(1):87–9.

39. John U, Kemper MJ. Urinary tract infections in children after renal transplantation. Pediatr Nephrol 2009;24:1129–36.

40. Lebovitch S, Mydlo J. HIV-AIDS—urologic considerations. Urol Clin North Am 2008;35:59–68.

41. Stapleton A. Urinary tract infections in patients with diabetes. Am J Med 2002;113(1A):80S–4S.

42. Sheiner E, Mazor-Drey E, Levy A. Asymptomatic bacteriuria during pregnancy. J Matern Fetal Neonatal Med 2009;22(5):423–7.

43. Wald H, Kramer A. Non-payment for harms resulting from medical care. Catheter-associated urinary tract infections. JAMA 2007;298(23):2782–4.

Vesicoureteral Reflux: Who Benefits from Correction

J. Christopher Austin, MD[a],*, Christopher S. Cooper, MD[b]

KEYWORDS

- Vesicoureteral reflux • Dimercaptosuccinic acid
- Urinary tract infections • Pyelonephritis

There has been an emergence of a therapeutic nihilistic attitude about the surgical treatment of vesicoureteral reflux (VUR). Evidence-based reviews have questioned whether surgical treatment is beneficial for children with VUR.[1,2] Even the use of prophylactic antibiotics, which have traditionally been the first-line therapy recommended for virtually all patients with VUR, has come under scrutiny after several randomized controlled trials found them to have no effect on decreasing the risk of urinary tract infections (UTIs) in children with VUR.[3–5] This issue is now the primary focus of the current randomized, double-blinded, placebo-controlled trial in children with VUR and UTIs in the United States—the RIVUR trial.[6] This nihilistic pattern challenges the effort that was put forth decades ago to evaluate children with UTIs for anatomic abnormalities, primarily VUR. Now more than ever, urologists treating VUR face a difficult decision process in deciding which patients should be followed conservatively and which should be offered operative correction. Factors influencing this decision include the risk of developing a UTI, and associated risk factors for UTIs such as voiding dysfunction, risk of development of new renal scars, and chance for spontaneous resolution. It is through consideration of these factors for each individual patient that the urologist tries to optimize the selection of patients who will benefit most from operative therapy. This review explores the important questions that guide the determination of who benefits from surgical treatment. The first question to be answered is, what does surgical correction of VUR do for patients?

BENEFITS OF SURGICAL TREATMENT OF VUR

In the 1990s, the first American Urological Association (AUA) panel to develop guidelines for the treatment of VUR was convened, and their summary statement was published in 1997.[7] This meta-analysis of multiple prior treatment options gave recommendations for the treatment of boys and girls with primary VUR from birth through age 10 years. The panel stratified their recommendations based on whether or not renal scarring was present. Surgical treatment was recommended for patients initially older than 1 year with grade V or bilateral grades III and IV if renal scarring was present. No consensus was reached as to what to do at the opposite end of the spectrum, such as those with persistent grades I to II VUR without renal scarring.

Surgical correction of VUR can be accomplished either by ureteral reimplantation or by endoscopically injecting a bulking agent at the ureterovesical junction. The success rates for ureteral reimplantation is routinely reported to be greater than 95% for grades I to IV, with slightly lower success rates for grade V.[8–11] Endoscopic treatment is a less successful but shorter outpatient procedure with minimal morbidity. Published success rates have been reported to be more

[a] Division of Pediatric Urology, Oregon Health and Sciences University, 3181 Southwest Sam Jackson Park Road, Portland, OR 97239, USA
[b] Department of Urology, Division of Pediatric Urology, University of Iowa, 200 Hawkins Drive, 3 RCP, Iowa City, IA 52242-1089, USA
* Corresponding author.
E-mail address: austin@ohsu.edu

Urol Clin N Am 37 (2010) 243–252
doi:10.1016/j.ucl.2010.03.012

than 90%,[12] but a recent meta-analysis probably gives a more realistic estimate. A single injection is successful for 67% of patients, and with a second injection the aggregate success rate increases to 87% of patients.[13] There is a significantly lower success rate for a third injection (34%); thus, after a second attempt at endoscopic injection, failures should be treated by other means. There is no debate that reflux can be corrected with surgery. More important are the benefits children may receive by no longer having VUR.

Only a few randomized studies compare observation on prophylactic antibiotics with surgical correction.[14–18] The largest study was the International Reflux Study. A summary of randomized studies of surgical correction of VUR is shown in **Table 1**. The main benefit demonstrated in these studies is that children are significantly less likely to develop pyelonephritis after surgical correction of VUR.[1] In the International Reflux Study, the overall rates of UTIs in the medical and surgical arm at 5 years were about 30%.[15] In the United States, the rate of pyelonephritis was 8% for the patients treated surgically versus 21% in those treated medically. In addition, only 10% of the medically treated patients had resolution of VUR at 5 years and only 47% at 10 years, whereas virtually all of the surgically treated patients were free of VUR.[19] Renal growth, the incidence of new renal scars, rates of hypertension, and progression to renal failure do not seem to be altered by surgical

treatment.[17,20–22] Although the benefits of surgical correction of VUR have not been what was initially hoped, the surgical treatment of VUR has a low complication rate, high success rate, and has not been harmful to renal function. There has been only one randomized study of patients treated endoscopically, which examined primarily rates of VUR present at 1 year after treatment.[18] In this study, 61 patients were randomized with 40 undergoing endoscopic treatment with dextranomer/hyaluronic acid (Dx/Ha). After 12 months, VUR was present in 62% of the medically treated patients and 31% of the patients treated endoscopically. UTIs were reported in 9 (22%) surgical patients and in none of the patients on prophylaxis; however, the details of the UTIs (pyelonephritis, cystitis, or asymptomatic bacteriuria) were not given. A meta-analysis of studies of endoscopic treatment shows a lower incidence of febrile UTIs after treatment.[13] Considering what is known about the benefits of surgical correction of VUR, the focus should be on selecting patients for treatment by identifying those at risk for recurrent pyelonephritis and those in whom VUR will not spontaneously resolve.

URETERAL REIMPLANTATION VERSUS ENDOSCOPIC INJECTION

The controversial topic of whether VUR should be treated with ureteral reimplantation or endoscopic

Table 1
Randomized controlled trials of surgical versus medical therapy for VUR

Study	Description	Summary of Results
Birmingham Reflux Study[14]	Randomized controlled trial (RCT) of severe VUR. Antibiotic prophylaxis vs ureteral reimplantation	No difference in rates of UTI, renal growth, new or progressive scarring after 5 years
International Reflux Study (Europe, United States)[5,16]	RCT of children age <11 y with grade III or IV VUR. Antibiotic prophylaxis vs ureteral reimplantation	No difference in overall rate of UTI or new scar formation at 5 years. Significantly lower rate of pyelonephritis in the surgical group
Smellie et al[17]	RCT of children age 1–12 years with bilateral grades III–V VUR with bilateral scarring. Antibiotic prophylaxis vs ureteral reimplantation	At 4 and 10 years no difference in renal function, rates of hypertension or renal failure, or renal growth in patients treated medically vs ureteral reimplantation
Capozza and Caione[18]	RCT of children age >1 year with grades II–IV VUR. Antibiotic prophylaxis vs endoscopic injection of Dx/Ha	More UTIs in the Dx/Ha-treated group. Reflux was resolved in 69% of the Dx/Ha-treated vs 38% treated with prophylactic antibiotics at 1 y

injection is one fueled with many divergent opinions and treatment philosophies. While the AUA Reflux Guidelines did not recommend endoscopic therapy as a surgical option, this was due to a lack of availability of a United States Food and Drug Administration approved agent[7] Since 2001, dextranomer/hyaluronic acid copolymer (Dx/Ha) (Deflux, Oceana Therapeutics, Edison, NJ) has been available in the United States. The guidelines are currently being revised and will likely include endoscopic injection as an option for surgical treatment. The choice of technique is one that needs to be individualized to the patient. Open ureteral reimplantation has a long track record of efficacy for all grades of VUR. Endoscopic correction success has been shown to be grade dependent, with most studies suggesting it is more effective for lower grades. **Table 2** shows the efficacies for a single injection based on grade of VUR.[13] There are few long-term studies of patients with endoscopic treatment. Recurrence of VUR seems to be partially dependent on the properties of the agent used. Long-term recurrence of VUR for bovine glutaraldehyde crosslike collagen was 87% at 3 years[23] versus a recurrence rate of 13% at a median of 3 years for Dx/Ha.[24] Most studies of endoscopic treatment of VUR report the success rate at 6 to 12 weeks. In 1 series of 246 ureters successfully treated endoscopically with Dx/Ha that were retested at 12 months, 27% showed recurrent VUR.[25] Most of those that recurred at 1 year were higher grades (III–V) of VUR. The only long-term follow-up study beyond 5 years was in patients treated with polytetrafluoroethylene. In this series there was a 5% recurrence at 10 years.[26] Studies have reported that febrile UTIs after successful endoscopic treatment with Dx/Ha is a predictor of recurrent VUR.[27,28] There is no consensus on which patients should undergo ureteral reimplantation or endoscopic

injection. One should consider the efficacy based on the individual's grade of VUR, age, infection history, and renal function. There have been no studies evaluating the risk of new scars in patients who have recurrent VUR and pyelonephritis after endoscopic therapy.

PYELONEPHRITIS IN PATIENTS WITH VUR

If the main benefit of treating VUR is the prevention of pyelonephritis and its associated sequelae, then the main focus in selecting patients for surgical correction of VUR should be those who present with recurrent pyelonephritis and those who are at greatest risk for recurrent pyelonephritis after diagnosis. Although the former can be selected at presentation after appropriate evaluation, it is difficult to predict which children will constitute the 10% to 20% of patients who will have a subsequent UTI per year. The presence of renal scarring, as detected on a dimercaptosuccinic acid (DMSA) renal scan, has been proposed as a way of identifying these patients. Patients with VUR and an abnormal renal scan have, in a retrospective series, been shown to have much higher likelihood of having a breakthrough infection if they also had dilating (grades III through V) VUR.[29] The incidence of breakthrough infections was 60% in those with an abnormal DMSA renal scan, versus only 6% of those with a normal DMSA scan. In addition, patients with an abnormal DMSA renal scan (renal scarring) in general have a lower likelihood of spontaneous resolution of VUR.[30,31] Whether the scarring is directly involved in this increased risk or is simply a marker of a worse anatomic defect at the ureterovesical junction is unknown. There have been limited studies of DMSA scans in lower grades of VUR; thus, whether scarring is as important in these grades is unknown.

VUR is typically present in less than 50% of patients who have acute pyelonephritis. In a meta-analysis of studies evaluating postpyelonephritic scarring, the incidence of permanent scarring in patients with an initial DMSA scan showing pyelonephritis was 41%.[32] There may be some geographic variations, with differing rates from 25% to 49% across the world. Renal scarring was strongly associated with VUR in patients after acute pyelonephritis. Renal scarring after acute pyelonephritis is a rare finding in patients without VUR. In the International Reflux Study, the risk of new renal scarring was low in children after the age of 6 years.[20] This finding is being challenged by reports of children with acute pyelonephritis presenting at all ages, showing that the risk of developing renal scars is present even at older ages.[33–36] Surprisingly, the risk was not increased

Table 2 Percentage of ureters with VUR resolved following a single endoscopic injection for VUR grades I to IV	
Grade of VUR	**% Success (Ureters)**
I	79%
II	79%
III	72%
IV	62%

Data from Elder JS, Diaz M, Caldamone AA, et al. Endoscopic therapy for vesicoureteral reflux: a meta-analysis. I. Reflux resolution and urinary tract infection. J Urol 2006;175:716–22.

in infants younger than 1 year. These findings may indicate that there is not a safe age after which there should be little concern for the development of new renal scars. In the International Reflux Study there was no difference in the progression and development of new scars in the medically and surgically corrected patients, despite a higher number of patients with pyelonephritis in the medically treated group. These contrary findings may be due to identifying preexisting scars in older patients or selection bias in the International Reflux Study that may have precluded older children with new scars from being enrolled.

Whereas it used to be widely believed that all scarring was postinfectious, it is now clear that renal abnormalities associated with VUR can precede infection. In patients with antenatal hydronephrosis and VUR, more than one-third have abnormalities detected on DMSA scans before the development of UTIs.[37] These areas of abnormality are believed to be regions of hypoplasia or dysplasia, which are postulated to be caused by abnormal embryogenesis of the kidney associated with the abnormal development of the ureterovesical junction that leads to VUR. There is currently no way to differentiate abnormalities that are postinfectious versus congenital on initial DMSA scan or intravenous pyelography. In patients with prenatal hydronephrosis, it is unclear whether the abnormal DMSA scans will predict the likelihood of subsequent episodes of pyelonephritis or decreased chances for spontaneous resolution. Because most of these patients are male, the risk of infection may be more influenced by other factors, such as circumcision status.[38]

EFFECT OF AGE AND SEX ON VUR RESOLUTION

Up until the widespread use of DMSA scanning to detect pyelonephritis and renal scarring in patients with febrile UTIs, it was generally believed that children younger than 6 years, particularly infants, were at the highest risk for pyelonephritis-induced scarring.[20] The scarring in these studies was typically detected by intravenous pyelogram, which may take years to become visible after the infectious event that triggered the scar. If the infant's kidneys are more susceptible to scarring, then why do the studies using DMSA fail to document permanent scarring more often in those with follow-up imaging after pyelonephritis? In a study by Garin and colleagues,[3] initial DMSA scan indicated pyelonephritis in all patients (median age 2), but scarring developed in only 6%. Most underwent a scan 6 months after the original but only repeated the scan if they had another UTI. While

this question remains unanswered, one can hypothesize that "new scars" that develop over time in patients followed with VUR simply are too tiny to detect radiographically when they form in the infant's kidney. The changes being detected by intravenous pyelograms may be the result of the abnormal growth of the kidney following injury from the infection. An infant's kidneys undergo significant growth over the first few years of life, and just as a small surgical scars grows larger with the child, it is likely that some small areas of renal scarring will become more noticeable with the child's growth and become apparent only after they are older. Because most recent studies have not repeated DMSA renal scans that were normal at presentation, it cannot be assuredly concluded that an initial normal DMSA is a guarantee of a patient being free from renal scarring throughout life and therefore not at risk for sequelae from VUR. Progression and new scar formation is one of the secondary outcomes being measured in the RIVUR trial, and will hopefully help answer whether the kidneys really are more susceptible to scarring in infancy.[6]

In cases of VUR presenting as antenatal hydronephrosis, boys are more commonly affected than girls.[39] Boys more often have bilateral and higher grade VUR at presentation. As noted previously, up to 40% of these patients may have preexisting abnormalities on DMSA scan in the absence of UTIs.[37] In patients presenting with UTIs, the majority are female.[40] Approximately 8% of females will experience a UTI before the age of 7 years versus only 2% of boys. Recurrence of infection will occur in up to 30% of these children.[41] Breakthrough infections are more common in females than males.[42] While in general the resolution rates for males and females with a given grade and laterality of VUR are similar, there have been studies that show a slightly better rate for resolution of low-grade VUR in males over time.[43] In addition, there is good evidence that boys with VUR who present in the first year of life have significantly better rates of resolution for high grades (IV and V) compared with older children and females. Rates of resolution of up to 29% at 1 year following diagnosis for grades IV and V have been reported.[44] After 1 year, the resolution rate drops significantly and is similar to females. One study compared the resolution of infants with normal kidneys to those with bilateral abnormal kidneys (defined as abnormal DMSA scan or renal ultrasound).[31] These investigators found that patients with the best chance for spontaneous resolution had normal kidneys, whereas none of those with bilateral abnormal kidneys resolved (100% vs 0%) at a mean age of 16 months. The patients with a single normal kidney had a 50% resolution rate at 16 months of age.

When the effect of age is considered independently, there is a decreasing chance for reflux resolution in patients with grade III reflux, particularly with bilateral VUR. In the 1997 AUA guidelines, the chances of spontaneous resolution over a 5-year period in a child younger than age 2 years with bilateral grade III VUR was reported to be approximately 50%, versus 15% if the child was older than 6 years.[7] In predicting early resolution of VUR (within 2 years of diagnosis), age younger than 2 years has been shown to be a significant factor independent of grade.[45] Given these data, patients with the highest likelihood of spontaneous resolution are young male children, younger than the age of 2, with normal kidneys.

GRADE OF VUR: THE STRONGEST PREDICTOR

There is no controversy regarding the importance of grade in predicting the chances of spontaneous resolution and likelihood of finding associated renal scarring. As the grade of VUR increases, the chances of spontaneous resolution decrease.[7,43,45,46] Multiple studies have shown that the rate of renal scaring increases with increasing grades of VUR.[29–31] The same is true with congenital renal abnormalities occurring in patients with VUR detected prenatally with no infection history.[37] Nondilating (grades I and II),

older age at presentation, and fewer episodes of pyelonephritis are associated with less risk of renal scarring at diagnosis and chances of developing progressive renal scarring.[20,34,35] **Fig. 1** shows the rate of spontaneous resolution in a published series examining multiple variables to predict VUR resolution.[45] **Fig. 1** clearly shows the consistent finding of high rates of spontaneous resolution for nondilating VUR (80%–90%) and the much lower likelihood of resolution of high grade VUR. Other associated factors that can help predict VUR resolution are reviewed below.

UNILATERAL VERSUS BILATERAL VUR

VUR occurs unilaterally and bilaterally. In patients who present with initial unilateral VUR, approximately 10%–20% will be found to have bilateral VUR on subsequent voiding cystourethrogram (VCUG) studies.[47] In their meta-analysis of spontaneous resolution, the AUA Reflux Guidelines panel found laterality was only significant for grades III and IV, where the presence of bilateral VUR was significantly less likely to resolve.[7] Bilateral VUR is often reported not to be an important factor in predicting resolution for lower grades of VUR; however, most series may be too small to be appropriately powered to detect this effect. A recent large series of 2462 patients found that bilateral VUR was less likely to resolve in females independent of grade.[46] Laterality was not a significant factor in males. The adjusted hazard ratio was 1.42 (95% confidence interval [CI] 1.26–1.59)

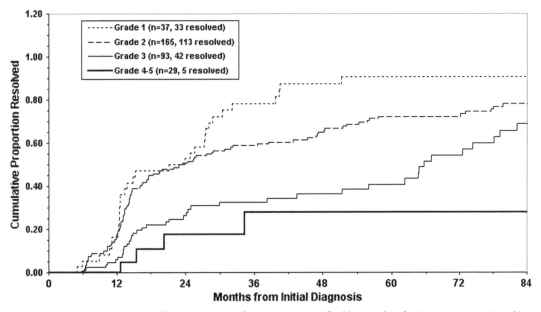

Fig. 1. Spontaneous resolution of VUR over time for patients stratified by grade of VUR at presentation. (*From* Knudson MJ, Austin JC, McMillan ZM, et al. Predictive factors of early spontaneous resolution in children with primary vesicoureteral reflux. J Urol 2007;178:1684–8; with permission.)

for males or females with unilateral reflux, indicating that males were 42% more likely to resolve their VUR than those females with bilateral VUR.

ASSOCIATED ANATOMIC ABNORMALITIES: DUPLICATION AND DIVERTICULUM

The root cause of primary VUR is an anatomic defect at the ureterovesical junction where there is a deficient tunnel length of the intramural ureter. While abnormal bladder dynamics may contribute to VUR, any surgeon who has corrected VUR has seen gaping, incompetent ureteral orifices during ureteral reimplantation. There really is no doubt that many patients who undergo surgical corrections have findings that are extremely unlikely to have ever spontaneously resolved. It is not surprising, then, that other associated anatomic anomalies may coexist with primary VUR and perhaps influence its natural history. Ureteral duplication is not an uncommon finding in patients with VUR. It may be diagnosed by noting the incomplete pyelogram (drooping lily) on a VCUG. Imaging of the kidney with ultrasound or renal scans may also show hints that there is also ureteral duplication. In patients with complete duplication, the VUR will virtually always occur only into the lower pole ureter.[48] While this predisposition is a well-known application of embryology of the genitourinary tract to clinical practice, the question of whether ureteral duplication is a significant negative prognostic factor for VUR resolution has been a subject of debate. There are series reporting no effect on resolution and others showing significant effects.[48–50] Many earlier series exclude following patients with higher grades of VUR. However, in studies where all patients with complete ureteral duplication were followed expectantly similar to patients with a single ureter, there did seem to be a lower likelihood of spontaneous resolution of higher grades of reflux with complete ureteral duplication.[48] In a large series from Boston Children's Hospital, the hazard ratio reported for the absence of duplication was 1.55 (95% CI 1.24–1.93) and indicates that single ureters are significantly more likely to resolve than duplicated ureters.[46] In our series of patients with VUR, duplication approached statistical significance but may not have been a significant factor due to it being underpowered.[45] It seems clear from larger studies that duplication is a significant factor in predicting reflux resolution and needs to be considered in the evaluation of these patients.

Para-ureteral diverticuli have traditionally been considered a marker of a severe defect at the ureterovesical junction that allows the mucosa of the bladder to prolapse through the bladder wall because of poor attachment of the ureter to detrusor muscle fibers. The defect has been considered an indication that the VUR is not likely to resolve and, by some investigators, an indication for ureteral reimplantation. Little has been published regarding this entity, however. There have been successful reports of endoscopic treatment of VUR associated with para-ureteral diverticuli with a cure rate of 80%.[51] Only a single series has recently evaluated the prognostic factor of a para-ureteral diverticulum on VUR resolution.[52] This study compared a cohort of 95 patients with primary VUR and a para-ureteral diverticulum with a control group of randomly selected patients with primary VUR. The groups were similar in age and VUR grade. The overall VUR resolution was similar in both groups, which strongly questions whether a para-ureteral diverticulum should be considered an indication for surgery and whether it has any effect on VUR resolution. When evaluating the VCUG in a child with a para-ureteral diverticulum, the size and involvement of the ureter needs to be considered. On occasion, there are instances where the ureteral attachment actually appears to protrude outside as the diverticulum expands outside the bladder. In those instances the chances for spontaneous resolution are likely minimal, and surgical correction should be considered. If there appears to be a para-ureteral diverticulum not involving the ureter, observation is a reasonable treatment choice.

EFFECTS OF BLADDER DYNAMICS ON VUR RESOLUTION

Rarely are bladder dynamics of children with VUR considered or evaluated during the routine evaluation of children with VUR. The time has come for this to end. Research during the last decade has greatly increased our understanding of the normal maturation of bladder dynamics from infancy and the associated bladder dysfunction seen in patients with VUR.[53–57] The bladder volume at the onset of VUR or timing of VUR (VUR during filling vs voiding only) are factors that influence the possibility of spontaneous resolution of VUR.[58–61] Intuitively, if the ureterovesical junction is anatomically abnormal, then the easier it is for urine to reflux. The more severe the abnormality, the lower is the chance for spontaneous resolution. Thus reflux, which occurs either early in filling or at low pressures, should be reflective of a more severe defect at the ureterovesical junction, and thus a lower likelihood for spontaneous resolution. Since 2000, children with VUR routinely have follow-up evaluation for VUR by nuclear cystometrograms at the University of Iowa.[62] Bladder pressure at the onset of VUR has been shown to be significantly lower in patients with persistent VUR than in those in whom it resolves, independent of grade.[62] Previous studies have demonstrated that reflux occurring at lower bladder volumes was also a negative prognostic factor for resolution.[44,58] Indeed VUR, which occurs only during voiding, has a much better chance to resolve than passive VUR during filling.[61] With further characterization of the timing of VUR during the filling phase of the VCUG, the volume instilled at the onset of VUR is recorded. To normalize this value for age, the volume at onset of reflux is converted to the percent of the predicted bladder capacity using the standard formula for predicted bladder capacity (2 + age × 30 mL). In a multivariate analysis controlled for grade of VUR, the volume at onset of VUR was the next most important factor in determining spontaneous VUR resolution. It was a stronger predictor than age, sex, laterality, and presentation. The authors' analysis focused on predictors for early resolution of VUR (1 and 2 years) rather than long-term resolution, as being able to predict early resolution may be more clinically relevant information for families trying to determine the choice of pursuing treatment over observation. The hazard ratio was 7.5 (95% CI 2.3–24) at 1 year and 3.9 (95% CI 2.1–7) at 2 years using a volume of greater than or less than 50% of the predicted bladder capacity.[45] Unfortunately, most radiologists do not note the bladder volume at onset of VUR during VCUGs; however, it is a value that can easily be obtained during VCUGs without the need for additional sophisticated urodynamic equipment. Routine reporting of this prognostic information should become standard practice for radiologists.

The voiding patterns in infants with VUR have been studied with urodynamics.[53,54,56,57] The findings can generally be divided into normal patterns (which we now know can include high voiding pressures and incomplete bladder emptying), large capacity with incomplete emptying, or bladder overactivity (OAB). Some investigators also describe a dyssynergic pattern.[54,57] The chances of spontaneous resolution are influenced by the presence or absence of bladder dysfunction.[31,53] The finding of bladder dysfunction along with and in the absence of abnormal kidneys has been associated with decreased chance for spontaneous resolution. The risk of breakthrough UTI is also higher in those patients with bladder dysfunction.[53]

The effects of correction of VUR on bladder dysfunction have not been extensively studied after ureteral reimplantation. In one study of school-age children treated at mean age of 4 years, most still had large bladder capacities but emptying was improved or complete in the majority.[63] In infants with high-grade VUR followed with serial urodynamic studies there seems to be a change in the pattern of bladder dysfunction. Males in particular seem to evolve from a pattern of decreased bladder capacity with high voiding pressures to a large-capacity bladder with lower voiding pressures and incomplete emptying over the first 2 years of life.[64]

Bladder dysfunction is also seen in older children with UTIs and VUR. The urodynamic patterns are similar to those seen in children with incontinence. Findings of dysfunctional voiding or OAB have been described; however, OAB seems to be more prevalent in patients with VUR.[53] Dysfunctional elimination (bladder dysfunction with associated bowel symptoms such as constipation or encopresis) is also found in older children with VUR.[65] Series have described that treatment of bladder dysfunction with anticholinergics, biofeedback, and laxatives for constipation can improve the resolution of VUR and decrease the need for surgical correction.[66–68] In a study of infants with high-grade VUR and poor bladder emptying, clean intermittent catheterization did not improve VUR resolution.[69] It makes sense to consider the effects of bladder dysfunction in patients with VUR, and if there are symptoms of bladder dysfunction or dysfunctional elimination syndrome, treatment of the dysfunction should be initiated before consideration of surgical correction.

COMPUTER MODELS AND NOMOGRAMS IN PREDICTING VUR RESOLUTION

Physicians now have ready access to computers in the clinic. Electronic medical records and medical informatics have changed the way medicine is practiced and information is retrieved. Computers are used for many aspects of patient care and have been studied as aids to decision making in urology.[70] Using a large database of VUR patients, a computer model for predicting VUR resolution has been created and is available online at http://godot.urol.uic.edu/web/svm_vur.html.[71] It can be used to predict VUR resolution at 2 years. Clinical variables that must be entered include age, sex, laterality, percent of predicted bladder capacity at onset of VUR, grade of VUR, timing of VUR, ureteral duplication, and the presence of voiding dysfunction. The model has a receiver-operating characteristic (ROC) of 0.86. The model was externally validated in a second study using patients from Japan.[72] The model was 81% accurate with an ROC value of 0.79. The model showed very good performance in patients from both the United States and abroad. In addition to predicting resolution or not at 2 years, the odds of resolution are given to help quantify the certainty of the prediction. Nomograms for VUR resolution have been published based on a large series of patients from the Boston Children's Hospital.[46] The nomograms use the age, sex, laterality, clinical presentation, ureter anatomy, and maximal grade of VUR to give the percentage of patients with VUR resolution at 1 to 5 years. A web-based calculator for these nomograms is available for use as well, at http://www.childrens hospital.org/vurcalculator. The data needed for the nomograms or VUR calculator are present in nearly all children diagnosed with VUR. The nomogram gives percentages of children who will resolve their VUR at a certain time over 1 to 5 years, but will not make an individual patient prediction. To use the computer model, the bladder volume of onset of VUR is needed to calculate the percent of the predicted bladder capacity. More recently another computer model has been generated, which incorporates all of the parameters noted in the first model and renal scan data.[73] This model is also located at http://godot.urol.uic.edu/web/vur2.html. The addition of the renal scan data improved the predictive accuracy of resolution at 2 years, with an ROC of 0.945. These new web-based computer models and nomograms should result in improved prognostic accuracy regarding the chance for spontaneous resolution, and permit better individualized patient management decisions.[74]

SUMMARY

The treatment of VUR primarily results in a decreased rate of pyelonephritis. There is a high rate of cure after ureteral reimplantation and a good but lower rate for endoscopic correction of VUR. High-grade VUR has poor long-term spontaneous resolution. There is no difference in the rate of renal scarring, renal growth, and UTIs in patients treated medically or surgically for dilating VUR. The patients who will benefit most from surgical correction of VUR are those with recurrent pyelonephritis and/or reflux that will not resolve spontaneously. Grade is the strongest predictor of VUR resolution, with high-grade VUR being much less likely to resolve. Other factors that negatively influence resolution include lower bladder volume or pressure at onset of reflux, older age, female sex, bilateral VUR, ureteral duplication, abnormal or scarred kidneys, and bladder dysfunction. These factors can be used, along with grade, in computer models or nomograms to improve the ability to predict spontaneous resolution.

REFERENCES

1. Wheeler D, Vimalachandra D, Hodson EM, et al. Antibiotics and surgery for vesicoureteral reflux: a meta-analysis of randomized controlled trials. Arch Dis Child 2003;88:688–94.

2. Craig JC, Irwig LM, Knight JF, et al. Does treatment of vesicoureteral reflux in childhood prevent end-stage renal disease attributable to reflux nephropathy? Pediatrics 2000;105:1236–41.

3. Garin EH, Olavarria F, Neito VG, et al. Clinical significance of primary vesicoureteral reflux and antibiotic prophylaxis after acute pyelonephritis: a multicenter, randomized, controlled study. Pediatrics 2006;117: 626–32.

4. Pennesi M, Travan L, Parotoner L, et al. Is antibiotic prophylaxis in children with vesicoureteral reflux effective in preventing pyelonephritis and renal scars? A randomized controlled trial. Pediatrics 2008;121:e1489–94.

5. Conway PH, Cnaan A, Zaoutis T, et al. Recurrent urinary tract infections in children: risk factors and association with prophylactic antimicrobials. JAMA 2007;298:179–86.

6. Keren R, Carpenter MA, Hoberman A, et al. Rationale and design issues of the randomized intervention for children with vesicoureteral reflux (RIVUR) study. Pediatrics 2008;122(Suppl 5):S240–50.

7. Elder JS, Peters CA, Arant BS Jr, et al. Pediatric vesicoureteral reflux guidelines panel summary report on the management of primary vesicoureteral reflux in children. J Urol 1991;157:1846–51.

8. Duckett JW, Walker RD, Weiss R. Surgical results: International Reflux Study in children—United States branch. J Urol 1992;148:1674–5.

9. Politano VA, Leadbetter WF. An operative technique for the correction of vesicoureteral reflux. J Urol 1958;79:932–41.

10. Glenn JF, Anderson EE. Distal tunnel ureteral reimplantation. J Urol 1967;97:623–6.

11. Wacksman J. Initial results with the Cohen cross-trigonal ureteroneocystotomy. J Urol 1983;129: 1198–9.

12. Kirsch AJ, Perez-Brayfield MR, Smtih EA, et al. The modified sting procedure to correct vesicoureteral reflux: improved results with submucosal implantation within the intramural ureter. J Urol 2004;171:2413–8.

13. Elder JS, Diaz M, Caldamone AA, et al. Endoscopic therapy for vesicoureteral reflux: a meta-analysis. I. Reflux resolution and urinary tract infection. J Urol 2006;175:716–22.

14. Birmingham Reflux Study Group. Prospective trial of operative versus non-operative treatment of severe

vesicoureteric reflux in children: five years' observation. Br Med J 1987;295:237–41.

15. Weiss R, Duckett J, Spitzer A. Results of a randomized clinical trial of medical versus surgical management of infants and children with grades III and IV primary vesicoureteral reflux (United States). J Urol 1992;148:1667–73.

16. Jodal U, Koskimies O, Hanson E, et al. Infection pattern in children with vesicoureteral reflux randomly allocated to operation or long-term antibacterial prophylaxis. J Urol 1992;148:1650–2.

17. Smellie JM, Barratt TM, Chantler C, et al. Medical versus surgical treatment in children with severe bilateral vesicoureteral reflux and bilateral nephropathy: a randomised trial. Lancet 2001; 357:1329–33.

18. Capozza N, Caione P. Dextranomer/hyaluronic acid copolymer implantation for vesico-ureteral reflux: a randomized comparison wit antibiotic prophylaxis. J Pediatr 2002;140:230–4.

19. Smellie JM, Jodal U, Lax H, et al. Outcome at 10 years of sever vesicoureteric reflux managed medically: report of the international reflux study in children. J Pediatr 2001;139:656–63.

20. Olbing H, Smellie JM, Jodal U, et al. New renal scars in children with severe VUR: a 10 year study of randomized treatment. Pediatr Nephrol 2003;18: 1128–31.

21. Jodal U, Smellie JM, Lax H, et al. Ten-year results of randomized treatment of children with severe vesicoureteral reflux. Final report of the International Reflux Study in children. Pediatr Nephrol 2006;21: 785–92.

22. Olbing H, Hirche H, Koskimies O, et al. Renal growth in children with severe vesicoureteral reflux: 10-year prospective study of medical and surgical treatment. Radiology 2000;216:731–7.

23. Haferkamp A, Contractor H, Mohring K, et al. Failure of subureteral bovine collagen injection for the endoscopic treatment of primary vesicoureteral reflux in long-term follow-up. Urology 2000; 55:759–63.

24. Lackgren G, Wahlin N, Skolenberg E, et al. Long-term followup of children treated with dextranomer/hyaluronic acid copolymer for vesicoureteral reflux. J Urol 2001;166:1887–92.

25. Lee EK, Gatti JM, DeMarco RT, et al. Long-term followup of dextranomer/hyaluronic acid injection for vesicoureteral reflux: late failure warrants continued followup. J Urol 2009;181:1869–75.

26. Chertin B, Colhoun E, Velayudham M, et al. Endoscopic treatment of vesicoureteral reflux: 11 to 17 years of followup. J Urol 2002;167:1443–6.

27. Traxel E, DeFoor W, Reddy P, et al. Risk factors for urinary tract infections after dextranomer/hyaluronic acid endoscopic injection. J Urol 2009;182: 1708–12.

28. Sedbarry-Ross S, Rice DC, Pohl HG, et al. Febrile urinary tract infections in children with an early negative voiding cystourethrogram after treatment of vesicoureteral reflux with dextranomer/hyaluronic acid. J Urol 2008;180:1605–9.

29. Mingin GC, Nguyen HT, Baskin LS. Abnormal dimercapto-succinic acid scans predict an increased risk of breakthrough infection in children with vesicoureteral reflux. J Urol 2004;172:1075–7.

30. Nepple KG, Knudson MJ, Austin JC, et al. Abnormal renal scans and decreased early resolution of low grade vesicoureteral reflux. J Urol 2008;180:1643–7.

31. Godley ML, Desai D, Yeung CK, et al. The relationship between early renal status, and the resolution of vesico-ureteral reflux and bladder function at 16 months. BJU Int 2001;87:457–62.

32. Faust WC, Diaz M, Pohl HG. Incidence of postpyelonephritic renal scarring: a meta-analysis of the dimercapto-succinic acid literature. J Urol 2009;181:290–8.

33. Pecile P, Miorin E, Romanello C, et al. Age-related renal parenchymal lesions in children with first febrile urinary tract infections. Pediatrics 2009;124: 23–9.

34. Martinell J, Hansson S, Claesson I, et al. Detection of urographic scars in girls with pyelonephritis followed for 13–38 years. Pediatr Nephrol 2000;14: 1006–10.

35. Wennerstrom M, Hansson S, Jodal U, et al. Primary and acquired renal scarring in boys and girls with urinary tract infection. J Pediatr 2000;136:30–4.

36. Kohler J, Thysell H, Tencer J, et al. Long-term follow up of reflux nephropathy in adults with vesicoureteral reflux- radiologic and pathoanatomical analysis. Acta Radiol 2001;42:355–64.

37. Nguyen HT, Bauer SB, Peters CA, et al. 99m-Technetium dimercapto-succinic acid renal scintigraphy abnormalities in infants with sterile high grade vesicoureteral reflux. J Urol 2000;164:1674–9.

38. Singh-Grewal D, Macdessi J, Craig J. Circumcision for the prevention of urinary tract infections in boys: a systematic review of randomized trials and observational studies. Arch Dis Child 2005; 90:853–8.

39. Farhat W, McLorie G, Geary D, et al. The natural history of neonatal vesicoureteral reflux associated with antenatal hydronephrosis. J Urol 2000;164: 1057–60.

40. Thompson RH, Chen JJ, Pugach J, et al. Cessation of prophylactic antibiotics for managing persistent vesicoureteral reflux. J Urol 2001;166:1465–9.

41. Williams G, Lee A, Craig J. Antibiotics for the prevention of urinary tract infection in children: a systematic review of randomized controlled trials. J Pediatr 2001;138:868–74.

42. Goldraich NP, Goldraich IH. Followup of conservatively treated children with high and low grade

vesicoureteral reflux: a prospective study. J Urol 1992;148:1688–92.

43. Schwab CW, Wu H, Selman H, et al. Spontaneous resolution of vesicoureteral reflux: a 15-year perspective. J Urol 2002;168:2594–9.

44. Sjostrom S, Sillen U, Bachelard M, et al. Spontaneous resolution of high grade infantile vesicoureteral reflux. J Urol 2004;172:694–9.

45. Knudson MJ, Austin JC, McMillan ZM, et al. Predictive factors of early spontaneous resolution in children with primary vesicoureteral reflux. J Urol 2007;178:1684–8.

46. Estrada CR, Passerotti CC, Graham DA, et al. Nomograms for predicting annual resolution rate of primary vesicoureteral reflux: results from 2,462 children. J Urol 2009;182:1535–41.

47. Sparr KE, Balcom AH, Mesrobian HO. Incidence and natural history of contralateral vesicoureteral reflux in patients presenting with unilateral disease. J Urol 1998;160:1023–5.

48. Afshar K, Papanikolaou R, Malek R, et al. Vesicoureteral reflux and complete duplication. Conservative or surgical management? J Urol 2004;173:1725–7.

49. Peppas DS, Skoog SJ, Canning DA, et al. Non-surgical management of primary vesicoureteral reflux in complete ureteral duplication: is it justified? J Urol 1991;146:1594–5.

50. Lee PH, Diamond DA, Duffy PG, et al. Duplex reflux: a study of 105 children. J Urol 1991;146:657–9.

51. Cerwinka WH, Scherz HC, Kirsch AJ. Endoscopic treatment of vesicoureteral reflux associated with a paraureteral diverticulum in children. J Urol 2007;178:1469–73.

52. Afshar K, Malek R, Bakhshi M, et al. Should the presence of congenital para-ureteral diverticulum affect the management of vesicoureteral reflux? J Urol 2005;174:1590–3.

53. Yeung CK, Sreedhar B, Sihoe JDY, et al. Renal and bladder functional status as diagnosis as predictive factors for the outcome of primary vesicoureteral reflux in children. J Urol 2006;176:1152–7.

54. Yeung CK, Godley ML, Dhillon HK, et al. Urodynamic patterns in infants with normal lower urinary tracts or primary vesico-ureteric reflux. Br J Urol 1998;81:461–7.

55. Jansson UB, Hanson M, Hanson E, et al. Voiding pattern in healthy children 0 to 3 years old: a longitudinal study. J Urol 2000;164:2050–4.

56. Sillen U, Hjalmas K, Aili M, et al. Pronounced detrusor hypercontractility in infants with gross bilateral reflux. J Urol 1992;148:598–9.

57. Sillen U, Bachelard M, Hermanson G, et al. Gross bilateral reflux in infants: gradual decrease of initial detrusor hypercontractility. J Urol 1996;155:668–72.

58. McMillan ZM, Austin JC, Knudson MJ, et al. Bladder volume at onset of reflux on initial cystogram predicts spontaneous resolution. J Urol 2006;176:1838–41.

59. Mozley PD, Heyman S, Duckett JW, et al. Direct vesicoureteral scintigraphy: quantifying early outcome predictors in children with primary reflux. J Nucl Med 1994;35:1602–8.

60. Papachristou F, Printza N, Doumas A, et al. Urinary bladder volume and pressure at reflux as prognostic factors of vesicoureteral reflux outcome. Pediatr Radiol 2004;34:556–9.

61. Arsanjani A, Alagiri M. Identification of filling versus voiding reflux as predictor of clinical outcome. Urol 2007;70:351–4.

62. Van Arendonk KJ, Madsen MT, Austin JC, et al. Nuclear cystometrogram-determined bladder pressure at onset of vesicoureteral reflux predicts spontaneous resolution. Urol 2007;69:767–70.

63. Sillen U, Mamoun A, Hellstrom AA, et al. Bladder dysfunction in infants with high grade reflux: does it persist at school-age after anti-reflux surgery. BJU Int 2003;91(Suppl I):s53–4.

64. Sjostrom S, Bachelard M, Sixt R, et al. Change of urodynamic patterns in infants with dilating vesicoureteral reflux: 3-year followup. J Urol 2009;182:2446–54.

65. Koff SA, Wagner TT, Jayanthi VR. The relationship among dysfunctional elimination syndromes, primary vesicoureteral reflux and urinary tract infections in children. J Urol 1998;160:1019–22.

66. Koff SA, Murtach DS. The uninhibited bladder in children: effect of treatment on recurrence of urinary infection and on vesicoureteral reflux resolution. J Urol 1983;130:1138–41.

67. Snodgrass W. The impact of treated dysfunctional voiding on the nonsurgical management of vesicoureteral reflux. J Urol 1998;160:1823–5.

68. Herndon CDA, DeCambre M, McKenna PH. Changing concepts concerning the management of vesicoureteral reflux. J Urol 2001;166:1439–43.

69. Sillen U, Holmdahl G, Hellstrom AL, et al. Treatment of bladder dysfunction and high grade vesicoureteral reflux does not influence the spontaneous resolution rate. J Urol 2007;177:325–30.

70. Niederberger C. Computational tools for the modern andrologist. J Androl 1996;17:462–6.

71. Knudson MJ, Austin JC, Wald M, et al. Computational model for predicting the chance of early resolution in children with vesicoureteral reflux. J Urol 2007;178:1824–7.

72. Shiraishi K, Matsuyama H, Nepple K, et al. Validation of a prognostic calculator for prediction of early vesicoureteral reflux resolution in children. J Urol 2009;182:687–91.

73. Nepple KG, Knudson MJ, Austin JC, et al. Adding renal scan data improved the accuracy of a computational model to predict vesicoureteral reflux resolution. J Urol 2008;180:1648–52.

74. Cooper CS. Diagnosis and management of vesicoureteral reflux in children. Nat Rev Urol 2009;6:481–9.

Contemporary Surgical Management of Pediatric Urolithiasis

Marc C. Smaldone, MD*, Steven G. Docimo, MD,
Michael C. Ost, MD

KEYWORDS

- Nephrolithiasis • Children • Endourology
- Ureteroscopy • Shock wave lithotripsy
- Percutaneous nephrolithotomy

Surgical management of urolithiasis in children has evolved dramatically over the past 2 decades. In the 1980s, the advent of shock wave lithotripsy (SWL) revolutionized pediatric stone management and is currently the procedure of choice in treating most upper tract calculi in industrialized nations. However, with miniaturization of equipment and refinement of technique, access to the entire pediatric urinary tract is now possible. In a growing number of centers, ureteroscopy (URS) is being performed in cases that previously would have been treated with SWL or percutaneous nephrolithotomy (PCNL). Recent data from large single-institution series demonstrate stone-free and complication rates for URS that are comparable with those for SWL, but prospective trials are necessary before consensus regarding the most effective primary treatment modality can be reached. This article provides a directed review of the literature, focusing on recent advances in the surgical management of pediatric stone disease.

INCIDENCE OF UROLITHIASIS IN CHILDREN

The incidence and characteristics of nephrolithiasis in children reflect a wide geographic variation, but stones occur in children of all ages without clear gender predominance.[1] Although uncommon in the western hemisphere, pediatric stone disease is considered endemic in developing nations including India, Turkey, Pakistan, and countries in the Far East. In these areas, ammonium acid urate and uric acid stones predominate, strongly implicating dietary factors.[2] Despite this discrepancy between hemispheres, nephrolithiasis in children is increasing in occurrence globally,[3] likely reflecting westernized lifestyle and dietary changes, including higher salt intake from processed foods, and decreased water consumption.

It is established that children with anatomic abnormalities, urinary tract infections, and metabolic disturbances are considered to be at high risk for stone development.[4] In developing nations, recent reports suggest that a metabolic risk factor can be found on urine studies in 84% to 87% of children, most commonly hypercalciuria or hypocitrauria.[5,6] However, evidence is accumulating that stones in a majority of westernized children are calcium based without any evidence of metabolic abnormality on 24-hour urine collection.[7] In a retrospective study of 1440 Pakistani children, Rivzi and colleagues[2] reported that while diet, dehydration, and poor nutrition remain the major causative factors of pediatric nephrolithiasis, there is an emerging predominance over the past decade of upper tract calculi more consistent with adult populations. Recent data support this trend: in a modern series of 150 children managed over an 8-year period, Kalorin and colleagues[8] reported that 57% of stones detected in children younger than 10 years were located in the upper tract.

Portions of this article were previously published in Smaldone MC, Gayed BA, Ost MC. The evolution of the endourologic management of pediatric stone disease. Indian J Urol 2009;25(3):302–11; with permission.
Division of Pediatric Urology, Children's Hospital of Pittsburgh, Department of Urology, University of Pittsburgh School of Medicine, 3471 5th Avenue, Suite 700, Pittsburgh, PA 15213-3232, USA
* Corresponding author.
E-mail address: smaldonemc@upmc.edu

DIAGNOSIS, METABOLIC EVALUATION, AND SURVEILLANCE

Renal calculi in neonates and younger children are often diagnosed with ultrasound. Although anatomic location and the associated presence of hydroureteronephrosis can be accurately assessed in a majority of children, up to 40% of calculi may be missed using ultrasound.[9] Despite the increased sensitivity of computed tomography (CT) compared with ultrasound,[10] concerns regarding radiation exposure limits its use in young children. Although speculative, risk as high as 1 fatal cancer for every 1000 CT scans performed in young children has been reported.[11] Investigators recently have begun to reassess diagnostic thresholds in an effort to reduce radiation exposure without sacrificing diagnostic efficacy, particularly in children with complex stone histories requiring serial imaging studies.[12]

In the authors' practice, asymptomatic calculi incidentally diagnosed with ultrasound are followed with serial ultrasound or plain abdominal films to minimize radiation exposure. Noncontrast helical CT is the diagnostic test of choice in older children presenting acutely with flank pain, but is reserved for younger children for whom plain films or ultrasound are nondiagnostic. Following definitive therapy, children are ideally followed in a multidisciplinary stone clinic including urologic, renal, nutrition, and endocrine evaluation if necessary. Routine evaluation includes urine culture, 24-hour urine collection, and office-based ultrasound or abdominal films to detect recurrence. While there is abundant reference material in the adult literature, data regarding standard 24-hour urine reference values for stone risk factors in children is just beginning to emerge,[13] and identifying normal 24-hour urine parameters for nonstone formers is currently is the subject of prospective evaluation in the authors' practice. Follow-up is individualized and is based on age, anatomy, stone burden, and any underlying metabolic abnormality.

CONSERVATIVE MANAGEMENT

Conservative management of pediatric nephrolithiasis closely mirrors that of adults. Even in very young children, renal calculi smaller than 3 mm are likely to spontaneously pass, and stones 4 mm or larger in the distal ureter are likely to require endourologic treatment.[14] In the authors' practice, if a child's pain is controlled with oral analgesia, clear liquids are tolerated, and there is no evidence of urinary tract infection, parents are offered a closely monitored trial of spontaneous passage for 4 to 6 weeks prior to definitive therapy. Based on efficacy demonstrated in the adult population,[15] tamsulosin may be offered on an individualized basis as adjunctive therapy to facilitate ureteral expulsion. A ureteral stent is placed acutely in children with evidence of an infected genitourinary system, refractory colic, or uncontrolled nausea and vomiting. Under these circumstances definitive therapy is delayed 7 to 14 days following stenting to allow for system decompression, ureteral orifice dilation, and resolution of edema before endourologic management is undertaken.

PEDIATRIC CONSIDERATIONS

Special considerations in the endourologic management of stone disease in children include preservation of renal development and function, prevention of radiation exposure, and minimizing the need for retreatment. Despite advances in endourologic equipment and technique, controversy remains regarding the contribution of SWL to future development of diabetes or hypertension, and whether ureteral orifice dilation during URS leads to ureteral stricture formation or development of vesicoureteral reflux. International consensus is lacking as to the most effective surgical management of pediatric stone disease because of the lack of prospective randomized trials comparing treatment modalities and disparity in the access to emerging technologies. Regardless of treatment modality, the presence of residual stone fragments is associated with adverse clinical outcome,[16] and every attempt should be made to achieve a stone-free status. Surgeon experience is paramount to facilitate complete stone clearance and minimize retreatment rates. The decision regarding the most efficacious primary treatment modality must be individualized per child based on age, anatomy, location, and composition of stone burden.

ANTIBIOTIC USE

Use of perioperative antibiotics in the management of pediatric urolithiasis closely mirrors that in adult patients. Per the 2008 American Urologic Association best practice statement on antibiotic prophylaxis, up to 24 hours of perioperative antibiotics are indicated in all patients undergoing upper tract instrumentation.[17] Appropriate agents include fluoroquinolones, trimethoprim-sulfamethazole, first- and second-generation cephalosporins, and ampicillin in combination with an aminoglycoside. A urine culture is mandatory before all upper tract procedures to determine if the urine is sterile, and culture results are used to guide preoperative antibiotic therapy, particularly for percutaneous procedures, patients with high-grade obstruction, or patients with an indwelling stent.[4] In the authors' practice, children with a negative urine culture undergoing uncomplicated SWL and URS procedures receive perioperative cefazolin, and all children undergoing a percutaneous procedure or that have a preexisting ureteral stent/nephrostomy tube receive a fluoroquinolone or ampicillin/gentamicin. Use of postoperative antibiotics is controversial and is determined on a per child basis, especially with recent data demonstrating an increased risk of developing resistant bacterial strains with prolonged use of antibiotic prophylactic therapy.[18]

SHOCK WAVE LITHOTRIPSY

The emergence of SWL revolutionized the minimally invasive treatment of urolithiasis during the early 1980s. Initially reported in children in 1986,[19] large series have reported complication, safety, and stone-free rates comparable with those of adults (**Table 1**).[20–27] When used as a primary treatment option for upper tract calculi, SWL efficacy ranges from 68% to 84%[20,23,28] and has become the preferred treatment modality for uncomplicated renal and proximal calculi of 15 mm or less. In a contemporary series of 216 children (mean age 6.6 years) with a mean stone size of 14.9 mm undergoing SWL with the Dornier HM3 lithotriptor, Landau and colleagues[29] reported a 3-month stone-free rate of 80%, demonstrating that efficacious stone-free rates can be achieved in appropriate candidates. Complications rates are minimal, and range in severity from hematuria and ecchymosis to obstruction with sepsis.[30] Although well tolerated in children, current stone-free rates with SWL are difficult to interpret from the existing body of data due to discrepancies between studies with regard to type of lithotriptor, number of shocks administered, and retreatment rates. Recent data suggest that stone-free rates in children with a history of urologic condition or urinary tract reconstruction are low (12.5%) and, with alternative surgical techniques available, may be better served with URS or PCNL.[31] Despite encouraging results, SWL has not been approved by the Food and Drug Administration for use in children, although it is a widely accepted treatment modality.

SWL Technique in Children

General anesthesia is administered in a majority of smaller children to avoid both patient and stone motion, and the need for repeated repositioning.

With modern lithotriptors, intravenous sedation has been successfully employed in select older children.[32] Bowel preparation is seldom utilized to avoid dehydration and electrolyte imbalance postoperatively. The number of shocks delivered and the kilovoltage used vary per lithotripter, but the current consensus is that low power settings (17–22 kV) be used to prevent stone migration during the procedure, with 3000 shock waves per session (<2000 in very young children).[30] A recent report assessed and compared the number and intensity of shock waves required for stone fragmentation in 44 children (mean age 5.9 years) and 562 adults (mean age 40.9 years). With an equivalent number of sessions (1.1 vs 1.1), the mean number of shockwaves (950 vs 1262, $P<.001$) and the kV required (11.8 vs 12.4, $P<.001$) were significantly reduced in the pediatric cohort.[33] Although still a controversial matter and dependent on stone burden and anatomy, the authors do not routinely stent children prior to SWL. However, ureteral catheters are occasionally employed to aid in the localization of radiolucent calculi.

Stone Size, Location, Composition, and Patient Age

Whereas early series focused primarily on the feasibility, safety, and efficacy of SWL in children, recent efforts have centered on identifying demographic, anatomic, and stone-related prognostic factors for treatment success. SWL is currently considered the primary treatment for upper tract calculi 15 mm or smaller in children,[30] but evidence supporting this stone size cut-off is lacking, Ather and Noor[24] analyzed the correlation between stone size and clearance in 105 children younger than 14 years. These investigators reported an overall stone-free rate of 95% after a mean of 1.7 treatments, with 5% of patients requiring additional procedures as adjuncts to SWL. With a maximum of 30 mm, mean stone size in the treatment success group was 14 mm compared with 16 mm in the treatment failure group. In contrast, Elsobky and colleagues[21] reported a 91% stone-free rate versus 75% stone-free rate for mean stone diameter less than and greater than 10 mm, respectively. Recently, Shouman and colleagues[34] reported a series of 24 children with a mean stone size of 31 mm undergoing SWL with the Dornier DoLi S device. In 53 sessions requiring a mean number of 3489 shock waves per session, stone-free and complication rates were 83.3% and 25%, respectively. While it is possible to treat very large stone burdens with SWL, concerns include the necessity of more shock treatments, more frequent retreatment sessions,

Table 1
Outcomes of shock wave lithotripsy in children

Report	Lithotripter	Children/Renal Units	Mean Age (y)	Stone Location (%)	Mean Size (mm)	Retreatment Rate (%)	Stone Free (%)	Complications (%)
Myers et al[20]	Siemans Lithostar	446	13.7 R 14.1 U	53.4 R 46.6 U	12.3 R 7.3 U	10.7 R 3.5 U	67.9 R 91.1 U	Sepsis 0.2
Muslumanoglu et al[22]	Siemans Lithostar	344	8.7	57.1 R 42.9 U	n/a	53.9	73.3	Overall 9.6 Steinstrausse 7.8 UTI 1.2 Colic 2.9
Rizvi et al[23]	EDAP LT02 Technomed	262	n/a	67.6 R 32.4 U	n/a	29.5	84.2 R 54.1 U	Colic 10.1 Fever 8.5 Steinstrausse 1.1 Hematuria 11.3
Aksoy et al[25]	Dornier MPL 9000	129/134	8.7	84.4 R 15.6 U	15.7	n/a	85%	Overall 14.7 Steinstrausse 5.4 UTI 7.8 Hematoma 0.8
Raza et al[26]	Piezolith 2300; Dornier Compact Delta	122/140	7.7	n/a	17.9	n/a	69	Fever 2.9 Colic 7.2 Steinstrausse 2.4
Demirkesen et al[27]	Siemans Lithostar	126/151	8 (median)	66.9 R 33.1 LP	10 R 6 LP	40	71.5	Overall 7.2 fever 0.8 Steinstrausse 6.4
Nelson et al[31]	Dornier Compact Delta	111	10.5	87.4 R 12.6 U	8	22	58.6	Overall 7 Obstruction 2 UTI 2 Hematoma 2
Landau et al[29]	Dornier HM3	216	6.6	72.7 R 27.3 U	14.9 R 9.5 U	19.7 R 22 U	80 R 78 U	Overall 2.8 Fever 0.5 Obstruction 0.5 UTI 0.5 Pain 0.9

Abbreviations: LP, lower pole; n/a, no data available; R, renal; S, staghorn; U, ureteral; UP, upper pole; UTI, urinary tract infection.
Adapted from Smaldone MC, Gayed BA, Ost MC. The evolution of the endourologic management of pediatric stone disease. Indian J Urol 2009;25(3):302–11; with permission.

and increased risk of postoperative obstruction. Further study delineating a clear size cut-off for uncomplicated upper tract stone burden is required to effectively counsel parents regarding the most effective first-line therapy for renal calculi between 1 and 1.5 cm.

Renal anatomy and stone location has been subject of recent interest. The subject of frequent debate in the adult population, the most effective management of lower pole calculi in children has yet to be determined. Stone-free rates from initial small retrospective SWL series range from 56% to 61%[35,36] with retreatment rates as high as 40%.[36] SWL failure and retreatment rates were associated with increased mean stone burden,[36] increased infundibular length,[35] and infundibulopelvic angle greater than 45°.[35] Staghorn calculi are uncommon in children and represent a management challenge. Although monotherapy success rates are low in adults, acceptable stone-free rates in children have been achieved with SWL. In 23 children stratified by age with a mean stone burden of 1.6 cm, Lottmann and colleagues[37] reported an overall stone-free rate of 82.6% with only one case of symptomatic obstruction. A ureteral stent was placed in 22% of children, and these investigators reported an 88% stone-free rate in children younger than 2 years compared with 71% in children aged 6 to 11 years. In 42 children with a mean stone burden of 3.2 cm stratified by ureteral stent placement, Al-Busaidy and colleagues[38] reported an overall stone-free rate of 79%. Although stent placement did not affect stone-free rates, the investigators found that stent placement significantly reduced the major complication rate. The superior success rates with SWL monotherapy in children compared with adults have been attributed to softer stone composition, smaller relative stone volume, increased ureteral compliance to accommodate stone fragments, and smaller body volume to facilitate shock transmission. SWL safety and efficacy have been demonstrated even in very young children. McLorie and colleagues[39] treated 34 children younger than 3.5 years (mean age 23 months) and reported an 86% overall stone-free rate (66% after one treatment) without major complications. Treatment of proximal ureteral stones has achieved similar success rates to renal stones in most pediatric series, although ureteral stenting is more commonly employed to aid in stone localization and clearance.[20] Treatment of mid to distal ureteral calculi have historically been avoided in children because of difficulties with localization over the sacroiliac joint and concern regarding possible injury to developing reproductive systems.

SWL success by stone composition is similar between the adult and pediatric populations. Cystine stones are uniquely challenging due to their durability and high recurrence rates. While SWL monotherapy has demonstrated variable results in adults, there are few reports on the pediatric population. In a small recent series, Slavkovic and colleagues[40] reported a 50% stone-free rate in 6 children with cystine stone burden ranging from 0.2 to 2.5 cm. Although stone-free rates were low, fragmentation was achieved in 100% of patients, and the stone dissolution was achieved with medical therapy in the remaining children following SWL. Investigators have proposed that cystine stones formed within 2 years of therapy may be more easily fragmented with SWL, and that stone number, and not diameter, may be more predictive of success.[30]

Limitations and Concerns

In children there is currently no consensus regarding the maximum size of residual stone fragments (RF) that are considered clinically significant,[4,30] and as a result there is no clear definition as to what constitutes "stone-free" status. While children have been shown to have a greater capacity to clear fragments than adults,[41] the presence of RFs has been correlated with adverse clinical outcome.[16] Afshar and colleagues[16] followed 26 renal units with RFs of 5 mm or smaller, and reported that while 31% were asymptomatic with no fragment growth, 69% had adverse clinical outcomes including RF growth or clinical symptoms. Patients with RF had a significant increase in adverse clinical outcome compared with stone-free subjects, and the presence of metabolic disorders was associated with RF growth. For these reasons, metabolic evaluations are now routinely being performed in children with a history of calculi, and every attempt should be made to achieve stone-free status. It is currently unclear whether placement of a ureteral stent prior to SWL facilitates fragment passage and improves stone-free outcomes. Although pre-stenting rates are not consistent across series, current relative indications include cases of solitary kidneys, staghorn calculi, large ureteral calculi, obstruction, and abnormal anatomy, not being based on total stone burden.

Although SWL is well tolerated in children with few complications, stone-free rates following single-session monotherapy remain as low as 44%.[22] As a result, children are subjected to multiple treatments requiring general anesthesia.[32] The need for multiple treatment sessions is concerning because the effects of shock waves on renal tissue are unclear. A growing body of evidence in adults indicates that shock waves result in renal vessel vasoconstriction, and that renal tubular injury and subcapsular hematoma from cavitation and shear forces are dependent on the kilovoltage applied.[42] In a large series of 340 adult patients with a mean follow-up of 19 years post SWL, Krambeck and colleagues[43] reported an increased risk of hypertension and diabetes mellitus related to bilateral treatment, number of administered shocks, and treatment intensity. Although these results are concerning, differences between pediatric and adult populations and limitations inherent to a questionnaire-based retrospective study make application of these data in children difficult. Retrospective studies with limited follow-up in children have reported that SWL and PCNL do not cause renal morphologic or functional alteration measured by glomerular filtration rate and serial dimercaptosuccinic acid functional studies,[44] but long-term data to date are unavailable. To eliminate confounding variables and fully address the risks of chronic renal damage from SWL, long-term prospective data in children are clearly required.

PERCUTANEOUS NEPHROLITHOTOMY

The safety and efficacy of PCNL for large stone burdens have been well established in adults.

Initially urologists were reluctant to perform PCNL in children due to concerns regarding the use of large instruments in pediatric kidneys, parenchymal damage and the associated effects on renal function, radiation exposure with fluoroscopy, and the risks of major complications including sepsis and bleeding. However, with increasing experience (**Table 2**),[23,45–51] PCNL is currently being used as monotherapy and in combination with SWL (sandwich therapy) in children achieving stone-free rates ranging from 68% to 100%.[23,52] Although there is no current international consensus, relative indications for PCNL as primary therapy in children include large upper tract stone burden (>1.5 cm), lower pole calculi greater than 1 cm, concurrent anatomic abnormality impairing urinary drainage and stone clearance, or known cystine or struvite composition.[4,30]

Initially described in children by Mor and colleagues[53] in 1997, early pediatric PCNL series described the use of adult-sized instruments. Although initial series avoided performing PCNL in very small children (<5 years of age) due to concerns regarding parenchymal damage, multiple series using adult-sized instruments have reported high efficacy rates with acceptable complication rates, even when dilating tract size

Table 2
Outcomes of percutaneous nephrolithotomy in children

Study	No. of Children/ Renal Units	Mean Age (y)	Stone Size (mm)	Transfusion (%)	Stone Free (%)	Sandwich Therapy (%)	Complications (%)
Badawy et al[45]	60	6	n/a	3.3	90	1.7	Fever 8.3 Colon injury 1.7 Urine leak 3.3 Open conversion 5
Zeren et al[46]	55/62	7.9	16.8	23.9	86.9	1.6	Fever 29.8 Open conversion 1.6
Rizvi et al[23]	62	n/a	47	25.3	67.7	27.4	Open conversion 4.8 Fever 46.8 Urine leak 6.4 Hydrothorax 1.6
Desai et al[47]	56	9.1	18.4	14.3	89.8	5.4	Urine leak 5.4
Salah et al[48]	135/138	8.9	22.5	0.7	98.6	0	Urine leak 8
Holman et al[49]	138	8.9	22.5	0.4	98.5	0	Fever 1.1 Urine leak 8
Samad et al[50]	169/188	8.2	27.2	4	59.3	34.5	Fever 42.8 Hyponatremia 0.1 Obstruction 0.1
Shokeir et al[51]	75/82	6.6	14.4	1.2	95.1	4.8	Urine leak 1.2

Abbreviations: EHL, electrohydraulic lithotripsy; HL, holmium laser; n/a, no data available; US, ultrasound.

Adapted from Smaldone MC, Gayed BA, Ost MC. The evolution of the endourologic management of pediatric stone disease. Indian J Urol 2009;25(3):302–11; with permission.

as high as 30 French (30F).[46,48,50,54] In fact, recent data have suggested that PCNL is possible in very young children using adult-size equipment.[55] Despite these successes, early efforts focused on developing technology to minimize percutaneous tract size without affecting PCNL efficacy. Jackman and colleagues[56] developed a novel percutaneous access technique ("mini-perc") using a 13F peel-away vascular access sheath, and reported an 85% stone-free rate for 11 procedures in 7 children with a mean age of 3.4 years. The benefits of minimal tract dilation include increased maneuverability, decreased blood loss, and shorter hospital stay. However, theoretical limitations including prolonged operative times and impaired visualization from bleeding imply that this technique may not be adequate for very large stone burdens. Recent advancements in instrumentation such as smaller nephroscopes (15–18F) and more efficient energy sources for intracorporeal lithotripsy, including holmium:YAG laser and smaller pneumatic lithoclast and ultrasound probes, have greatly facilitated percutaneous treatment techniques. As a result, PCNL has now replaced open surgery as the treatment of choice for large stone burdens in children of all ages.

Percutaneous Nephrolithotomy Technique in Children

All percutaneous procedures are performed using general anesthesia and antibiotic prophylaxis. A warm operating room, body temperature isotonic irrigation solution, brief anesthetic induction, short operative times, proper draping, and monitoring of body temperature should decrease the incidence of hypothermia and hyponatremia. After induction of anesthesia with the patient in the lithotomy position, a retrograde pyelogram is performed to outline the collecting system and an occlusive balloon catheter is left in situ. The patient is then repositioned in the prone position with the torso elevated at 30° from the table surface with a towel roll.[30]

Circumstances that require special consideration involve children with spinal anomalies such as spina bifida. In these patients, positioning can be a challenge due to existing spinal hardware and limb contracture.[57] Patients who have had prior spinal surgery consisting of vertebral fusion or Harrington rod placement will have restricted spinal mobility, spinal curvature, and/or atrophic or contracted extremities. Assessing the degree of mobility in the trunk and extremities is crucial in planning for PCNL in these patients. These patients must be placed in the most comfortable position possible, without excessive contortion or flexion of the joints. Special attention must be paid to latex precautions in the myelomeningocele population and, as in all cases, proper padding of pressure points is mandatory.

After selection of the desired calyx, an 18-gauge spinal needle is placed with the assistance of fluoroscopy in 2 planes. The ideal tract is one that provides the shortest and most direct access to the stone. For complex calculi occupying multiple calices including the lower pole, a supracostal posterior access is preferred to provide visualization of the superior calyx and pelvis, access to the pelvis and ureter, and straight access to the inferior calices allowing easier manipulation of the working instruments and minimizing torque on the collecting system.[58] Following initial puncture, no attempt should be made to redirect the needle while it is located within the cortex of the kidney to avoid trauma. After access is confirmed with urine or irrigation return, a flexible guide wire is placed into the collecting system through the needle and directed down the ureter into the bladder. A small skin incision is made with a No. 11 scalpel, and 8F and 10F coaxial dilators are passed over the guide wire into the collecting system. Once in place, an Amplatz Super Stiff guide wire is placed as a working wire.

Tract dilation can be performed by several techniques. Serial dilation with Amplatz dilators over working wires and subsequent sheath placement under fluoroscopic guidance is the most common technique employed. Alternatively, a 13F peel-away sheath (Docimo Mini-Perc, Cook Urological Inc, Spencer, IN, USA) and trocar are passed over the wire into the calyx under fluoroscopic guidance and the trocar is removed. The authors have had success using the NephroMax High Pressure Nephrostomy Balloon Catheter (Boston Scientific, Natick, MA, USA), which facilitates dilation to 30F at a pressure of 17 atmospheres. This technique permits dilation and sheath placement in a single step, thereby minimizing potential parenchymal trauma and bleeding from sequential dilation with metal dilators. While the decision to proceed with mini-perc or dilation is individualized based on child's age, anatomy, and stone burden, familiarity with all of the above techniques facilitates complete access with minimal morbidity.

Once access is obtained, nephroscopy and nephrolithotomy can be performed with a variety of energy sources for stone fragmentation. The outer diameter of nephroscopes ranges from 17 to 26F, and a 15F flexible nephroscope with a 6F working channel has also been developed. In addition, 7F and 8F offset cystoscopes with 5F working ports and 7F to 9F flexible ureteroscopes can be used through an 11F access sheath, with enough clearance to allow low-pressure irrigation.[4] Energy sources currently used include ultrasonic lithotripsy, electrohydraulic lithotripsy (EHL), and the holmium laser, although individual preference is determined by availability and surgeon experience. Postoperative stenting and/or placement of a nephrostomy tube are both patient and surgeon dependent, and vary between series. Similar to adult procedures, tubeless PCNL has theoretical advantages including decreased postoperative pain and a short hospital stay, but currently data are limited in the pediatric population.[59]

Percutaneous Nephrolithotomy Outcomes

Recent large retrospective series of PCNL monotherapy have demonstrated high efficacy rates approaching 90%.[46,47,54] In 56 children (mean age 9.1 years) with a mean stone burden of 337.5 mm^2, Desai and colleagues[47] reported a stone-free rate of 89.8% using EHL through a 14F nephroscope and a 20F to 24F sheath. Of these, 61% required multiple tracts and 45% were staged procedures. Findings demonstrated that the number and size of tracts were significantly associated with postoperative hemoglobin decrease (mean 1.9 g/dL) and overall transfusion rate (14%). In 52 children with a mean age of 7.9 years and a mean stone burden of 282 mm^2, Zeren and colleagues[46] reported an 87% stone-free rate using ultrasound and EHL for fragmentation and tract dilation from 18 to 30Fr. Complications included post operative fever (30%) and need for transfusion (24%). Transfusion was associated with operative time, sheath size, and stone burden. In 135 children aged 8.9 years with a mean stone burden of 507 mm^2, Salah and colleagues[48] reported a 98.5% stone-free rate using ultrasound through a 26F nephroscope. Complications were low (8% urine leak rate and 0.7% transfusion rate), with only one patient requiring a second procedure. In a recent series of 46 children with a mean stone burden of 332 mm^2, Bilen and colleagues[54] reported an 88% stone-free rate using EHL, ultrasound, and the holmium laser. When stratified by tract size (14F, 20F, and 24F), efficacy rates were similar in all groups, but there were no complications or transfusions in the 14F tract group.

In an effort to reduce the number of tracts and associated morbidity, some centers have chosen to follow primary PCNL with adjunctive SWL therapy to clear RFs. In a small series of 29 children with a mean age of 3.8 years and a mean stone burden of 2.4 cm, Mahmud and Zaidi[52] reported a 60% stone-free rate after PCNL

monotherapy using EHL through a 17F angled nephroscope. Only one tract was used in all patients, and after SWL sandwich therapy the stone-free rate increased to 100%. In a larger series of 169 children with a mean stone burden of 3.1 cm, Samad and colleagues[50] reported a 59% monotherapy stone-free rate with 96% of cases performed through a single tract. Approximately one-third (34.5%) of primary failures were treated with SWL; the cumulative stone-free rate in all patients was 93.8% with a 3.6% transfusion rate. When stratified by age, anatomy, bilaterality, and renal function, stone-free outcomes were equivalent in all groups. The decision to follow PCNL with SWL is related to operator experience with percutaneous technique and available technology. It is the authors' preference to perform a second-look nephroscopy through the original tract to ensure stone-free status during the initial hospital admission rather than progress to SWL sandwich therapy. Endoscopic surveillance during the initial procedure can determine the need for second-look nephroscopy without relying on additional imaging and the associated risks of radiation exposure.[60] With continued improvement in technology and technique, the indications for PCNL in children will continue to increase. Technically challenging in nature, surgeon experience with PCNL is paramount in developing individualized treatment plans to optimize efficacy with minimal morbidity.

URETEROSCOPY

Adoption of URS for the treatment of pediatric stone disease has lagged behind that of adults due to concerns regarding the use of large ureteroscopes in small-caliber ureters, a higher post-SWL stone fragment clearance rate compared with adults,[41] and the low incidence of stone formation in children. Since the mid 1980s, with the acceptance of SWL as primary therapy for upper tract calculi smaller than 1.5 cm, URS has been historically used for calculi below the iliac crests, and for upper tract calculi after SWL failure.[4] URS was not considered primary therapy for upper tract stones in children because of concern for ureteral ischemia, perforation, stricture formation, and development of vesicoureteral reflux as a result of dilation of small-caliber ureteral orifices.

With significant improvements in both the miniaturization and durability of endoscopic equipment and the acceptance of the holmium laser, URS has become a more attractive option in young children. First described by Ritchey and colleagues[61] in 1988, early series using rigid URS for distal ureteral stones reported stone-free rates ranging from 86% to 100%, with low complication rates.[14,23,62–65] In a comparison of 31 children randomized to URS or SWL as primary therapy for distal ureteral stones, De Dominicis and colleagues[63] reported a significantly higher stone-free rate after one treatment (94% vs 43%) for children treated with URS. The results of these retrospective studies have begun to refute the notion that dilation of the pediatric ureter will result in vesicoureteral reflux or the development of ureteral strictures. In a systematic review of the literature encompassing 221 pediatric ureteroscopies, Schuster and colleagues[62] noted only 2 ureteral strictures and a minimal incidence of vesicoureteral reflux.

Early successes with treatment of distal calculi in children[66–68] have led to several centers expanding their use of URS to the treatment of upper tract calculi (**Table 3**). Findings from the first series treating upper tract calculi have recently become available, and demonstrate stone-free rates between 88% and 100% with complication rates similar to that of the adult population.[65,69–75] Lesani and Palmer[69] reported their experience using 4.5F, 6F, and 8F rigid URS in treating proximal ureteral stones in 24 children with a mean age of 10.7 years. Lesani and Palmer did not perform ureteral dilation in any cases, and 100% of children were rendered stone free. In a large series of 100 children with a mean stone diameter of 8.3 mm, of whom 52% had upper tract calculi, Smaldone and colleagues[70] reported a 91% stone-free rate with 9% of children undergoing staged procedures. With a mean follow-up of 10 months, they reported a 4.2% perforation rate managed with ureteral stenting and one distal ureteral stricture requiring open neocystostomy. Corcoran and colleagues[71] reviewed their cohort of 47 children (mean age 9.4 years) with upper tract calculi managed with flexible URS and holmium laser lithotripsy. With a mean stone burden of 10.2 mm, they reported an 88% stone-free rate with 26% requiring staged procedures. In the largest series to date, Kim and colleagues[74] reported their results in 167 children undergoing 170 flexible URS treatments. Choosing to pre-stent to allow passive dilation in 95 children (57%) if retrograde access could not be obtained, they reported 100% stone clearance for stone burdens 10 mm or less and 97% for stone burdens greater than 10 mm (mean stone burden 6.1 mm).

As the indications for URS in children continue to expand, acceptable stone-free rates have been reported for increasingly large stone burdens. In 23 children with a mean stone size of 17 mm, Dave and colleagues[73] reported stone-free rates of 75% for renal pelvis calculi and

100% for polar stones. However, in 7 children with partial staghorn stones, the stone-free rate was only 14%, implying that complex stone burdens involving more than one calyx may be more amenable to PCNL. Supporting this notion, a recent report observed that 71% of upper tract calculi greater than 10 mm in diameter required more than one procedure to achieve stone-free status,[75] indicating that there still is room for improvement in the ureteroscopic management of the upper tract. Adoption of techniques used in the adult population, most notably sequential coaxial and balloon dilation of the ureteral orifice and use of ureteral access sheaths, may facilitate the treatment of larger stone burdens during a single session. Initially described in 8 children by Singh and colleagues,[76] ureteral access sheaths have been shown to facilitate repetitive upper tract access, reduce intrarenal pressures, decrease operative time, and improve stone-free rates in adults. In the authors' experience, use of ureteral access sheaths and the 6.9F flexible ureteroscope has made possible treatment of lower pole calculi that would have previously required SWL or PCNL. Cannon and colleagues[72] reported a 76% stone-free rate in 21 children with lower pole calculi and a mean stone diameter of 12.2 cm. After a mean of 11.4 months, no major complications were observed. With the transition from SWL to URS as a primary treatment modality at the authors' institution, current relative contraindications to ureteroscopic management include staghorn stones in recurrent stone formers more amenable to PCNL, anatomic anomalies making retrograde access difficult, and previous endoscopic failure.

Ureteroscopic Technique in Children

All ureteroscopic procedures are performed under general anesthesia to prevent patient movement and minimize the risk of ureteral perforation. Following antibiotic prophylaxis, patients are placed in the lithotomy position and rigid cystoscopy (7.5F, 11F, or 18F) is performed to place a safety or working wire. Under fluoroscopic guidance, the guide wire is advanced into the renal pelvis or beyond the level of the stone. Ureteral orifice dilation is performed with 8/10F coaxial dilators in ureters that have not been pre-stented, or when the rigid/flexible ureteroscope cannot easily be advanced. The authors generally do not use balloon dilation of the ureteral orifice because of concern for development of ureteral stricture from ischemia. The bias is that use of the 8/10 dilator allows for tactile feedback regarding the tightness of the ureter, which is not available with

Table 3
Outcomes of rigid and flexible ureteroscopy in children

Study	Number of Children/No. of Procedures	Mean Age (y)	Stone Size (mm)	Stone Location (%)	Ureteral Orifice Dilation (%)	Stone Free (%)	Staged (%)	Postoperative Stenting (%)	Complications (%)
Rigid ureteroscopy for mid to distal ureteral calculi									
Al-Busaidy et al[66]	43/47	6.2	12.6	100 U	n/a	93	n/a	n/a	Ureteral perforation 4, Ureteral stricture 2, Fever/VUR 12
Bassiri et al[67]	66/66	9	8	100 U	37.9	88	n/a	n/a	Renal colic 1.5, Gross hematuria 16.7, Pyelonephritis 4.5
Raza et al[68]	35/52	5.9	9.4	100 U	3.9	79.3	28.6	n/a	Ureteral stricture 2, Fever 10, Ureteral perforation 6
Rigid and flexible ureteroscopy for upper tract and renal calculi									
Minevich et al[65]	58/65	7.5	n/a	64.6 U, 35.4 P	30	98	n/a	85	Ureteral stricture 1.3
Smaldone et al[70]	100/115	13.2	8.3	52 R, 48 U	70	91	9	75	Ureteral perforation 4.2, Ureteral stricture 1
Cannon et al[72]	21/21	15.1	12.2	100 LP	81	76	14	71	0
Corcoran et al[71]	47/61	9.4	10.2	100 R	91	88	26	70	Ureteral perforation 9
Kim et. al[74]	167/170	5.2	6.1	60 P, 40 U	0	77.3	N/A	98.2	0
Tanaka et al[75]	50/52	7.9	8.0	75 R, 25 LP	35	76	34.6	98	Nausea/pain 2

Abbreviations: EHL, electrohydraulic lithotripsy; HL, holmium laser; LP, lower pole; n/a, no data available; P, proximal; R, renal; U, ureteral.
Adapted from Smaldone MC, Gayed BA, Ost MC. The evolution of the endourologic management of pediatric stone disease. Indian J Urol 2009;25(3):302–11; with permission.

balloon dilation. If the authors encounter difficulty with the 8/10 dilator, preference is to place a stent and return for a second procedure rather than dilate more aggressively.

The decision to use a flexible (6.9F) or semirigid (7.5F) ureteroscope is made depending on size and location of stone, anatomic factors, and individual surgeon preference. A 4.5F rigid ureteroscope is also currently available for use, although the authors' experience with this device is limited. Rigid or semirigid ureteroscopy is routinely performed with a safety wire in place while flexible ureteroscopy is performed with both a safety and working wire in place. Ureteral access sheaths (internal diameter of 9.5F or 12F) are used in select cases to facilitate flexible URS in cases of large proximal ureteral or renal pelvis stone burdens. Irrigating fluid, which may be used under pressure, should be isotonic and at body temperature to avoid hypothermia and hyponatremia. Calculi are extracted with a basket when feasible or fragmented using the holmium:YAG laser to facilitate removal. Other energy sources for fragmentation available include ultrasound lithotripsy and EHL. The decision to place a ureteral stent postoperatively is made based on the duration of the procedure, number of passes with the ureteroscope, and degree of visible ureteral trauma or edema at the conclusion of the procedure. If the patient can tolerate leaving a urethral string in place for 3 days to 1 week, the patient's parents are asked to remove the stent at home; otherwise the stent is removed under brief anesthetic after 7 days.

Concerns and Limitations

With smaller, more durable ureteroscopes and improved optics for visualization, URS is becoming more prominent in the pediatric endourologist's armamentarium of stone management techniques. However, many unanswered questions still need to be addressed. In postpubertal children with an adult body mass, ureteroscopic access is technically similar to that for the adult population. In the small prepubertal child, questions regarding whether to attempt primary treatment without ureteral orifice dilation, perform dilation at the time of definitive therapy, or to place a stent and allow the ureter to passively dilate prior to definitive therapy remain. In 29 children with a mean age of 11 years, Herndon and colleagues[77] performed semirigid URS with 4.5F and 6.5F ureteroscopes for distal ureteral calculi. Fourteen percent of children were pre-stented, but no child was actively dilated. The ureter was accessed in 100% of cases for a stone-free rate of 96%. Because the authors' flexible and semirigid

ureteroscopes are 6.9F and 7.5F, respectively, it is their preference to sequentially dilate with the 8/10 coaxial dilator even in very young children, but if difficulty is encountered a stent is placed rather than dilating more aggressively. While the authors believe this approach minimizes long-term complication rates, particularly in the management of upper tract calculi, it increases the number of children who require a second anesthetic and procedure to achieve stone-free status. The authors' recent finding that 40% of pediatric patients will require at least 2 procedures to treat upper tract calculi ureteroscopically suggests that with the current equipment, the likelihood of achieving a stone-free state after one ureteroscopic procedure may not be significantly better than with SWL.[71] Another area of contention is the necessity of placing a post-URS stent in all children. Whereas the tendency in large series has been to leave a stent in place after ureteroscopic manipulation in a majority of children,[70] some investigators have reported no acute or long-term sequelae despite leaving a post-URS stent in less than 20% of cases.[71] In the authors' experience, the decision to place a post-URS stent is made on an individual patient basis, and is dependent on surgeon experience and degree of visible ureteral trauma at the conclusion of the procedure.

LAPAROSCOPIC AND ROBOTIC-ASSISTED PYELOLITHOTOMY

Treatment of large stone burdens in children is technically challenging, often requiring multiple procedures. Laparoscopy and robotic-assisted laparoscopy has been used successfully in adults for treatment of calculi during the concomitant treatment of ureteropelvic junction obstruction and in the primary treatment of staghorn calculi. Small series using these techniques in children have only recently been described. In 8 children (mean age 4 years) with a mean stone burden of 2.9 cm undergoing transperitoneal laparoscopic pyelolithotomy, Casale and colleagues[78] reported a 100% success rate, a mean hospital stay of 2.15 days, and a mean operative time of 1.6 hours with no major complications. In the first report of robotic-assisted laparoscopic pyelolithotomy, Lee and colleagues[79] described their experience of 5 patients; 4 with cystine staghorn calculi refractory to PCNL and SWL and 1 with calcium oxalate calculi and concurrent ureteropelvic junction obstruction. Of these cases, 4 were completed robotically, with 1 patient having a residual 6-mm lower pole stone and 1 patient requiring conversion to an open procedure. Mean operative time in this series was 315 minutes, mean estimated blood loss was less than 20 mL, and the mean hospital length of stay was 3.8 days. These early experiences demonstrate that laparoscopic pyelolithotomy is feasible, safe, and efficacious as an alternative to open pyelolithotomy in children, and warrants further study. However, due to their demanding technical nature, these procedures will likely be limited to endourologic management failures in academic centers with abundant expertise in laparoscopic and robotic pediatric surgery.

DETERMINATION OF STONE-FREE STATUS

As the surgical management of pediatric stone disease evolves, the lack of a consistent definition of "stone-free" following definitive therapy is an issue that remains unaddressed. Although controversial, in select adult patients all stone fragments can be considered clinically significant and can lead to stone recurrence.[80] Likewise, the presence of RFs in children has been associated with poor outcomes,[16] and any size of stone fragment in a young stone former may result in the need for repeat surgical procedures. However, these fragments often are not detected on ultrasound or kidney-ureter-bladder radiography, necessitating reliance on CT imaging in select children.

Balancing the risks of radiation exposure for posttreatment stone detection and the risks of anesthesia for secondary procedures is a challenging dilemma for contemporary pediatric endourologists. Newer, high-speed helical CT scanners reduce radiation exposure and rarely require intravenous sedation. In addition, maximizing intraoperative fragment detection by direct visualization in URS and PCNL and continued development of high-resolution real-time fluoroscopy may result in less reliance on postoperative imaging and may decrease the need for second-look nephroscopy/URS, SWL, or sandwich therapy.[81] Until the risks of radiation exposure in children are more clearly defined, surveillance in these children will be individualized based on age, anatomy, stone burden, and underlying metabolic abnormalities.

SUMMARY

Evolution of technique and miniaturization of instruments have changed the management of pediatric stone disease. However, despite encouraging results, concern remains regarding safety of endourologic treatment in smaller patients and its subsequent effects on the growing kidney. While SWL is still considered first-line therapy for upper tract calculi smaller than 1.5 cm, evidence is accumulating that URS may be more efficacious in treating upper tract stone disease in children. While PCNL remains the most effective technique for large upper tract stone burdens, there are now reports of laparoscopic and robotic-assisted laparoscopic pyelolithotomy in major pediatric academic centers with extensive laparoscopic and robotic experience. Prospective randomized studies designed to evaluate the endourologic management of upper tract calculi in children are sorely needed, and until these data are available, individual surgeon experience is the most important factor in determining the appropriate treatment modality. Similar to endourologic management in the adult population, familiarity with the full spectrum of endourologic techniques facilitates a minimally invasive approach to the entire pediatric urinary tract.

REFERENCES

1. Novak TE, Lakshmanan Y, Trock BJ, et al. Sex prevalence of pediatric kidney stone disease in the United States: an epidemiologic investigation. Urology 2009;74(1):104–7.
2. Rizvi SA, Naqvi SA, Hussain Z, et al. Pediatric urolithiasis: developing nation perspectives. J Urol 2002;168(4 Pt 1):1522–5.
3. Hesse A, Brandle E, Wilbert D, et al. Study on the prevalence and incidence of urolithiasis in Germany comparing the years 1979 vs. 2000. Eur Urol 2003; 44(6):709–13.
4. Wu HY, Docimo SG. Surgical management of children with urolithiasis. Urol Clin North Am 2004; 31(3):589–94, xi.
5. Alpay H, Ozen A, Gokce I, et al. Clinical and metabolic features of urolithiasis and microlithiasis in children. Pediatr Nephrol 2009;24(11):2203–9.
6. Spivacow FR, Negri AL, del Valle EE, et al. Metabolic risk factors in children with kidney stone disease. Pediatr Nephrol 2008;23(7):1129–33.
7. Sternberg K, Greenfield SP, Williot P, et al. Pediatric stone disease: an evolving experience. J Urol 2005; 174(4 Pt 2):1711–4 [discussion: 1714].
8. Kalorin CM, Zabinski A, Okpareke I, et al. Pediatric urinary stone disease—does age matter? J Urol 2009;181(5):2267–71 [discussion: 2271].
9. Palmer JS, Donaher ER, O'Riordan MA, et al. Diagnosis of pediatric urolithiasis: role of ultrasound and computerized tomography. J Urol 2005;174(4 Pt 1):1413–6.
10. Oner S, Oto A, Tekgul S, et al. Comparison of spiral CT and US in the evaluation of pediatric urolithiasis. JBR-BTR 2004;87(5):219–23.
11. Rice HE, Frush DP, Farmer D, et al. Review of radiation risks from computed tomography: essentials for

the pediatric surgeon. J Pediatr Surg 2007;42(4): 603–7.

12. Karmazyn B, Frush DP, Applegate KE, et al. CT with a computer-simulated dose reduction technique for detection of pediatric nephroureterolithiasis: comparison of standard and reduced radiation doses. AJR Am J Roentgenol 2009;192(1):143–9.

13. Borawski KM, Sur RL, Miller OF, et al. Urinary reference values for stone risk factors in children. J Urol 2008;179(1):290–4 [discussion: 294].

14. Van Savage JG, Palanca LG, Andersen RD, et al. Treatment of distal ureteral stones in children: similarities to the American Urological Association guidelines in adults. J Urol 2000;164(3 Pt 2):1089–93.

15. Porpiglia F, Ghignone G, Fiori C, et al. Nifedipine versus tamsulosin for the management of lower ureteral stones. J Urol 2004;172(2):568–71.

16. Afshar K, McLorie G, Papanikolaou F, et al. Outcome of small residual stone fragments following shock wave lithotripsy in children. J Urol 2004;172(4 Pt 2):1600–3.

17. Wolf JS Jr, Bennett CJ, Dmochowski RR, et al. Best practice policy statement on urologic surgery antimicrobial prophylaxis. J Urol 2008;179(4):1379–90.

18. Conway PH, Cnaan A, Zaoutis T, et al. Recurrent urinary tract infections in children: risk factors and association with prophylactic antimicrobials. JAMA 2007;298(2):179–86.

19. Newman DM, Coury T, Lingeman JE, et al. Extracorporeal shock wave lithotripsy experience in children. J Urol 1986;136(1 Pt 2):238–40.

20. Myers DA, Mobley TB, Jenkins JM, et al. Pediatric low energy lithotripsy with the Lithostar. J Urol 1995;153(2):453–7.

21. Elsobky E, Sheir KZ, Madbouly K, et al. Extracorporeal shock wave lithotripsy in children: experience using two second-generation lithotripters. BJU Int 2000;86(7):851–6.

22. Muslumanoglu AY, Tefekli A, Sarilar O, et al. Extracorporeal shock wave lithotripsy as first line treatment alternative for urinary tract stones in children: a large scale retrospective analysis. J Urol 2003; 170(6 Pt 1):2405–8.

23. Rizvi SA, Naqvi SA, Hussain Z, et al. Management of pediatric urolithiasis in Pakistan: experience with 1,440 children. J Urol 2003;169(2):634–7.

24. Ather MH, Noor MA. Does size and site matter for renal stones up to 30-mm in size in children treated by extracorporeal lithotripsy? Urology 2003;61(1): 212–5 [discussion: 215].

25. Aksoy Y, Ozbey I, Atmaca AF, et al. Extracorporeal shock wave lithotripsy in children: experience using a mpl-9000 lithotriptor. World J Urol 2004;22(2):115–9.

26. Raza A, Turna B, Smith G, et al. Pediatric urolithiasis: 15 years of local experience with minimally invasive endourological management of pediatric calculi. J Urol 2005;174(2):682–5.

27. Demirkesen O, Onal B, Tansu N, et al. Efficacy of extracorporeal shock wave lithotripsy for isolated lower caliceal stones in children compared with stones in other renal locations. Urology 2006;67(1): 170–4 [discussion: 174–5].

28. Defoor W, Dharamsi N, Smith P, et al. Use of mobile extracorporeal shock wave lithotripter: experience in a pediatric institution. Urology 2005;65(4):778–81.

29. Landau EH, Shenfeld OZ, Pode D, et al. Extracorporeal shock wave lithotripsy in prepubertal children: 22-year experience at a single institution with a single lithotriptor. J Urol 2009;182(Suppl 4): 1835–9.

30. Farhat WA, Kropp BP. Surgical treatment of pediatric urinary stones. AUA Update Series 2007;26(3):22–7.

31. Nelson CP, Diamond DA, Cendron M, et al. Extracorporeal shock wave lithotripsy in pediatric patients using a late generation portable lithotriptor: experience at Children's Hospital Boston. J Urol 2008; 180(4 Suppl):1865–8.

32. Aldridge RD, Aldridge RC, Aldridge LM. Anesthesia for pediatric lithotripsy. Paediatr Anaesth 2006; 16(3):236–41.

33. Kurien A, Symons S, Manohar T, et al. Extracorporeal shock wave lithotripsy in children: equivalent clearance rates to adults is achieved with fewer and lower energy shock waves. BJU Int 2009; 103(1):81–4.

34. Shouman AM, Ziada AM, Ghoneim IA, et al. Extracorporeal shock wave lithotripsy monotherapy for renal stones >25 mm in children. Urology 2009; 74(1):109–11.

35. Ozgur Tan M, Karaoglan U, Sen I, et al. The impact of radiological anatomy in clearance of lower caliceal stones after shock wave lithotripsy in paediatric patients. Eur Urol 2003;43(2):188–93.

36. Onal B, Demirkesen O, Tansu N, et al. The impact of caliceal pelvic anatomy on stone clearance after shock wave lithotripsy for pediatric lower pole stones. J Urol 2004;172(3):1082–6.

37. Lottmann HB, Traxer O, Archambaud F, et al. Monotherapy extracorporeal shock wave lithotripsy for the treatment of staghorn calculi in children. J Urol 2001; 165(6 Pt 2):2324–7.

38. Al-Busaidy SS, Prem AR, Medhat M. Pediatric staghorn calculi: the role of extracorporeal shock wave lithotripsy monotherapy with special reference to ureteral stenting. J Urol 2003;169(2):629–33.

39. McLorie GA, Pugach J, Pode D, et al. Safety and efficacy of extracorporeal shock wave lithotripsy in infants. Can J Urol 2003;10(6):2051–5.

40. Slavkovic A, Radovanovic M, Siric Z, et al. Extracorporeal shock wave lithotripsy for cystine urolithiasis in children: outcome and complications. Int Urol Nephrol 2002;34(4):457–61.

41. Gofrit ON, Pode D, Meretyk S, et al. Is the pediatric ureter as efficient as the adult ureter in transporting

fragments following extracorporeal shock wave lithotripsy for renal calculi larger than 10 mm.? J Urol
2001;166(5):1862–4.

42. Lingeman JE, Kim SC, Kuo RL, et al. Shockwave lithotripsy: anecdotes and insights. J Endourol 2003;
17(9):687–93.

43. Krambeck AE, Gettman MT, Rohlinger AL, et al. Diabetes mellitus and hypertension associated with
shock wave lithotripsy of renal and proximal ureteral
stones at 19 years of followup. J Urol 2006;175(5):
1742–7.

44. Wadhwa P, Aron M, Bal CS, et al. Critical prospective appraisal of renal morphology and function in
children undergoing shockwave lithotripsy and
percutaneous nephrolithotomy. J Endourol 2007;
21(9):961–6.

45. Badawy H, Salama A, Eissa M, et al. Percutaneous
management of renal calculi: experience with percutaneous nephrolithotomy in 60 children. J Urol 1999;
162(5):1710–3.

46. Zeren S, Satar N, Bayazit Y, et al. Percutaneous
nephrolithotomy in the management of pediatric
renal calculi. J Endourol 2002;16(2):75–8.

47. Desai MR, Kukreja RA, Patel SH, et al. Percutaneous
nephrolithotomy for complex pediatric renal calculus
disease. J Endourol 2004;18(1):23–7.

48. Salah MA, Toth C, Khan AM, et al. Percutaneous
nephrolithotomy in children: experience with 138
cases in a developing country. World J Urol 2004;
22(4):277–80.

49. Holman E, Khan AM, Flasko T, et al. Endoscopic
management of pediatric urolithiasis in a developing
country. Urology 2004;63(1):159–62 [discussion:
162].

50. Samad L, Aquil S, Zaidi Z. Paediatric percutaneous
nephrolithotomy: setting new frontiers. BJU Int 2006;
97(2):359–63.

51. Shokeir AA, Sheir KZ, El-Nahas AR, et al. Treatment
of renal stones in children: a comparison between
percutaneous nephrolithotomy and shock wave lithotripsy. J Urol 2006;176(2):706–10.

52. Mahmud M, Zaidi Z. Percutaneous nephrolithotomy
in children before school age: experience of a Pakistani centre. BJU Int 2004;94(9):1352–4.

53. Mor Y, Elmasry YE, Kellett MJ, et al. The role of
percutaneous nephrolithotomy in the management
of pediatric renal calculi. J Urol 1997;158(3 Pt 2):
1319–21.

54. Bilen CY, Kocak B, Kitirci G, et al. Percutaneous nephrolithotomy in children: lessons learned in 5 years at
a single institution. J Urol 2007;177(5):1867–71.

55. Nouralizadeh A, Basiri A, Javaherforooshzadeh A,
et al. Experience of percutaneous nephrolithotomy
using adult-size instruments in children less than 5
years old. J Pediatr Urol 2009;5(5):351–4.

56. Jackman SV, Hedican SP, Peters CA, et al. Percutaneous nephrolithotomy in infants and preschool age

children: experience with a new technique. Urology
1998;52(4):697–701.

57. Ost MC, Lee BR. Urolithiasis in patients with spinal
cord injuries: risk factors, management, and
outcomes. Curr Opin Urol 2006;16(2):93–9.

58. El-Nahas AR, Shokeir AA, El-Kenawy MR, et al.
Safety and efficacy of supracostal percutaneous
nephrolithotomy in pediatric patients. J Urol 2008;
180(2):676–80.

59. Khairy Salem H, Morsi HA, Omran A, et al. Tubeless
percutaneous nephrolithotomy in children. J Pediatr
Urol 2007;3(3):235–8.

60. Roth CC, Donovan BO, Adams JM, et al. Use of
second look nephroscopy in children undergoing
percutaneous nephrolithotomy. J Urol 2009;181(2):
796–800.

61. Ritchey M, Patterson DE, Kelalis PP, et al. A case of
pediatric ureteroscopic lasertripsy. J Urol 1988;
139(6):1272–4.

62. Schuster TG, Russell KY, Bloom DA, et al. Ureteroscopy for the treatment of urolithiasis in children.
J Urol 2002;167(4):1813 [discussion: 1815–6].

63. De Dominicis M, Matarazzo E, Capozza N, et al.
Retrograde ureteroscopy for distal ureteric stone
removal in children. BJU Int 2005;95(7):1049–52.

64. Tan AH, Al-Omar M, Denstedt JD, et al. Ureteroscopy for pediatric urolithiasis: an evolving first-line
therapy. Urology 2005;65(1):153–6.

65. Minevich E, Defoor W, Reddy P, et al. Ureteroscopy
is safe and effective in prepubertal children. J Urol
2005;174(1):276–9 [discussion: 279].

66. Al-Busaidy SS, Prem AR, Medhat M. Paediatric ureteroscopy for ureteric calculi: a 4-year experience.
Br J Urol 1997;80(5):797–801.

67. Bassiri A, Ahmadnia H, Darabi MR, et al. Transure-
teral lithotripsy in pediatric practice. J Endourol
2002;16(4):257–60.

68. Raza A, Smith G, Moussa S, et al. Ureteroscopy in
the management of pediatric urinary tract calculi.
J Endourol 2005;19(2):151–8.

69. Lesani OA, Palmer JS. Retrograde proximal rigid
ureteroscopy and pyeloscopy in prepubertal children: safe and effective. J Urol 2006;176(4 Pt 1):
1570–3.

70. Smaldone MC, Cannon GM Jr, Wu HY, et al. Is ureteroscopy first line treatment for pediatric stone
disease? J Urol 2007;178(5):2128–31 [discussion:
2131].

71. Corcoran AT, Smaldone MC, Mally D, et al. When is
prior ureteral stent placement necessary to access
the upper urinary tract in prepubertal children? J
Urol 2008;180(4 Suppl):1861–3 [discussion: 1863–4].

72. Cannon GM, Smaldone MC, Wu HY, et al. Ureteroscopic management of lower-pole stones in a pediatric population. J Endourol 2007;21(10):1179–82.

73. Dave S, Khoury AE, Braga L, et al. Single-institu-
tional study on role of ureteroscopy and retrograde

intrarenal surgery in treatment of pediatric renal calculi. Urology 2008;72(5):1018–21.

74. Kim SS, Kolon TF, Canter D, et al. Pediatric flexible ureteroscopic lithotripsy: the children's hospital of Philadelphia experience. J Urol 2008;180(6): 2616–9 [discussion: 2619].

75. Tanaka ST, Makari JH, Pope JC, et al. Pediatric ureteroscopic management of intrarenal calculi. J Urol 2008;180(5):2150–3 [discussion: 2153–4].

76. Singh A, Shah G, Young J, et al. Ureteral access sheath for the management of pediatric renal and ureteral stones: a single center experience. J Urol 2006;175(3 Pt 1):1080–2 [discussion: 1082].

77. Herndon CD, Viamonte L, Joseph DB. Ureteroscopy in children: is there a need for ureteral dilation and postoperative stenting? J Pediatr Urol 2006;2(4): 290–3.

78. Casale P, Grady RW, Joyner BD, et al. Transperitoneal laparoscopic pyelolithotomy after failed percutaneous access in the pediatric patient. J Urol 2004;172(2):680–3 [discussion: 683].

79. Lee RS, Passerotti CC, Cendron M, et al. Early results of robot assisted laparoscopic lithotomy in adolescents. J Urol 2007;177(6):2306–9 [discussion: 2309–10].

80. Krambeck AE, LeRoy AJ, Patterson DE, et al. Long-term outcomes of percutaneous nephrolithotomy compared to shock wave lithotripsy and conservative management. J Urol 2008;179(6):2233–7.

81. Ost MC, Smith AD. Editorial comment: intraoperative fragment detection during percutaneous nephrolithotomy: evaluation of high magnification rotational fluoroscopy combined with aggressive nephroscopy. J Urol 2006;175(1):165–6.

Treatment Strategy for the Adolescent Varicocele

Samuel P. Robinson, MD, Lance J. Hampton, MD,
Harry P. Koo, MD*

KEYWORDS

• Varicocele • Adolescent • Infertility

A varicocele is a dilatation of the testicular vein and the pampiniform venous plexus within the spermatic cord. Although rare in pediatric populations, the prevalence of varicoceles markedly increases with pubertal development to approximately 15% by the late teenage years, a rate similar to that in adult populations.[1,2] Varicoceles are progressive lesions that may hinder testicular growth and function over time and are the most common and correctable cause of male infertility. The incidence of varicocele in men with abnormal semen is 25% compared with almost 12% in men with normal semen.[3] Approximately 40% of men with primary infertility have a varicocele, and more than half of them experience improvements in semen parameters after varicocelectomy.[4–6] However, experts continue to debate the efficacy of surgical intervention in improving fertility as evidenced by a recent Cochrane review, which suggested that "there is no evidence that treatment of varicoceles in men from couples with otherwise unexplained subfertility improves the couple's chance of conception."[7] Furthermore, as only 20% of men with a documented varicocele suffer from infertility,[3] care must be taken in the clinical evaluation of a varicocele, and treatment must be tailored to the specific subgroup of individuals most likely to benefit from a surgical intervention.

The decision to treat adolescents with varicocele is a controversial one. Most physicians agree that treating all adolescent boys with varicocele, thus subjecting a large percentage of boys to potentially unnecessary surgery, would be inappropriate, costly, and not without ethical considerations. However, waiting until patients present themselves as adults with possible irreversible infertility would be equally unacceptable. The task for pediatricians and urologists is to identify those adolescents who are at greatest risk for infertility in adulthood, in an effort to offer early surgical intervention to those most likely to benefit.

ANATOMY AND VARICOCELE FORMATION

The formation of a varicocele has been attributed predominantly to anatomic variance, increased pressure in the left renal vein, and incompetent or congenitally absent valves. Approximately 90% of varicoceles are left sided. Several anatomic differences between the right and left testicular (internal spermatic) veins are thought to contribute to this predominance. Although highly variable, the left system usually consists of 1 or more veins within the spermatic cord that coalesce in the retroperitoneal space to become the testicular vein. The left testicular vein inserts into the left renal vein at a right angle, whereas the right testicular vein joins the inferior vena cava at an oblique angle. The relative greater blood flow in the inferior vena cava is thought to augment drainage on the right.[8] The left testicular vein, however, is 8 to 10 cm longer (more craniad) than the right, with a proportional increase in pressure head.

Increases in left renal vein pressure also have been noted secondary to 2 nutcracker phenomenon mechanisms.[9] The proximal nutcracker

Division of Urology, Virginia Commonwealth University School of Medicine, 1200 East Broad Street, Richmond, VA 23298-0118, USA
* Corresponding author.
E-mail address: hpkoo@vcu.edu

Urol Clin N Am 37 (2010) 269–278
doi:10.1016/j.ucl.2010.03.011
0094-0143/10/$ – see front matter © 2010 Published by Elsevier Inc.

phenomenon describes compression of the left renal vein as it passes between the aorta and superior mesenteric arteries. The distal mechanism involves retrograde blood flow through the deferential and external spermatic veins caused by compression of the left common iliac vein as it courses under the left common iliac artery.

Congenitally absent or incompetent valves have classically been thought to be the primary cause of varicocele formation. Subsequent research has shown that there are males without varicocele who have incompetent or absent testicular vein valves and males with varicocele who have competent valves.[10,11] Even with normal valves, dilation of the testicular vein can cause functional incompetence as a result of loss of coaptation.[12] Valve pathology may not be a sole cause, but it certainly contributes to varicocele formation and severity. Alterations in venous architecture at the microscopic level may also play a role in the pathogenesis of varicocele. However, it remains difficult to differentiate between cause and effect in anatomic analysis, as evidenced by several recent studies, which documented significant histologic changes in the amount of connective tissue present in the vein wall of the pampiniform plexus that appeared to have a linear correlation with varicocele grade.[13,14]

Although the exact mechanisms have yet to be elucidated, several physical findings have been found to be associated with an increased risk for developing varicocele in adolescence. A low body mass index has been found to be associated with the development of varicocele in adolescence. Increased penile length and circumference as well as rapid pubertal development were also found to be the independent risk factors for the development of varicocele.[15,16]

PATHOLOGIC FINDINGS RELATED TO TESTICULAR DYSFUNCTION IN ASSOCIATION WITH VARICOCELE

The association between varicocele and testicular dysfunction has been observed by scientists and physicians for nearly 2000 years, dating back to the Greek physician, Celsus, who noted a testicular size discrepancy in the face of dilated veins within the scrotum, suggesting that the discrepancy resulted in impaired testicular nutrition. Since the idea resurfaced in medical texts in the late 1800s, varicocele has been documented in association with a variety of conditions including testicular hypotrophy, an abnormal gonadotropin axis, histologic changes within the testicle, abnormal spermatogenesis, and ultimately, infertility.[17] However, despite the existence of a growing body of literature defining these associations, a direct causal relationship has yet to be confirmed conclusively. As such, debate continues on the pathologic effects of varicocele.

Testicular Hypotrophy

The most well-documented abnormality associated with clinical varicocele is testicular hypotrophy. A large multicenter study[3] performed by the World Health Organization found an association between varicocele and ipsilateral testicular volume; Mori and colleagues[18] took it a step further to define a relationship between varicocele grade and incidence of testicular hypotrophy in adolescents. Although testicular size remains an easily observable clinical phenomenon in the presence of varicocele, its relationship to testicular dysfunction, as defined by abnormal semen analysis results, remains more difficult to quantify in adolescents.

Impaired Spermatogenesis

In adults, the most common findings on semen analysis are decreased motility, decreased sperm density, and increased number of pathologic sperm forms.[3,19] Furthermore, a variety of histologic changes related to testicular dysfunction have been documented in the results of testicular biopsy in males with varicocele, including Leydig cell hyperplasia, decreased number of spermatogonia per tubule, decreased spermatogenesis and maturation arrest, sloughing of germinal epithelium, and interstitial fibrosis.[20,21] Because the adult testicle is composed mostly of seminiferous and germinal cells, it is not surprising to find a correlation between testicular volume and function as defined by semen analysis in this group.[22,23] This correlation seems to be consistent when related to dysfunction and postoperative improvement.[24,25] Although a wealth of research describes abnormal semen analysis results in the presence of varicocele, the heterogeneity of parameters used to define abnormal and the relatively large number of confounding factors related to the desired outcome (successful pregnancy) continue to complicate the debate.

Identifying Pathology in Adolescents

Although the toxic effect of varicocele on semen parameters has been demonstrated in adolescents,[19] the correlation between testicular hypotrophy and abnormal spermatogenesis in this age group has historically been harder to quantify. Haans and colleagues[26] reported that adolescents with pronounced left testicular growth failure had significantly reduced sperm count, but concentration, motility, and morphology were unaffected. This lack of clear association in adolescents could potentially be explained in part by the fact that left testicular growth failure occurs before significant decreases occur in semen parameters. Furthermore, there were relatively few studies to compare semen analysis in adolescents, given the difficulty in obtaining specimens in this age group and ethical questions regarding the psychological impact of their procurement. Researchers have defined a statistically significant correlation between sonographic testicular volume and decreased sperm concentration and total motile sperm counts in adolescents as well as a relation with varicocele grade.[18,27] Addressing the subject of molecular dysfunction, another study documented an increase in the number of sperm with abnormal DNA and a decrease in the number of sperm with normal DNA in adolescents with high-grade varicocele, even when semen analysis result was normal.[28]

PROPOSED PATHOLOGIC MECHANISMS

Although the association of clinically detectable varicocele with testicular hypotrophy, an abnormal gonadotropin axis, histologic changes, abnormal spermatogenesis, and infertility has been clearly documented in the literature, the exact mechanism whereby varicocele induces pathologic change has yet to be elucidated. Many theories have been postulated on the subject, including increased testicular temperature, hypoxia, reflux of adrenal and renal metabolites, and generation of reactive oxygen species (ROS).

Hyperthermia

Elevated scrotal and testicular temperature is the most widely accepted mechanism for testicular dysfunction. Experimentally induced varicocele increases scrotal temperature and is reversible with surgical correction.[29,30] Hyperthermia has consistently been shown to negatively affect germ cell function, proliferation, and subsequent fertility.[31] Furthermore, scrotal cooling and, consequently, testicular cooling have been documented to improve semen quality.[32] Varicocelectomy in human studies has been shown to normalize temperature, with subsequent increases in sperm count.[33–35] When comparing infertile men with varicocele to normal controls, as well as to men with varicocele and normal fertility, infertile men with varicocele were shown to have increased intrascrotal temperatures.[36,37] Several studies have sought to define the molecular basis for infertility in association with elevated testicular temperatures in both adult and adolescent males with varicocele. It would seem that the downregulation of heat shock proteins may be associated with infertility in these groups.[38,39] Furthermore, an increase in the expression of heat shock proteins after varicocelectomy has been documented.[39,40]

Hypoxia

Although early studies did not support the proposal that venous stasis and reduced blood flow of the testicular vessels resulted in hypoxia, several recent publications have proposed a direct link between impaired testicular drainage and tissue hypoxia. These studies suggest that tissue damage is the result of impaired testicular microcirculation secondary to increased hydrostatic pressure rather than global hypoxia.[41] This proposal has been supported by studies identifying increased expression of hypoxia-inducible factor-1 alpha in association with varicocele in human and animal models.[42]

Reflux of Renal and Adrenal Metabolites

Reflux of adrenal and renal metabolites has been proposed as a mechanism for testicular damage in men with varicocele. Research has been inconclusive, and experimental studies have shown that toxic effects of varicocele do not require adrenal contribution and that reflux may not occur.[43] Adrenomedullin, a potent vasodilator expressed in adrenal and kidney tissues but not in the testes, has been isolated in blood samples from the testicular veins of men with varicocele.[44] In rat models, varicocele-induced testicular damage was found to be enhanced in subjects with viable adrenal glands when compared with those in whom a unilateral adrenalectomy was performed before varicocele induction.[45] Further research is required to determine if adrenomedullin plays a role in the formation of or toxicity associated with varicocele.

ROS and Oxidative Stress

Venous blood from varicoceles of infertile men has shown increased production of nitric oxide, its active metabolites, and ROS that are known to play a role in sperm dysfunction.[46–48] These increased levels have been shown to correlate with the severity of varicocele.[48] Varicocele also reduces antioxidant defenses, potentially adding to the localized oxidative stress (OS).[49] Several studies reported a decrease in markers of ROS-associated damage and an improvement in antioxidant levels after varicocelectomy.[50,51] Although the relation between varicocele and OS is clear, the exact cause of OS in this case has yet to be clearly defined. Nevertheless, numerous mechanisms have been proposed to identify the origin of OS in patients with varicocele, including the role of cytokines (interleukin 1); increased expression of leptin receptors; increased nitric oxide levels resulting from hypoxia, as an inducer of apoptosis and precursor of oxidants; and downregulation of glial cell line derived–neurotrophic factor receptor (factor involved in spermatogenesis).[48] Whether these complex mechanisms are the final common pathway for varicocele-induced infertility or an effect of testicular injury is still unknown. Although few reports exploring the administration of antioxidants in subfertile men with varicocele have been produced, the use of zinc, glutathione, and Chinese herbal remedies containing a variety of antioxidants have shown some promise.[48]

DIAGNOSIS

Typically, varicoceles are asymptomatic and detected in adolescents during routine physical examination. Occasionally, scrotal mass evaluations referred from primary care physicians are found to be varicoceles. Differential diagnoses for generally painless scrotal masses in adolescence include communicating hydrocele, hydrocele of the spermatic cord, inguinal hernia, epididymal cyst, and spermatocele.

Patients should be examined in a warm room in standing and supine positions and with and without a Valsalva maneuver. Classically, varicoceles are graded according to the following criteria:

Grade 1 (small): palpable only with Valsalva maneuver
Grade 2 (medium): palpable with the patient standing
Grade 3 (large): visible through scrotal skin, palpable with the patient standing.

After examining in an upright position, the patient should be reexamined in the supine position. Idiopathic varicocele is more prominent in the upright position and disappears in the supine position. Secondary varicoceles, especially on the right side, can be caused by retroperitoneal tumors or lymphadenopathy and do not change size as noticeably as in the supine position.

An important part of the physical examination in all boys with varicocele is an accurate assessment of testicular consistency (firmness) and volume. Although the assessment of testicular consistency is subjective, a careful simultaneous comparison of both testes may give the clinician additional

qualitative information about the overall condition of the ipsilateral testis. Several methods are available to measure the size of the testis, including visual comparison, calipers, Prader orchidometer (comparative ovoids), Takahira orchidometer (disc elliptical rings), and ultrasonography. Measurement of testis volume has been reported to be assessed accurately and reproducibly by using either a Prader or a disc orchidometer.[52] However, ultrasonography should be considered the standard criterion for assessing testicular volume. Results of ultrasonography have consistently shown high correlation with actual testis volume and have been highly reproducible, with improved detection of bilateral varicoceles and increased sensitivity in the evaluation of volume differentials as compared with orchidometer.[53,54]

In a clinical study comparing Prader orchidometer and ultrasonography in adolescents with a varicocele, Costabile and colleagues[55] found that 24% of patients with growth arrest would have been missed and 14% would have been identified falsely to have a significant size discrepancy if measured by Prader orchidometer alone. Diamond and colleagues[53] noted similar superiority of ultrasonography for measuring testicular volume; they recommend annual ultrasonography of testis in adolescents with varicocele.

IDENTIFYING PATIENTS AT RISK

Left untreated, with time, in a subset of patients, the varicocele will continue to affect testicular growth, with loss of volume and progressive deterioration in semen parameters.[56,57] In adults, treatment is straightforward and is proposed whenever (1) there is a palpable varicocele, (2) there is documented infertility, (3) it has been confirmed that there is no female infertility problem, and (4) there is at least 1 abnormality found on semen analysis.[58] In the adolescents, significant controversy exists regarding the appropriate methods of evaluation for surgery. The diagnosis of varicocele leads to additional questions about possible infertility and the need to establish clinical criteria for varicocele repair. Currently, a variety of clinical tests are available for identifying adolescents at risk for infertility associated with varicocele. However, a consensus has yet to be reached on the most appropriate combination of tests in evaluation of adolescent varicocele. This topic remains at the forefront of debate and research. Currently, clinical tests proposed in evaluation for surgical intervention in adolescents with varicocele include (1) physical examination and radiologic evaluation, (2) biochemical tests, and (3) semen analysis.

Physical Examination and Radiologic Evaluation

Physical examination includes identification of varicocele grade and the measurement of testicular volume, as well as some novel approaches to ultrasound imaging to measure retrograde flow in the spermatic venous plexus. There remain conflicting opinions about the correlation between the grade of varicocele and its ultimate effect on the testis. Some investigators have found no correlation between varicocele grade and testicular size or semen parameters,[27] whereas others have noticed that boys with severe varicoceles have smaller ipsilateral testis and increasingly abnormal findings in semen analysis in comparison with those adolescents with lower-grade varicoceles.[18,55,59] In an early study involving adolescent boys and young men aged 12 to 25 years, 34% of subjects with a grade-2 varicocele had testicular changes, compared with 81% of those with grade-3 varicocele. Within the grade-3 group, the percentage of subjects aged 18 to 25 years with testicular change reached almost 98%, illustrating the progressive nature of varicocele-induced testicular damage and indicating that testicular hypotrophy is almost inevitable in males with grade-3 varicocele.[60] Although the higher-grade varicoceles seem more concerning, varicocele grade should not be a sole determinant in recommending treatment.[61]

There is abundant literature confirming that varicocele is associated with testicular growth arrest in adolescents and that varicocele repair results in testicular catch-up growth.[62–65] The risk for testicular growth arrest also has been shown to be time dependent and to correlate with varicocele and reflux grade.[66,67] However, according to a study by Zampieri and associates,[68] involving 465 patients, only 32% of patients had complete catch-up growth. Also, Preston and colleagues[69] determined that a statistically significant number of adolescents with varicocele and testicular-size discrepancy experience testicular catch-up growth as a normal function of development. Nevertheless, the relationship between testicular hypotrophy and infertility remains clear, and a recent study confirmed that size differentials greater than 10% between normal and hypotrophic testicles correlated with a decreased sperm concentration and total motile-sperm count.[27] Furthermore, this difference was found to increase dramatically when the size differential reached 20%. These data would suggest that patients with a persistent size differential of greater than 20% should be offered surgical intervention without further investigation. Although a waiting period is recommended for adolescents to assess for resolution of size discrepancy, a recent study proposed that peak retrograde flow velocities of greater than 38 cm/s (found to be a predictor of persistent asymmetry), when combined with a size differential of 20% or greater, negated the need for such a waiting period.

Biochemical Tests

Biochemical tests are based on the integrity of the testis and any effect of the varicocele on the hypothalamic-pituitary axis. At the testis level, serum inhibin levels reflect the integrity of the seminiferous tubules and the function of Sertoli cells. A recent study suggests that in adolescents, inhibin B levels are elevated in untreated varicocele and directly correlate with testicular volume.[70] Because inhibin levels have been shown to improve in men whose semen analysis improved after varicocelectomy, inhibin may have a role postoperatively as well.[71] However, contradictions exist among the studies, and there are not enough data to support the use of serum inhibin levels in stratifying adolescents with varicoceles.[72,73]

The gonadotropin-releasing hormone (GnRH) stimulation test is based on the theory that damage to germinal epithelium results in compensatory stimulation of the pituitary gland and subsequent increase in the production of follicle-stimulating hormone (FSH) and luteinizing hormone (LH) by gonadotrophs. Several studies demonstrate an abnormal gonadotropin axis in men with varicocele as evidenced by increased FSH or LH response to administration of GnRH.[72,74] Although some would recommend the GnRH stimulation test for adolescents as part of a standardized evaluation for surgery, the GnRH stimulation test has not been conclusively shown to be a good predictor of postsurgical improvement in adolescents.[75–77]

Semen Analysis

Semen analysis in men with varicoceles reveals decreased motility, decreased sperm density, and more pathologic forms. By applying strict morphologic criteria to semen analysis, varicocele repair improves the seminal parameters in approximately 70% of patients, with the improvement in motility being the most common.[24,25]

Over the last several years, researchers have increasingly come to use semen analysis in the evaluation of testicular dysfunction associated with adolescent varicoceles.[78] Studies suggest that the effect of varicocele on semen quality is similar in adults and adolescents.[79] In a study of

88 boys, Laven and colleagues[62] found a statistically significant increase in sperm concentration values 1 year after varicocele repair. No differences in total sperm count, sperm motility, or morphology were observed among postoperative varicocele patients, normal healthy boys, and in controls with untreated varicoceles. However, difficulties remain because established norms for adolescent semen analysis have yet to be defined. Semen analysis cannot adequately be performed until the subjects have progressed to the point in pubertal development necessary for adequate ejaculation, and sample procurement continues to raise several ethical questions.[19,80] Nevertheless, it would seem from current trends in the literature that recommendations for the role of semen analysis in evaluation of adolescent varicocele are forthcoming.

MANAGEMENT

Prophylactic surgery for every adolescent with varicocele is not advisable. Understanding the limitations in predicting future fertility potential, several reproducible parameters would be helpful in identifying individuals who would benefit most from treatment. Testicular volume discrepancy of more than 20%, as assessed by ultrasonography, is the most common indication for treatment. However, as described in previous sections, size differentials seem to provide the most accurate assessment of impaired fertility to date. The authors prefer to follow testicular volume with ultrasonography. Still, several studies have shown a strong linear relationship between testicular volume measurements using either Prader orchidometer or scrotal ultrasonography.[54,81] Although it is recommended that the clinicians use the method in which they have the most experience, ultrasonography has become the standard method and provides a significant benefit over orchidometer in regard to size differentials.

Symptoms such as pain, fullness, or swelling not relieved by conservative measures may be another possible indicator for treatment. However, correlation between symptoms and pathology has not been evaluated in a controlled manner to date.[82] Because it would be difficult to have a normal contralateral testis as a comparison, adolescents with bilateral varicoceles should be considered for therapy. For the older adolescent, the physician may discuss the possibility of semen analysis to aid in decision making. A patient with abnormal semen analysis with high-grade varicocele, even without testicular hypotrophy, should be considered for treatment.

TREATMENT OPTIONS

The best method for treatment of adolescent varicocele has yet to be established. There have been no randomized, controlled, prospective clinical studies that compare the various techniques in adolescents or adults. Treatment options include open surgical approaches, laparoscopic varicocele ligation, and percutaneous transvenous embolization. Several investigators have described innovative minimally invasive surgical approaches for the treatment of adolescent varicocele, including laparoscopic single-port surgery[83] and robotic-assisted techniques.[84]

Open Surgery and Arterial Sparing

Open surgery remains the mainstay of varicocele treatment in adolescents. Based on a review of the literature and the results of a survey of pediatric urologists in the United States, Paduch and Skoog[65] found that high retroperitoneal ligation of the testicular artery and veins (Palomo procedure) is the treatment of choice in adolescents. Kass and Marcol[85] demonstrated that the classic Palomo repair was associated with a statistically significant decrease in surgical failure rate compared with artery sparing or inguinal varicocele ligation. In addition, no patient exhibited testis atrophy after high ligation of internal spermatic artery and vein, which is consistent with findings by other investigators.[86,87]

The issue of preserving the testicular artery has been questioned in adults, in whom inadvertent arterial ligation during inguinal dissection for varicocele ligation led to poorer postoperative sperm quality compared with artery-preserved cohorts.[63] Zampieri and colleagues[88] compared semen analysis from adolescents with prior laparoscopic varicocelectomy using either testicular artery preservation or artery ligation. They showed that patients with artery-sparing procedures had semen analyses with higher sperm concentration, better motility, increased semen volume, and a higher rate of morphologically normal sperm than those with prior artery ligation.[88]

Microscopic inguinal or subinguinal approach with arterial preservation should also be considered as a viable option for adolescent varicocele treatment. The microsurgical low inguinal or subinguinal approach has been reported in the adult infertility literature as the method with the highest success rate (99%) and the lowest morbidity (0% hydrocele). The main potential disadvantage of this approach is the need for an operating microscope to spare the arteries and lymphatics and the increased number of veins at this level.

Laparoscopic and Robotic Varicocelectomy

Laparoscopic varicocelectomy is an appealing option in that the patient is spared the morbidity of a groin incision. The transabdominal intraperitoneal approach also offers the possibility of bilateral repair through the same small incisions. There is 1 report of a randomized controlled trial of laparoscopic and open repair that found that the rate of varicocele relapse was statistically similar (1.84% vs 1.35%, respectively) between laparoscopic and open varicocelectomy but that the likelihood of wound complications, scrotal edema, and necessity of analgesia were all increased significantly in the open repair group. The laparoscopic group also had a decreased length of stay and shorter operative time.[89] In terms of varicocele recurrence, Barroso and colleagues[90] recently reported a comparison of 1344 patients who underwent open varicocelectomy with 496 patients who underwent laparoscopic varicocelectomy and noted that recurrence was seen in 2.9% and 4.4%, respectively.

One of the drawbacks to laparoscopic varicocelectomy is that the patient traditionally was required to have 3 incisions to facilitate a laparoscopic camera and 2 working instruments. Link and colleagues[91] described a technique for 2-trocar laparoscopic varicocelectomy, which uses two 5-mm ports only. After obtaining pneumoperitoneum with a Veress needle, a 5-mm port was placed supraumbilically. A second 5-mm port was placed in the contralateral lower quadrant. Ten varicoceles in 9 patients were identified and operated on by using this technique. A harmonic scalpel was used to fulgurate and divide the entire spermatic cord above the inguinal ring. No attempt was made to spare the testicular artery or lymphatics. At short (6 weeks postoperation) follow-up, there was no evidence of recurrence or hydrocele.

An evolutionary step forward was also reported by Kaouk and Palmer[83] with their series of single-port laparoscopic varicocelectomy. This procedure was completed in 3 adolescents using Uni-X Single Port Access Laparoscopic System (Pnavel Systems, Morganville, NJ, USA), a unique 20-mm laparoscopic port, placed transumbilically. This port, in combination with both rigid and articulating instruments, allows for single-port laparoscopic varicocelectomy.

With the advent of the robotic da Vinci Surgical System (Intuitive Surgical, Inc, Sunnyvale, CA, USA), the use of a robotic platform for minimally invasive surgery has expanded. Robotic varicocelectomy has been reported by 2 groups using 2 different techniques. Shu and colleagues[84] reported their technique with 8 patients using the da Vinci robot to perform a magnified subinguinal varicocelectomy, whereas Corcione and colleagues[92] performed a standard transperitoneal bilateral varicocelectomy on 2 patients.

Percutaneous Varicocele Ablation

Transvenous percutaneous varicocele ablation has the advantages of a quick recovery and minimal pain. The success rate ranges from 89% to 95%, with approximately 6% complications, in addition to the issue of radiologic exposure of the testes. Many urologists reserve this approach for cases of surgical failure.[93]

THE FUTURE

The past several years have seen explosive growth in the literature about minimally invasive varicocelectomy including laparoscopic, robotic, and percutaneous techniques. This has enabled surgeons to offer multiple options to young patients to maximize surgical outcomes and minimize morbidity.

There is also a great need for further research to improve selection of patients who may most benefit from surgical correction of varicocele. Advanced molecular biology techniques used for the evaluation of the infertile men have increased the understanding of the physiology of spermatogenesis. It is estimated that 13% of men with azoospermia carry microdeletions of the long arm of chromosome Y.[94–96] Men with varicocele and azoospermia or severe oligoasthenospermia may suffer from point mutation or deletion of genes important in spermatogenesis. Y-chromosome microdeletion analysis is not universally available, and the assay technique has not been standardized fully. In the near future, by screening for aberrations of genes involved in regulation of spermatogenesis, better criteria for management of patients with varicocele may be established.[17,65]

REFERENCES

1. Akbay E, Cayan S, Doruk E, et al. The prevalence of varicocele and varicocele-related testicular atrophy in Turkish children and adolescents. BJU Int 2000; 86:490–3.
2. Skoog S, Roberts K, Goldstein M, et al. The adolescent varicocele: what's new with an old problem in new patients? Pediatrics 1997;100:112–21.
3. The influence of varicocele on parameters of fertility in a large group of men presenting to infertility clinics. World Health Organization. Fertil Steril 1992;57:1289–93.

4. Dubin L, Amelar R. Etiologic factors in 1294 consecutive cases of male infertility. Fertil Steril 1971;22: 469–74.

5. Rigau L, Weiss D, Zukerman Z, et al. A possible mechanism for the detrimental effect of varicocele on testicular function in man. Fertil Steril 1978;30:577–85.

6. Vermeulen A, Vandeweghe M, Deslypere J. Prognosis of subfertility in men with corrected or uncorrected varicocele. J Androl 1986;7:147–55.

7. Evers J, Collins J, Clarke J. Surgery or embolisation for varicoceles in subfertile men. Cochrane Database Syst Rev 2009;(1):CD000479.

8. Shafik A, Moftah A, Olfat S, et al. Testicular veins: anatomy and role in varicocelogenesis and other pathologic conditions. Urology 1990;35:175–82.

9. Coolsaet B. The varicocele syndrome: venography determining the optimal level for surgical management. Urology 1980;124:833–9.

10. Wishahi M. Anatomy of the spermatic venous plexus (pampiniform plexus) in men with and without varicocele: intraoperative venographic study. Urology 1992;147:1285–9.

11. Braedel H, Steffens J, Ziegler M, et al. A possible ontogenic etiology for idiopathic left varicocele. Urology 1994;151:62–6.

12. Gorenstein A, Katz S, Schiller M. Varicocele in children: "to treat or not to treat"—venographic and manometric studies. Pediatr Surg 1986;21:1046–50.

13. Iafrate M, Galfano A, Macchi V, et al. Varicocele is associated with an increase of connective tissue of the pampiniform plexus vein wall. World J Urol 2009;27(3):363–9.

14. Macchi V, Porzionato A, Iafrate M, et al. Morphological characteristics of the wall of pampiniform plexus veins and modifications in patients with varicocele. Ital J Anat Embryol 2008;113(1):1–8.

15. Kumanov P, Robeva RN, Tomova A. Adolescent varicocele: who is at risk. Pediatrics 2008;121:53–7.

16. May M, Taymoorian K, Beutner S, et al. Body size and weight as predisposing factors in varicocele. Scand J Urol Nephrol 2006;40:45–8.

17. Sigman M, Jarrow JP. Male infertility. In: Wein AJ, Kavoussi LR, Novick AC, et al, editors. Campbell-Walsh urology. Philadelphia: Saunders Elsevier; 2007. p. 609–53.

18. Mori M, Bertolla R, Fraietta R, et al. Does varicocele grade determine extent of alteration to spermatogenesis in adolescents? Fertil Steril 2008;90(5):1769–73.

19. Paduch DA, Niedzielski J. Semen analysis in young men with varicocele: preliminary study. J Urol 1996; 156:788–90.

20. Turek P, Lipshultz L. The varicocele controversies I. Etiology and pathophysiology. AUA Update 1995; XIV(13):114–9.

21. Castro-Magana M, Angulo M, Canas A, et al. Leydig cell function in adolescent boys with varicocele. Arch Androl 1990;24:73–9.

22. Takihara H, Cosentino M, Sakatoku J, et al. Significance of testicular size measurement in andrology: II correlation of testicular size with testicular function. J Urol 1987;137:416–9.

23. Sigman M, Jarow J. Ipsilateral testicular hypotrophy is associated with decreased sperm counts in infertile men with varicoceles. J Urol 1997;158:605–7.

24. Sakamoto H, Saito K, Ogawa Y, et al. Effects of varicocele repair in adults on ultrasonographically determined testicular volume and on semen profile. Urology 2008;71(3):485–9.

25. Zucchi A, Mearini L, Mearini E, et al. Varicocele and fertility: relationship between testicular volume and seminal parameters before and after treatment. J Androl 2006;4(27):548–51.

26. Haans L, Laven J, Mali W, et al. Testis volumes, semen quality, and hormonal patterns in adolescents with and without a varicocele. Fertil Steril 1991;56:731–6.

27. Diamond D, Zurakowski D, Bauer S, et al. Relationship of varicocele grade and testicular hypotrophy to semen parameters in adolescents. J Urol 2007; 178:1584–8.

28. Bertolla RP, Cedenho A, Hassun Filho P, et al. Sperm nuclear DNA fragmentation in adolescents with varicocele. Fertil Steril 2006;85:625–8.

29. Saypol D, Howards S, Turner T, et al. Influence of surgically induced varicocele on testicular blood flow, temperature, and histology in adult rats and dogs. J Clin Invest 1981;68:39–45.

30. Goldstein M, Eid J. Elevation of intratesticular and scrotal skin surface temperature in men with varicocele. J Urol 1989;142:743–5.

31. Paul C, Teng S, Philippa T, et al. A single, mild, transient scrotal heat stress causes hypoxia and oxidative stress in mouse testes, which induces germ cell death. Biol Reprod 2009;80:913–9.

32. Jung A, Eberl M, Schill W. Improvement of semen quality by nocturnal scrotal cooling and moderate behavioral change to reduce genital heat stress in men with oligoasthenoteratozoospermia. Reproduction 2001;121:595–603.

33. Merla A, Ledda A, Di Donato L, et al. Assessment of the effects of varicocelectomy on the thermoregulatory control of the scrotum. Fertil Steril 2004;81: 471–2.

34. Agger P. Scrotal and testicular temperature: its relation to sperm count before and after operation for varicocele. Fertil Steril 1971;22:286–97.

35. Wright E, Young G, Goldstein M. Reduction in testicular temperature after varicocelectomy in infertile men. Urology 1997;50:257–9.

36. Zorgniotti A, Macleod J. Studies in temperature, human semen quality, and varicocele. Fertil Steril 1973;24:854–63.

37. Lund L, Nielsen K. Varicocele testis and testicular temperature. Br J Urol 1996;78:113–5.

38. Lima S, Cenedeze M, Bertolla R, et al. Expression of the HSPA2 gene in ejaculated spermatozoa from adolescents with and without varicocele. Fertil Steril 2006;86:1659–63.

39. Yeşilli C, Mungan G, Seçkiner I, et al. Effect of varicocelectomy on sperm creatine kinase, HspA2 chaperone protein (creatine kinase-M type), LDH, LDH-X, and lipid peroxidation product levels in infertile men with varicocele. Urology 2005;66:610–5.

40. Marmar J, Agarwal A, Prabakaran S, et al. Reassessing the value of varicocelectomy as a treatment for male subfertility with a new meta-analysis. Fertil Steril 2007;88:639–48.

41. Gat Y, Zukerman Z, Chakraborty J, et al. Varicocele, hypoxia and male infertility. Fluid mechanics analysis of the impaired testicular venous drainage system. Humanit Rep 2005;20:2614–9.

42. Lee J, Jeng S, Lee T. Increased expression of hypoxia-inducible factor-1alpha in the internal spermatic vein of patients with varicocele. J Urol 2006; 175:1045–8.

43. Turner T, Lopez T. Effects of experimental varicocele require neither adrenal contribution nor venous reflux. J Urol 1989;142:1372–5.

44. Ozbek E, Yurekli M, Soylu A, et al. The role of adrenomedullin in varicocele and impotence. BJU Int 2000;86:694–8.

45. Camoglio F, Zampieri N, Corroppolo M, et al. Varicocele and retrograde adrenal metabolites flow. An experimental study on rats. Urol Int 2004;73:337–42.

46. Koksal I, Tefekli A, Usta M, et al. The role of reactive oxygen species in testicular dysfunction associated with varicocele. BJU Int 2000;86:549–52.

47. Romeo C, Ientile R, Impellizzeri P, et al. Preliminary report on nitric oxide-mediated oxidative damage in adolescent varicocele. Humanit Rep 2003;18: 26–9.

48. Agarwal A, Sharma R, Desai N, et al. Role of oxidative stress in pathogenesis of varicocele and infertility. Urology 2009;73:461–9.

49. Barbieri E, Hidalgo M, Venegas A, et al. Varicocele-associated decrease in antioxidant defenses. J Androl 1999;20:713–7.

50. Mostafa T, Anis T, El-Nashar A, et al. Varicocelectomy reduces reactive oxygen species levels and increases antioxidant activity of seminal plasma from infertile men with varicocele. Int J Androl 2001;24:261–5.

51. Chen S, Huang W, Chang L, et al. Attenuation of oxidative stress after varicocelectomy in subfertile patients with varicocele. J Urol 2008;179:639–42.

52. Nagu T, Takahira H. A new apparatus for the measurement of testicular volume. Jpn J Fertil Steril 1979;24:12.

53. Diamond D, Paltiel H, DiCanzio J, et al. Comparative assessment of pediatric testicular volume: orchidometer versus ultrasound. J Urol 2000;164:1111–4.

54. Cayan S, Akbay E, Bozlu M, et al. Diagnosis of pediatric varicoceles by physical examination and ultrasonography and measurement of the testicular volume: using the Prader orchidometer versus ultrasonography. Urol Int 2002;69:293–6.

55. Costabile R, Skoog S, Radowich M. Testicular volume assessment in the adolescent with a varicocele. J Urol 1992;147:1348–50.

56. Gorelick J, Goldstein M. Loss of fertility in men with varicocele. Fertil Steril 1993;59:613–6.

57. Sayfan J, Siplovich L, Koltun L, et al. Varicocele treatment in pubertal boys prevents testicular growth arrest. J Urol 1997;157:1456–7.

58. Wagner L, Tostain J, d'Urologie C, et al. Varicocele and male infertility: AFU 2006 guidelines. Prog Urol 2007;17:12–7.

59. Lyon R, Marshall S, Scott M. Varicocele in childhood and adolescence: implication in adulthood infertility? Urology 1982;19:641–4.

60. Steeno O, Knops J, Declerck L, et al. Prevention of fertility disorders by detection and treatment of varicocele at school and college age. Andrologia 1976; 8:47–53.

61. Kozakowski K, Gjertson C, Decastro G, et al. Peak retrograde flow: a novel predictor of persistent, progressive and new onset asymmetry in adolescent varicocele. J Urol 2009;181:2717–22.

62. Laven J, Haans L, Mali W, et al. Effects of varicocele treatment in adolescents: a randomized study. Fertil Steril 1992;58(4):756–62.

63. Turek P, Lipshultz L. The varicocele controversies II. Diagnosis and management. AUA Update 1995;XIV: 114–9.

64. Paduch D, Niedzielski J. Repair versus observation in adolescent varicocele: a prospective study. J Urol 1997;158:1128–32.

65. Paduch D, Skoog S. Current management of adolescent varicocele. Rev Urol 2001;3:120–33.

66. Thomas J, Elder J. Testicular growth arrest and adolescent varicocele: does varicocele size make a difference? J Urol 2002;168:1689–91.

67. Zampieri N, Zuin V, Corroppolo M, et al. Relationship between varicocele grade, vein reflux and testicular growth arrest. Pediatr Surg Int 2008;24:727–30.

68. Zampieri N, Mantovani A, Ottolenghi A, et al. Testicular catch-up growth after varicocelectomy: does surgical technique make a difference? Urology 2009;73:289–92.

69. Preston M, Carnat T, Flood T, et al. Conservative management of adolescent varicoceles: a retrospective review. Urology 2008;72:77–80.

70. Romeo C, Arrigo T, Impellizzeri P, et al. Altered serum inhibin B levels in adolescents with varicocele. J Pediatr Surg 2007;42:390–4.

71. Ozden C, Ozdal O, Bulut S, et al. Effect of varicocelectomy on serum inhibin B levels in infertile patients with varicocele. Scand J Urol Nephrol 2008;42:441–3.

72. Plymate S, Paulsen C, McLachlan R. Relationship of serum inhibin levels to serum follicle stimulating hormone and sperm production in normal men and men with varicoceles. J Clin Endocrinol Metab 1992;74:859–64.

73. Basar M, Kisa U, Tuglu D, et al. The effect of varicocele on seminal plasma and serum inhibin-B levels in adolescent and adult men. Int Urol Nephrol 2010;42:47–51.

74. Bickel A, Dickstein G. Factors predicting the outcome of varicocele repair for subfertility: the value of the luteinizing hormone-releasing hormone test. J Urol 1989;142:1230–4.

75. Nagao R, Plymate S, Berger R, et al. Comparison of gonadal function between fertile and infertile men with varicoceles. Fertil Steril 1986;46:930–3.

76. Guarino N, Tadini B, Bianchi M. The adolescent varicocele: the crucial role of hormonal tests in selecting patients with testicular dysfunction. J Pediatr Surg 2003;38(1):120–3.

77. Fisch H, Hyun G, Hensle T. Testicular growth and gonadotrophin response associated with varicocele repair in adolescent males. BJU Int 2003;91:75–8.

78. Diamond D. Adolescent versus adult varicoceles-how do evaluation and management differ? J Urol 2009;181:2418–9.

79. Pasqualotto F. Semen analysis: role of age and varicocele. J Postgrad Med 2007;53:1–2.

80. Zampieri N, Corroppolo M, Zuin V, et al. Longitudinal study of semen quality in adolescents with varicocele: to treat or not? Urology 2007;70:989–93.

81. Behre H, Nashan D, Nieschlag E. Objective measurement of testicular volume by ultrasonography: evaluation of the technique and comparison with orchidometer estimates. Int J Urol 1989;12:395–403.

82. Zampieri N, Ottolenghi A, Camoglio F. Painful varicocele in pediatric age: is there a correlation between pain, testicular damage and hormonal values to justify surgery. Pediatr Surg 2008;24:1235–8.

83. Kaouk J, Palmer J. Single-port laparoscopic surgery: initial experience in children for varicocelectomy. BJU Int 2008;102:97–9.

84. Shu T, Taghechian S, Wang R. Initial experience with robot-assisted varicocelectomy. Asian J Androl 2008;10:146–8.

85. Kass E, Marcol B. Results of varicocele surgery in adolescents: a comparison of techniques. J Urol 1992;148:694–6.

86. Okuyama A, Nakamura M, Namiki M, et al. Surgical repair of varicocele at puberty: preventive treatment for fertility improvement. J Urol 1988;139:562–4.

87. Marsuda T, Horii Y, Yoshida O. Should the testicular artery be preserved at varicocelectomy? J Urol 1993;149:1357–60.

88. Zampieri N, Zuin V, Corroppolo M, et al. Varicocele and adolescents: semen quality after 2 different laparoscopic procedures. J Androl 2007;28:727–33.

89. Podkamenev V, Stalmakhovich V, Urkov P, et al. Laparoscopic surgery for pediatric varicoceles: randomized controlled trial. J Pediatr Surg 2002;37:727–9.

90. Barroso U, Andrade D, Novaes H, et al. Surgical treatment of varicocele in children with open and laparoscopic Palomo technique: a systematic review of the literature. J Urol 2009;181:2724–8.

91. Link B, Kruska J, Wong C, et al. Two trocar laparoscopic varicocelectomy: approach and outcomes. JSLS 2006;10:151–4.

92. Corcione F, Esposito C, Cuccurullo D, et al. Advantages and limits of robot-assisted laparoscopic surgery. Surg Endosc 2005;19:117–9.

93. Fretz P, Sandlow J. Varicocele: current concepts in pathophysiology, diagnosis, and treatment. Urol Clin North Am 2002;29:921–37.

94. Nakahori Y, Kuroki Y, Komaki R, et al. The Y chromosome region essential for spermatogenesis. Horm Res 1996;46:20–3.

95. Pryor J, Kent-First M, Muallem A, et al. Microdeletions in the Y chromosome of infertile men. N Engl J Med 1997;336:534–9.

96. Seifer I, Amat S, Delgado-Viscogliosi P, et al. Screening for microdeletions on the long arm of chromosome Y in 53 infertile men. Int J Androl 1999;22:148–54.

Laparoscopic and Robotic Approach to Genitourinary Anomalies in Children

Pasquale Casale, MD

KEYWORDS

- Minimally invasive • Child • Robot • Laparoscopy
- Testis • Kidney • Ureter • Bladder

Laparoscopy has its origins in the use of the cystoscope to inspect the peritoneal cavity. Within urology and pediatric surgery, the first widely accepted use of laparoscopy was for inspection of the gonads in a child with ambiguous genitalia, rather than using open abdominal exploration.

From these roots, laparoscopy has taken on a greater role in the surgical solutions for urologic disease in pediatric patients. Minimally invasive laparoscopic procedures have become widely available for several ablative and reconstructive operations in children. The small incisions used for open surgery on large organs such as the kidney in pediatric urology typically require a large amount of dissection. The organ system is then brought up to the skin or even out of the wound to perform the operation when an open approach is used. With minimally invasive surgery (MIS) the exposure to internal organs and allowing surrounding tissue to remain in situ can only be paralleled by large open incisions. There is minimal tissue manipulation with MIS when done properly.

In the past decade, technical advances such as smaller endoscopic instruments and high-resolution cameras have contributed to the widespread use of MIS in children.[1,2] The introduction of robotic surgical systems represents a further step in the evolution of endoscopic instrumentation. These computer-enhanced systems offer three-dimensional visualization and significantly improved instrumentation with motion scaling and a wrist mechanism that allows surgeons to perform complex reconstructive procedures.

Although these specific advantages might benefit pediatric patients, the number of reports of robotic repairs performed in children is increasing. Initially, the robot was thought to be bulky for children, but the delicate robotic movements are ideal for the reconstructive surgeries children require; hence, pediatric urology has embraced robotic technology.

THE LEARNING CURVE

The learning curve for MIS in children must be addressed. The skill set requires thinking regarding placement of incisions, different presentation of anatomy, and the operating room staff must learn to use new and ever-changing equipment. The technical surgical skills require mastery. The time constraints for experienced surgeons to move from the comfort of the proficient master to join the ranks of the novice surgeon make the task daunting. For those in academic training centers, training residents and fellows can present an unfamiliar challenge, particularly if their exposure is otherwise limited. Deliberate practice is a term introduced by K. Anders Ericcson to describe the methods by which expert performers in many fields (eg, sports, music, sculpture) achieve the highest levels of ability. Deliberate practice, although time consuming, is essential for obtaining proficiency in MIS and needs to be done in a mentored environment. It is erroneous to assume that experience is synonymous with expertise. Practicing the same mistakes creates an experienced, but poorly

Division of Pediatric Urology, Children's Hospital of Philadelphia, 34th Street and Civic Center Boulevard, Philadelphia, PA 19104, USA
E-mail address: Casale@email.chop.edu

Urol Clin N Am 37 (2010) 279–286
doi:10.1016/j.ucl.2010.03.005

skilled surgeon. The learning curve entails a kinesi-ology of MIS where surgeons need to learn how their body works for and against the task at hand; for example, tendencies that are disadvantageous in surgery such as upward retraction, tunnel vision, and nondominant hand neglect. Overcoming these errors requires training them away.

EQUIPMENT

As a new field with constantly emerging new tech-nology, an institutional commitment to the purchase and upgrading of instrumentation is required, and the surgeons must understand the equipment. MIS requires mastery of the tech-nology of surgery to proficiently and safely use the instrument; the surgeon needs to know exactly how the tools work, the way the engineers de-signed them to work, and why they work. For example, surgeons should understand how elec-trosurgery generators actually work; what wave-forms are generated; and how voltage changes with impedance, the tissue, and the patient size.

PATIENT PHYSICS AND PHYSIOLOGY

Children present a small working environment compared with adults. For instance, an adult pneumoperitoneum will typically provide a 5- to 6-L working space, whereas a 1-year old will present a 1-L intra-abdominal space. Also, the body surface area is smaller and the chance of port site conflicts, such as instrument crossing or trocar headpiece collisions, is greater for children.

Children are considered more sensitive to pres-sure in the working space than adults, and have a greater chance of developing crepitation and dissection of insufflation gas. In the author's expe-rience, working pressures in infants (aged 0–2 years) are 8 to 10 mm Hg; with older children and adolescents pressures of 10 to 12 mm Hg are typically sufficient. The abdominal wall of chil-dren has less resistance (or tone), so there is little change in the working space afforded by increasing the pressure beyond these levels. A benefit can be realized in increasing the pressure to 15 to 20 mm Hg for trocar insertion. Although the added pressure does not increase the working space, it does increase the resistance of the wall to deformation, easing safe trocar insertion.

Because of the more abdominal position of the bladder in infants, a Foley or straight catheter should be placed before access in all infants to reduce the possibility of bladder injury. Placement is also recommended for all children during pelvic procedures to aid visualization of pelvic structures. Because of the greater incidence of aerophagia

and inflation of the stomach with air during induc-tion of anesthesia in children, tube decompression of the stomach is an advantage.

ACCESS IN CHILDREN
Open Access

The Hasson technique where an incision is made in an open fashion and carried down to expose the peritoneum, which is then opened, allows the initial port to be placed in the peritoneal cavity under direct vision. This technique has been rec-ommended safer for children because of the decreased anterior-posterior diameter of the abdomen, and hence, closer proximity to the great vessels. Large multicenter analyses of complica-tions associated with laparoscopy have shown a substantial reduction in the incidence of major vascular injuries with open access.[3–7] The risk of major vascular injury during access is low but not zero with open techniques. The risk of bowel injury was higher with open methods in these studies. The frequency of injuries with access has decreased with time (earlier studies report higher complication rates) and decreases with operator experience.[3–7]

Needle Access

The Veress technique uses a needle with a spring-loaded safety insert that is placed blindly into the abdomen. The abdomen is inflated and then the ports are placed. The risk of injury is perceived to be higher. There are numerous case reports published describing a trocar or Veress needle injury, proposing open access as the means to avoid that injury. However, large multicenter anal-yses document similar rates of injury with all methods.[3–7]

Direct Access

Direct access implies the use of optical or special bladeless trocars. The trocar is placed directly through the abdominal wall without insufflation. For optical trocars, progress through the abdom-inal wall is observed directly as the port transits the wall. Anecdotally, this seems to be the least used in pediatric access techniques.

PROCEDURES
Diagnostic Laparoscopy

Initial applications of laparoscopy were used for diagnostic purposes. For example, laparoscopy can be used for evaluation of the impalpable testis; it is currently used for laparoscopic orchiopexy rather than for diagnosis alone. The benefit of diagnostic laparoscopy is that it can be done with needle scopes typically 2 mm in diameter that fit through a Veress needle containing a sheath for the endoscope. Diagnostic laparoscopy also plays a role in the child with intersex conditions when conventional imaging is insufficient or not possible.

For hernia surgery, laparoscopic assessment of the contralateral inguinal ring at the time of inguinal hernia repair has been well described with large series demonstrating its utility,[8] although controversy exists in its clinical relevance when a contralateral patent processus vaginalis is noted.[9] Access is gained via the ipsilateral open hernia sac. Either a 3- to 5-mm trocar or a 16-gauge angiocatheter is placed into the abdominal cavity via the sac. Insufflation at 8 mm Hg is used and then a 70° endoscope is placed through the access. The size of the scope varies with the type of access used. The ring is easily visualized and then one can determine if the contralateral side warrants repair.

Orchiopexy

Laparoscopic orchiopexy is the most widely performed laparoscopic technique in pediatric urology, and is used for correction of intra-abdominal testis (**Fig. 1**). This technique is performed either by a single stage or primary orchiopexy that leaves the spermatic vessels intact, or by a staged Fowler-Stephens orchiopexy where the vessels are ligated and transected. In the latter method, the spermatic vessels are occluded, usually with a clip, suture, or by fulguration. The testis is left in place, and at a second sitting, 4 to 6 months later, the testis is mobilized to the scrotum on a pedicle of the vas deferens and peritoneum with the spermatic vessels transected. Robotic surgery can be used in difficult cases such as high intra-abdominal testicles, and in particular for second-stage surgeries. The patient

is placed supine in the Trendelenburg position with the ipsilateral side elevated 30° to 40°. The bladder is emptied to aid in access and visualization. Port placement entails the camera port in the umbilicus and 2 working ports or stab incisions made with a number 11-blade scalpel: one on the same side of the testicle above the umbilicus in the midclavicular line, and the other contralaterally below the umbilicus, also in the midclavicular line. Although available, I have not found the robot to be useful in orchiopexies because reconstruction is not a part of the procedure.

Nephrectomy

As with robotic orchiopexy, simple nephrectomy is somewhat of an overkill of robotic technology; however, robotic advantages such as the three-dimensional images, increased dexterity, and decreased learning curve can be advantageous for beginners.[10] Nephrectomy can be performed using transperitoneal or retroperitoneal approaches, but in robotics the transperitoneal operation is the most readily accomplished because of the size of the ports and the arms, especially in the infant population. The choice of the transperitoneal or retroperitoneal approach depends on the surgeon's experience. The choice may be influenced by the need for additional procedures such as complete nephroureterectomy and bladder access if ureteral reimplantation is required. Retroperitoneal access is distinct in port placement and patient positioning. Ports are placed posteriorly or laterally depending on the surgeon's preference. The size of the robotic arms makes a posterior approach more difficult except in older children (ie, >12 years). Appropriate placement of the trocars is of utmost importance, and 3 to 4 laparoscopic ports are inserted at the surgeon's discretion.

Retroperitoneal access is achieved through the first trocar incision, 15-mm long and 10-mm from the lower border of the tip of the 12th rib (**Fig. 2**A). A working space is created by gas insufflation dissection, and the first trocar is fixed with a purse-string suture applied around the deep fascia to ensure an airtight seal. Another approach to create the retroperitoneal space uses 2 index fingers of a powder-free surgical glove placed one inside the other and ligated onto the 5- or 10-mm trocar sheath. The dissection is then performed by instilling 500 mL of warm saline through the insufflation channel of the trocar. After completed dissection, the trocar is reinserted without the balloon and pneumoretroperitoneum is established (maximum pressure 12 mm Hg or age dependent). A 5- or 10-mm 0° telescope is

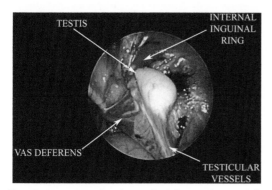

TESTIS — INTERNAL INGUINAL RING

VAS DEFERENS — TESTICULAR VESSELS

Fig. 1. Laparoscopic view of right testis at right internal inguinal ring.

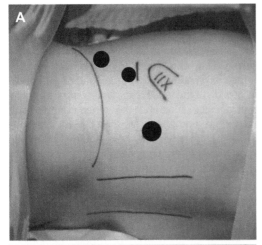

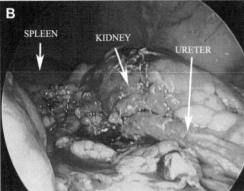

Fig. 2. (A) Retroperitoneal port placement for renal access. (B) Transperitoneal view of kidney and ureter after left colonic mobilization.

inserted through the first trocar. A second 3-mm trocar is inserted posteriorly near the costovertebral angle; the third 3-mm trocar is inserted 10 mm above the top of the iliac crest at the anterior axillary line. To avoid transperitoneal insertion of this trocar, the working space is fully developed and the deep surface of the anterior wall muscles are identified before the trocar is inserted. The insufflation pressure is less than 12 mm Hg and the flow rate of CO_2 is progressively increased from 1 to 5 L/min The kidney is approached posteriorly, Gerota fascia is incised parallel to the psoas muscle, the perirenal fat is dissected to reveal the lower pole of the kidney in which the renal pelvis is first identified, and then mobilized (see **Fig. 2B**). The ureter should be identified first and transected because it can be used as a handle and guide to reach the hilum.

In the transabdominal approach, the patient is placed in a modified flank position with a 60° elevation of the flank. Ports are placed in the umbilicus for the camera port and in the midline above the umbilicus and midclavicular line below the umbilicus for the working ports. In infants, the upper working port should be placed subxyphoid in the midline and the lower working port as lateral as possible to the rectus muscle. The robot, if used, is docked over the ipsilateral shoulder.

Heminephroureterectomy

Heminephroureterectomy (HNU) may also be performed transperitoneally or retroperitoneally in a manner similar to nephrectomy. HNU is similar to complete nephrectomy with regard to port placement and initial exposure of the ureters and hilum. The transection of the affected moiety may be done either with the hook or scissor cautery. Before patient positioning, it might be beneficial to cystoscopically place an open-ended ureteral catheter in the unaffected moiety to inject methylene blue after moiety transection to ensure there is no leakage. The procedure is performed as described for the laparoscopic nephrectomy approach. The poles can be separated using either cautery or the harmonic scalpel (**Fig. 3**). I prefer the transperitoneal approach because if bladder access is needed one can readily turn to the bladder for repair. The robot typically needs to be redocked from the foot of the bed in this case. A bladder catheter is kept in place overnight and the patient can be discharged the same or next day.

Pyeloplasty

Laparoscopic or robotic-assisted pyeloplasty can also be performed by a trans- or retroperitoneal approach. I typically use a 6-0 monofilament absorbable suture, but one can use any 5-0 or 6-0 absorbable suture depending on the size of the patient. Sutures larger than 6-0 for small children and infants are not recommended. The

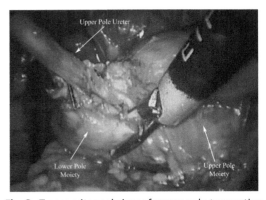

Fig. 3. Transperitoneal view of upper pole transection from lower pole moiety.

patient is placed in the same position and robotic docking, if needed, is performed as for nephrectomy. The uteropelvic junction (UPJ) is exposed transmesenterically on the left or by mobilizing the colon on the right for the transperitoneal approach. If one chooses colonic mobilization on the left, it must be taken medially over the aorta. In the retroperitoneal approach, the kidney is approached posteriorly, Gerota fascia is incised parallel to the psoas muscle, the perinephric fat is dissected to reveal the lower pole of the kidney where the renal pelvis is first identified and then mobilized. The UPJ is identified and minimally dissected to free it from connective tissue so that the anterior surface is seen to identify crossing vessel pathology, if present.

A hitch stitch can be passed through the abdominal wall and is placed to elevate and stabilize the pelvis if so desired (**Fig. 4**). I use a hitch stitch if a pyelolithotomy is necessary. After the pelvis is incised, the ureter is spatulated laterally and the anastomosis is performed using a running suture. A double-pigtail stent can be placed after the posterior wall closure is complete; otherwise before pyeloplasty positioning, an opened-ended catheter can be placed cystoscopically if one wishes to remove it on the first postoperative day. This is performed by placing an 18-gauge angiocatheter through the anterior abdominal wall. A guide wire is then placed in an antegrade fashion. The stent is then passed over the guide wire. It might be beneficial to fill the bladder with saline or methylene blue so that one can observe the efflux of urine when there is access into the bladder by the stent. The stent can also be placed retrograde to use a dangling string to allow removal in the orifice. Postoperatively, a urethral catheter is left overnight and the double-J stent, if used, is removed in 2 to 4 weeks. The results described in the literature report a success rate of 95% similar to that of the open procedure, which is the gold standard.[11–14]

URETERAL REIMPLANTATION
Vesicoscopic

The laparoscopic Cohen procedure using a pneumovesicum was first described in a pig model in 2003.[15] The limitations of this procedure have been described and this approach is not advocated for bladder that has a capacity less than 130 mL in voiding cystourethrogram studies.[16–18] The patient is placed in the supine position with legs apart. The bladder is filled with saline solution through the urethra. Using an open technique or visualization via a flexible pediatric cystoscope, the camera port is placed in the midline at the bladder dome. A 3-0 absorbable suture secures the bladder wall and skin to the trocar. The working ports are positioned midway between the umbilicus and pubis at the midclavicular line. Ports are fixed to the abdominal wall using a stitch, which is also used to close the bladder. The bladder is filled with CO_2 to drain the saline, and the robotic device, if used, is brought over the patient's feet. Similar to the open technique, ureteral dissection starts after placement of a 6-cm segment of a 5-F feeding tube or 4-F open-ended ureteral catheter, secured to the ureter with a 4-0 absorbable suture. Mobilization of the ureters is done by using the hook or scissor cautery. (**Fig. 5**) The submucosal tunnels are created by dissecting with scissors from the original hiatus to the other side of the trigone, and

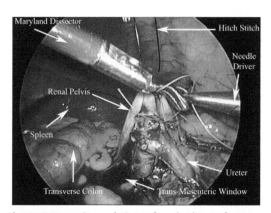

Fig. 4. Transperitoneal view of pyeloplasty after pyelolithotomy via a transmesenteric approach, with hitch stitch in place.

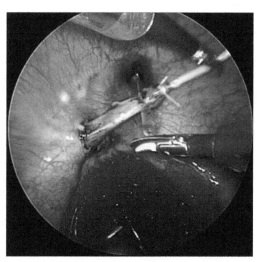

Fig. 5. Vesicoscopic view of left ureter being dissected with open-ended ureteral catheter secured in the ureter.

incising the mucosa at the site of the new mucosal hiatus. Anastomosis of the ureters is performed after bringing them through the mucosal tunnel. Anchoring sutures (4-0 absorbable suture) are used to secure the ureter to the bladder musculature, and the mucosal cuff is attached with 5-0 absorbable suture. The mucosa over the original hiatus is closed with running 5-0 absorbable suture.

The working ports are removed and the bladder holding stitches are then tied. The flexible cystoscope is used to inspect the inside of the bladder. The port sites are also closed at the fascial level. The bladder catheter is kept overnight. This technique is extremely challenging. The visualization and control are excellent and we must continue to develop this approach.

Extravesical Ureteral Reimplantation

The extravesical approach can be performed unilaterally or bilaterally, following the same steps as the open Lich-Gregoir technique. Cystoscopy can be performed to place open-ended ureteral catheters to aid in the dissection. With the patient in the supine position an open technique is used to place the first trocar in the umbilicus. The working ports are positioned in the midclavicular line bilaterally, about 1 cm below the umbilical line. If the robot is used and the child has a puboumbilical length less than 8 cm, then the midline camera port should be placed above the umbilicus between the xyphoid and umbilicus to prevent robotic arm collision. The robot, if used, is docked over the patient's feet.

The technique follows the same steps as the open Lich-Gregoir procedure, and starts by dissecting the ureter after opening the peritoneum, anterior to the uterus and just over the posterior bladder wall. The ureter is freed from the surrounding tissue keeping its vessels intact. The pelvic plexus is readily identified medial and caudal to the ureter. Approximately 4 to 5 cm is dissected to permit mobility and to prevent kinking as the bladder tunnel is created for the ureter (**Fig. 6**). A hitch stitch through the posterior bladder wall can be used to improve the exposure of the ureteral hiatus if the bladder is large. A detrusor trough is created by incising the muscularis of the bladder for about 3 cm and developing flaps with the cautery scissors. Any perforations of the mucosa are closed using a 5-0 absorbable suture before trough closure. The bladder muscularis is then closed over the ureter, using a 4-0 absorbable interrupted suture. Care must be taken to avoid any kinking or excessive compression of the ureter to prevent obstruction. Closure is performed

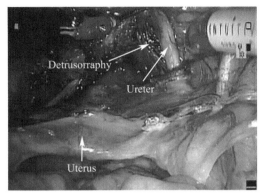

Fig. 6. Transperitoneal view of robotic extravesical reimplantation (right side view).

proximal to distal or vice versa. In the latter, the ureter is well visualized but the needle needs to be passed under the ureter each time the suture is placed. I catch the adventitia of the ureter with each suture to ensure it does not slip back during the healing process. The urethral catheter is removed the next morning and the child is discharged after voiding.

Appendicovesicostomy and Augmentation

There is 1 case report of a robotically assisted Mitrofanoff procedure[19] and one report of a laparoscopic procedure in a child.[18] As the author of the purely laparoscopic procedure, I can subjectively state the procedure is extremely facilitated with robotics. The patient is placed in the supine position in Trendelenburg. Three ports are used. The camera port is placed lateral to the umbilicus, and the other 2 working ports, on the right and left sides in the midclavicular line at the level of the umbilicus.

The procedure commences with cecal mobilization. Care is taken to protect the appendiceal mesentery and mobilize with an adequate length. Once the cecum is mobilized, the appendix is separated from the cecum, leaving a small cuff of cecum with the appendix (**Fig. 7**). The bladder is filled with saline after measuring the best position for the appendix due to its length, mobility of the bladder, and location of the stoma. A 4-cm detrusorhaphy is made. The appendix is anastomosed to a small mucosal opening in the apex of the detrusor trough and the defect is closed using 4-0 absorbable interrupted suture (**Figs. 8** and **9**). The base of the appendix is brought up to reach the umbilicus or the right lower quadrant (see **Fig. 8**).

Although initial reports of conventional laparoscopic bladder augmentation generally involved laparoscopic bowel mobilization and harvesting

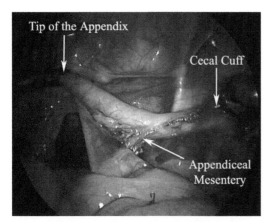

Fig. 7. Mobilization of the appendix from the cecum, maintaining the integrity of the mesentery.

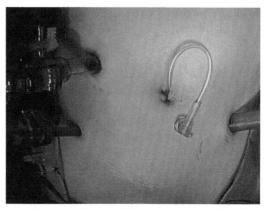

Fig. 9. View of matured appendicovesicostomy in umbilicus with feeding tube in place.

followed by extracorporeal bowel reconstruction, the current laparoscopic and robotic procedures have been successfully performed in a completely intracorporeal manner.[20,21] Conventional laparoscopic bladder augmentation is possible but not practical because of some difficulties with suturing for reconstruction and long operative time; however, robotic bladder augmentation is expected to overcome these difficulties and allow shorter operative times.

Cystoscopy can be performed, and open-ended ureteral catheters should be placed for easy intraoperative identification of ureters. The patient's position and port placement are basically the same as those in robotic appendicovesicostomy. Additional robotic and/or laparoscopic assistant ports are placed to introduce sutures easily into the abdomen and assist with retraction. A 20-cm ileal segment should be chosen 15 cm proximal to the ileocecal valve, and it is then isolated and detubularized. An endoscopic stapler device,

which is introduced through a laparoscopic assistant port, may be useful for isolation of ileum. Care is taken to protect the ileal mesentery and mobilize with an adequate length. Intracorporeal irrigation of the ileal segment with sterile saline can be done after detubularization of ileum. Bowel continuity is reestablished in 2 layers with an end-to-end ileoileostomy using intracorporeal running 3-0 absorbable sutures followed by a Lembert suture, and the mesenteric window is closed. After opening the native bladder, the anastomosis of the simple ileal onlay patch[21] or U-shaped configuration[20] to the native bladder is performed from a posterior to anterior direction using complete intracorporeal 4-0 absorbable running sutures. Care must be taken to avoid twisting the ileal mesentery as the ileal segment is brought down to the bladder. If an appendicovesicostomy is needed, the appendix is anastomosed to the posterior wall of the native bladder in an extravesical fashion, as described earlier. A suprapubic catheter is usually placed. A watertight anastomosis is confirmed by irrigation with sterile saline through the Foley catheter. Open-ended ureteral catheters can be removed after surgery.

OTHER PROCEDURES

A variety of other procedures, such as pyelolithotomy, adrenalectomy, bladder neck sling, ureteropyelostomy, excision of müllerian duct remnants, sacrocolpopexy, and so forth, have been performed using robotics in children. Situations with abnormal müllerian structures such as seminal vesicle cysts are well managed with laparoscopic excision.[22] These cases also indicate the potential flexibility of this system for varied case challenges, particularly in pediatric urology where a large

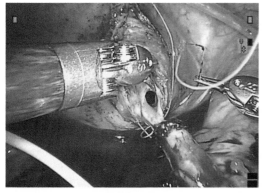

Fig. 8. Transperitoneal view of the appendix anastomosed to a mucosal opening in the apex of the detrusor trough.

variety of surgical procedures are needed in the care of patients.

SUMMARY

Minimally invasive procedures have revolutionized surgery for urologic disorders in pediatric patients. The success rates have paralleled the results of open surgery and provide the benefit of smaller incisions and less manipulation of tissue during the procedures. Robotics has enhanced these factors, coupled with increased dexterity, better visualization, and less fatigue, allowing greater precision. We must continue to evolve with the ever-changing advancements in technology. The true visionaries in this domain are focusing on the surgical robot as an information system, one that can be fused with other information systems.

One example of this fusion might be image-guided surgery where surgeons will be able to see real-time, three-dimensional scanner images electronically superimposed over the operative field that is displayed on the monitor. This can be taken a step further into the realm of simulation and training where surgeons or trainees can robotically practice their patient's surgery the night before. Also, the maneuvers could theoretically be programmed into the robot to help avoid injury. The surgery and training can be specific to that patient's anatomy. Telesurgery is another exciting frontier that will undoubtedly be part of the robotic future, and would allow equal care everywhere for everyone. We must take a keen interest in its growth so that we can influence its development.

REFERENCES

1. Garcia-Ruiz A, Smedira NG, Loop FD, et al. Robotic surgical instruments for dexterity enhancement in thoracoscopic coronary artery bypass graft. J Laparoendosc Adv Surg Tech A 1997;7:277–83.
2. Kavoussi LR, Moore RG, Adams JB, et al. Comparison of robotic versus human laparoscopic camera control. J Urol 1995;154:2134–6.
3. Paterson-Brown S. The acute abdomen: the role of laparoscopy. Baillieres Clin Gastroenterol 1991; 5(3):691–703.
4. Hakki-Siren P, Kurki T. A nationwide analysis of laparoscopic complications. Obstet Gynecol 1997;89: 108–12.
5. Jones KD, Fan A, Sutton CJG. Safe entry during laparoscopy. Gynaecol Endosc 2002;11:327–34.
6. Larobina M, Nottle P. Complete evidence regarding major visceral injuries during laparoscopic access. Surg Laprosc Endosc Percutan Tech 2005;5(3): 119–23.
7. Catarci M, Carlini M, Santioro E. Major and minor injuries during creation of pneumoperitoneum, a multicenter study of 12,919 cases. Surg Endosc 2001;15:566–9.
8. Holcomb GW 3rd. Diagnostic laparoscopy for congenital inguinal hernia. Semin Laparosc Surg 1998;5(1):55–9.
9. Miltenburg DM, Nuchtern JG, Jaksic T, et al. Laparoscopic evaluation of the pediatric inguinal hernia— a meta-analysis. J Pediatr Surg 1998;33(6):874–9.
10. Koyle MA, Woo HH, Kavoussi LR. Laparoscopic nephrectomy in the first year of life. J Pediatr Surg 1993;28(5):693–5.
11. Atug F, Woods M, Burgess SV, et al. Robotic assisted laparoscopic pyeloplasty in children. J Urol 2005;174(4 Pt 1):1440–2.
12. Kutikov A, Nguyen M, Guzzo T, et al. Robot assisted pyeloplasty in the infant-lessons learned. J Urol 2006;176(5):2237–9 [discussion: 2239–40].
13. Lee RS, Retik AB, Borer JG, et al. Pediatric robot assisted laparoscopic dismembered pyeloplasty: comparison with a cohort of open surgery. J Urol 2006;175(2):683–7.
14. Olsen LH, Jorgensen TM. Computer assisted pyeloplasty in children: the retroperitoneal approach. J Urol 2004;171(6 Pt 2):2629–31.
15. Olsen LH, Deding D, Yeung CK, et al. Computer assisted laparoscopic pneumovesical ureter reimplantation a.m. Cohen: initial experience in a pig model. APMIS Suppl 2003;109:23–5.
16. Peters CA, Woo R. Intravesical robotically assisted bilateral ureteral reimplantation. J Endourol 2005; 19(6):618–21 [discussion: 621–2].
17. Casale P, Feng WC, Grady RW, et al. Intracorporeal laparoscopic appendicovesicostomy: a case report of a novel approach. J Urol 2004;171(5):1899–900.
18. Kutikov A, Guzzo TJ, Canter DJ, et al. Initial experience with laparoscopic transvesicle ureteral reimplantation at the Children's Hospital of Philadelphia. J Urol 2006;176(5):2222–5 [discussion: 2225–6].
19. Pedraza R, Weiser A, Franco I. Laparoscopic appendicovesicostomy (Mitrofanoff procedure) in a child using the da Vinci robotic system. J Urol 2004;171(4):1652–3.
20. Lorenzo AJ, Cerveira J, Farhat WA. Pediatric laparoscopic ileal cystoplasty: complete intracorporeal surgical technique. Urology 2007;69:977–81.
21. Gundeti MS, Eng MK, Reynolds WS, et al. Pediatric robotic-assisted laparoscopic augmentation ileocystoplasty and Mitrofanoff appendicovesicostomy: complete intracorporeal—initial case report. Urology 2008;72:1144–7.
22. Carmignani G, Gallucci M, Puppo P, et al. Video laparoscopic excision of a seminal vesicle cyst associated with ipsilateral renal agenesis [comments]. J Urol 1995;153(2):437–9.

Pediatric Urologic Oncology: Organ-Sparing Surgery in Kidney and Testis

John H. Makari, MD, MHA, MA[a,b],
Puneeta Ramachandra, MD[a],
Fernando A. Ferrer Jr, MD[a,b],*

KEYWORDS

- Wilms tumor • Nephron-sparing surgery
- Testis-sparing surgery • Teratoma

NEPHRON-SPARING SURGERY
Partial Nephrectomy for Wilms Tumor: Introduction

Current accepted indications for renal-sparing surgery in the setting of Wilms tumor are bilateral Wilms tumor (BWT), Wilms tumor in a solitary kidney, and multicentric, unilateral Wilms tumor in patients at risk for metachronous tumors. Renal-sparing surgery in unilateral Wilms tumor in patients who are not at risk for metachronous tumors remains controversial. In this section, studies regarding partial nephrectomy in patients with BWT, solitary kidneys, or Wilms tumor-associated syndromes are reviewed. The current ongoing Children's Oncology Group (COG) protocol for bilateral Wilms tumor is outlined and the current literature on nephron-sparing surgery in unilateral Wilms tumor patients is discussed. Finally, several surgical techniques for performing a partial nephrectomy in the setting of Wilms tumor are described.

Bilateral Wilms Tumor

For more than 20 years, the National Wilms Tumor Study Group (NWTSG) has recommended preoperative chemotherapy for patients with BWT, with the goal of avoiding total nephrectomy at initial surgery. In reviewing prior NWTSG trials, 9.1% of patients with BWT eventually developed renal failure; in almost three-fourths of these patients, the cause of renal failure was a contralateral nephrectomy for recurrent or persistent tumor after initial nephrectomy.[1] BWT patients also have had significantly worse outcomes than similar patients with unilateral Wilms tumor. In NWTS-3 and -4, 344 patients with BWT had a 10-year relapse-free survival rate of only 65% and a 10-year overall survival rate of 78%, compared with unilateral stage I to IV favorable histology Wilms tumor (recurrence-free survival 86% and overall survival 92%). Poor outcomes in patients with BWT may have various contributing factors including delay in local control, understaging and undertreatment, or increased incidence of

---

Equal contribution (JHM, PR).

[a] Division of Urology, Department of Surgery, University of Connecticut School of Medicine, 263 Farmington Avenue, Farmington, CT 06030, USA

[b] Division of Pediatric Urology, Connecticut Children's Medical Center, 282 Washington Street, Suite 2E, Hartford, CT 06106, USA

* Corresponding author. Division of Urology, Department of Surgery, University of Connecticut School of Medicine, 263 Farmington Avenue, Farmington, CT 06030.

E-mail address: fferrer@connecticutchildrens.org

Urol Clin N Am 37 (2010) 287–298
doi:10.1016/j.ucl.2010.03.008

unfavorable histology (ie, >10% have anaplasia). Of the 145 patients enrolled in NWTS-2 and -3, total excision of tumor was possible in less than 40.[2] In NWTS-4, complete removal of all gross tumor using a nephron-sparing approach was possible in 88% of kidneys, but local recurrence occurred in 8.2% of the remaining kidneys.[3] In comparison, patients with unilateral tumors of favorable histology who underwent complete nephrectomy only had a 3% incidence of local recurrence.[4] This higher rate of local recurrence in patients with bilateral tumors may be due in part to surgical technique; surgeons may accept a higher rate of positive margins to spare a normal kidney. More intensive up-front preoperative chemotherapy may reduce tumor burden in these patients, facilitating nephron-sparing surgery. The current COG protocol aims to improve outcomes in BWT patients while decreasing treatment-related morbidity.

Role of Initial Biopsy in Bilateral Tumors

Two reasons are typically given for performing preoperative biopsy. The first reason is to avoid misdiagnosis. In patients with bilateral renal lesions on imaging, misdiagnosis of BWT is very unlikely because most non-Wilms malignancies and benign renal entities present with unilateral lesions. Furthermore, in the collective experience of NWTS, Societé Internationale D'Oncologie Pédiatrique (SIOP), and German and United Kingdom cancer studies, no patient with bilateral tumors has been found not to have Wilms in either kidney. The second often-quoted rationale is to detect anaplasia. Experience from NWTS-4 has demonstrated that needle biopsy is inaccurate for the detection of anaplasia.[5] This failure rate is not substantially improved through open biopsy whereby the detection rate was 1 in 3 in the same study. Furthermore, in prior NWTSG studies, tumor biopsy was considered local spill, in effect upstaging of the tumor. Local spill was associated with an increased rate of abdominal recurrence in NWTS-4.[4] For these reasons, neither open surgical biopsy nor needle biopsy at initial presentation is recommended for most patients as part of the current protocol.

Overview of Bilateral Wilms Tumor Treatment Strategy

In patients with bilateral tumors, a baseline abdominal computed tomographic (CT) scan or magnetic resonance imaging (MRI) is performed, with follow-up imaging at 6 and 12 weeks, as well as at the end of therapy. Intensive up-front chemotherapy with vincristine, dactinomycin, and doxorubicin is then administered for 6 weeks. Patients are reimaged after 6 weeks of chemotherapy; at this point, those tumors that are amenable to partial nephrectomy are completely excised. The use of MR angiography and venography is frequently helpful if surgery is contemplated. Patients with tumors that are not amenable to renal-sparing surgery undergo an open renal biopsy, followed by 6 more weeks of chemotherapy driven by tumor-specific histology. At 12 weeks tumors are reassessed, and partial nephrectomy is performed if feasible. Radical nephrectomy is performed if partial nephrectomy is still not possible at this point (**Fig. 1**). Delaying surgical resection is not advisable, as prolonging chemotherapy may not lead to a better response and may even jeopardize outcomes in patients with progressive or nonresponsive disease.[6] Patients with Wilms tumor of high-risk histology, such as those with anaplasia, benefit from early resection and histology-guided chemotherapy.

Nephron-Sparing Surgery for Unilateral Tumors

Nephron-sparing surgery in the setting of unilateral Wilms tumor (UWT) is controversial for several reasons. Previously, reasons for considering partial nephrectomy in these children were the 2% to 3% risk of metachronous contralateral Wilms tumor and the risk of developing renal failure in the future. The incidence of renal failure in patients with UWT is reported to be very low. In 1996, the NWTS reported that children with UWT had only a 0.25% incidence of renal failure. Most of the patients in that study experiencing renal failure had Denys-Drash syndrome (DDS), making them more prone to medical renal disease.[1] Only a very small number of patients in this study were observed for more than 20 years, making it difficult to determine long-term effects of complete unilateral nephrectomy in most patients. Patients with DDS or aniridia and UWT are at increased risk of renal failure due to a mutation in the WT1 gene.[7] In the NWTSG Late Effects Study, patients with DDS had the highest risk of early renal failure, but children with the WAGR syndrome (Wilms tumor, aniridia, genitourinary anomalies, and mental retardation) had somewhat higher rates in later years.[7] Renal-sparing surgery for unilateral lesions can be considered in this cohort of patients.

Most unilateral Wilms tumors will not be amenable to partial nephrectomy at diagnosis, with the occasional exception of tumors found on screening ultrasound for children with Wilms tumor-related syndromes. Therefore, preoperative

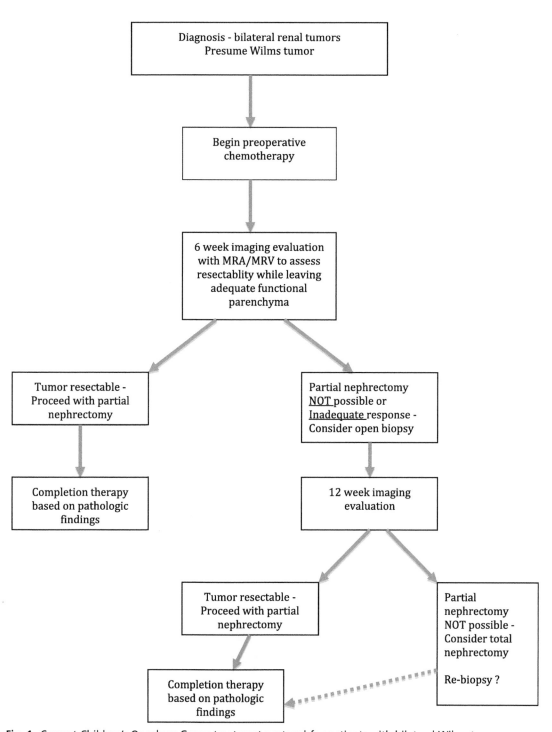

Fig. 1. Current Children's Oncology Group treatment protocol for patients with bilateral Wilms tumor.

chemotherapy may be necessary to reduce tumor burden enough to facilitate partial nephrectomy. In 2003, Haeker and colleagues[8] reviewed the results of partial nephrectomy in unilateral Wilms tumor from SIOP 93-01/GPOH. Between 1994 and 2001, 37 partial nephrectomies were performed compared with 770 total nephrectomies for unilateral Wilms tumor. Of these 37 patients, 15 underwent partial nephrectomy prior to chemotherapy; 4 of these 37 patients had tumor recurrence, 2 of whom subsequently died. One patient who died had metastatic disease after a partial nephrectomy; the other had a malignant rhabdoid tumor. The other 2 patients had local recurrence, which was completely resected at re-operation. Overall, there was an 8.1% rate of local recurrence after partial nephrectomy compared with only 3.1% in patients who underwent total nephrectomy. Despite the higher rate of relapse after partial nephrectomy, tumor stage, overall survival, and relapse-free survival were not different between those who underwent partial nephrectomy and those who underwent total nephrectomy. There did appear to be a trend, although not statistically significant, toward poor outcomes in those patients with "high-risk" histology after partial nephrectomy. Also, there was a trend toward improved outcomes in those who underwent partial nephrectomy after chemo-therapy. Based on these results, the investigators recommended that partial nephrectomy only be considered after chemotherapy for stage I, low-risk or intermediate-risk patients in whom complete tumor resection is possible and in whom tumor-free margins can be confirmed on in-traoperative frozen section. Excellent outcomes after nephron-sparing surgery in patients with stage I tumors were also reported by Zani and colleagues[9] in 2005. In their retrospective series, 10 patients with stage I Wilms tumor had under-gone nephron-sparing surgery, and at a mean follow-up of 75.3 months, all patients were alive and event-free.

In an earlier retrospective series of 90 patients with Wilms tumor diagnosed between 1982 and 1992, partial nephrectomy was performed in 7 patients with unilateral lesions. Selection criteria for performing a partial nephrectomy were tumor confined to 1 pole of a functioning kidney, occu-pying less than a third of that kidney, and absence of invasion into the renal vein or collecting system. Of these 7 patients 2 died of metastatic disease, but no patient had evidence of local recurrence at a median follow-up of 101 months. The kidney remnant appeared to have excellent differential kidney function at follow-up.[10]

Current COG protocols do not allow for partial nephrectomy in cases of unilateral Wilms where a predisposition syndrome does not exist.

Diffuse Hyperplastic Perilobar Nephrogenic Rests

Diffuse hyperplastic perilobar nephrogenic rests (DHPLNR) represent a unique variant of nephro-genic rest (NR) in which the entire cortical surface of the kidney is composed of a hyperplastic NR.

These lesions can be quite confusing because they can be very large and appear identical to a Wilms tumor. Imaging with MR or CT scan can be helpful in distinguishing NR from Wilms tumor. NRs appear homogeneous compared with the cortex on contrast-enhanced CT scan (**Fig. 2**). On MRI, the NR is seen as isointense or slightly hy-pointense when compared with the cortex on T1-weighted images; the intensity does not change with gadolinium administration. Wilms tumor, on the other hand, has a mixed echogenicity and inhomogeneity.[11–13] Large rests can respond dramatically to chemotherapy, leaving a rind around the kidney (**Fig. 3**). When confusion exists, biopsy may be appropriate. Because of the risk of subsequent Wilms tumor development, these patients should undergo a renal-sparing approach (**Fig. 4**). A discussion of chemotherapy for treat-ment of DHPLNRs is beyond the scope of this article.

Surgical Technique

In this section the authors describe their preferred technique used for performing partial nephrec-tomy, as well as a more traditional technique that may be employed at other centers.

At the authors' institution, surgical planning begins with preoperative MR arteriography and venography. Identifying accessory vessels preop-eratively can often facilitate a successful partial resection. One patient at the authors' institution with bilateral Wilms tumors underwent a left total nephrectomy and right lower pole partial nephrec-tomy. **Fig. 5** demonstrates a right accessory lower

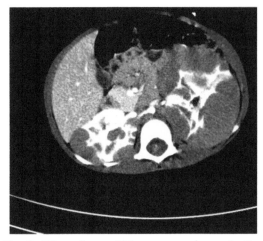

Fig. 2. MR angiogram/MR venogram demonstrating right accessory lower pole artery and vein in a patient with bilateral Wilms tumors. The patient eventually underwent right partial nephrectomy of the lower pole and left total nephrectomy.

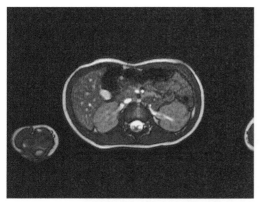

Fig. 3. CT scan demonstrating diffuse hyperplastic perilobar nephrogenic rests.

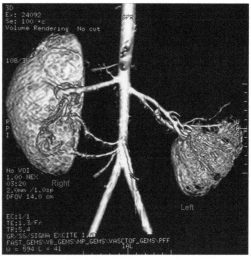

Fig. 5. Intraoperative photograph of patient from **Fig. 3** demonstrating multiple open renal biopsies after chemotherapy for DHPLNRs. The kidney has a thick rind of pale tissue encasing the entire kidney.

pole artery in this patient. Intraoperatively, the lower pole vessels were dissected and ligated, demarcating the parenchyma. This procedure allowed for resection of the lower pole including the tumor and adequate rim of normal parenchyma in a relatively bloodless field. The main renal vessels supplying the upper and midpole of the right kidney did not need to be clamped.

The following is a description of the operative technique. The patient is placed in a supine position after induction of general anesthesia. Wide exposure of the kidney is obtained via a transperitoneal approach. The renal vessels are carefully exposed and encircled with vessel loops and then polar vessels are divided as appropriate. Routine clamping of renal vessels is not performed. Recently, the authors have successfully used the TissueLink device (Salient Surgical Technologies, Portsmouth, NH, USA), a saline-coupled radiofrequency device, to perform simple polar partial nephrectomies and more complex midpolar procedures. Used as a hand device, it works by

concentrating sound waves into a conductive fluid, generating heat that seals blood vessels. Proceeding slowly through the renal parenchyma has allowed for a near bloodless field. Given the potential for creating tissue artifact, it is imperative that generous margins be obtained. Intraoperative ultrasound and spinal needle placement have been used to select appropriate planes for dissection, ensuring that the entire lesion is removed with a rim of normal tissue. Pathologic frozen section must be done to ensure that a border of normal tissue is removed. Despite the generation of heat extending into the remaining parenchyma, postoperative radionucleotide imaging has confirmed the preservation of functional parenchyma in the patients after use of TissueLink for partial nephrectomy (**Fig. 6**). Entry into the collecting system is repaired with 5-0 or 6-0 polydioxanone sutures, and a double-J stent is placed from above. Placement of an omental patch or fibrin sealant is often used to cover the repair and reduce the incidence of urinary leaks. In both cases, postoperative imaging will need to be interpreted with caution, taking into consideration how the repair was performed.

While one can routinely obtain access to the renal vasculature, with modern hemostatic techniques occlusion of the renal artery is not necessary in most cases. Preparation of all patients undergoing partial nephrectomy should include suprahydration, avoidance of unnecessary traction on the renal vasculature, and prevention of periods of hypotension. If renal artery occlusion is required, the administration of 20% mannitol is

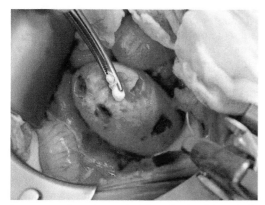

Fig. 4. MRI of patient with diffuse hyperplastic perilobar nephrogenic rests from **Fig. 3** after chemotherapy.

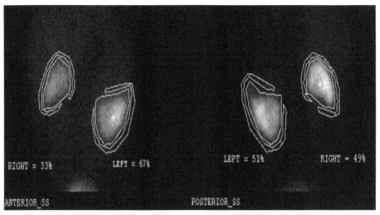

Fig. 6. DMSA scan after right partial nephrectomy using TissueLink device demonstrating preserved functioning right renal parenchyma.

recommended. For periods of ischemia exceeding 30 minutes, hypothermia is recommended. Lowering renal temperature to 20°C to 25°C decreases cellular activity, providing a protective window of up to 3 hours during renal occlusion. Surface cooling with ice-slush is accomplished by mobilizing the kidney, and then surrounding it with bowel bags into which ice-slush is poured. Full immersion of the kidney to rapidly lower temperature should be maintained for 15 to 20 minutes after occlusion for maximum protective benefit. Thereafter, it is presumed that portions of the kidney may not be fully immersed at certain times. The authors do not prefer infusion of a cooling solution into the renal artery to cool the kidney because this technique risks injury to the vessel.

Another approach may be to position the patient in a lateral position over the kidney rest for dissection of unilateral lesions. A supracostal incision may be best for adolescents, whereas a partial anterior transverse incision could be used in a smaller child. Gerota fascia is opened laterally, and the entire kidney is freed from the surrounding attachments. Perirenal fat around the tumor is left in place. The vascular pedicle is dissected sufficiently to allow the placement of vascular clamps. The renal capsule is then incised. Occlusion of the renal artery with a rubber-shod clamp may be done; occlusion of the renal vein is not necessary if the main renal artery is occluded. The parenchyma is then bluntly dissected away from normal tissue. Arcuate vessels are sharply divided and suture-ligated using 4-0 or 5-0 chromic sutures. An argon beam laser may be used for coagulation if available. The vascular clamp may be released temporarily to identify bleeding vessels. The collecting system should be closed in a running fashion. The kidney is then closed using 3-0 or 4-0 chromic mattress sutures. Gerota fascia is

then reapproximated. A frozen-section examination should be performed to assess for negative margins. A closed suction drain is left in place.

Enucleation of very small tumors may be considered for patients with multicentric tumors in a solitary kidney. A layer of normal parenchyma should be included in the resection when possible. Vascular control is usually not needed. The kidney is mobilized as mentioned previously. After the renal capsule is incised sharply, the tumor is bluntly enucleated by following the plane outside the compressed pseudocapsule of tumor. The collecting system should be avoided if possible. The resection bed is fulgurated with an argon beam laser and packed with oxidized cellulose or omentum for hemostasis. Finally, the capsule is closed.

Ex Vivo Surgery and Autotransplantation

Bench surgery or ex vivo partial nephrectomy followed by autotransplantation is an alternative surgical technique that may be considered. As described in 1975 by Lilly and colleagues,[14] ex vivo surgery may permit performance of partial nephrectomy that may not be possible in situ. According to these investigators, extracorporeal kidney surgery allows "careful definitive tumor excision" in a bloodless field. Removing the kidney from the renal fossa provides the opportunity for a proper regional lymph node sampling. A nephrectomy is performed either via a flank incision or transperitoneally and autotransplanted in the iliac fossa or back into the renal fossa. The iliac fossa provides a convenient place for transplantation because of the relative ease of performing the vascular anastomoses. The ureter may be left intact or may be transected and reimplanted into the bladder. Once outside the body, the kidney is flushed with chilled hyperosmolar electrolyte solution to prolong ischemia time. Ischemic injury is a result of depletion of adenosine triphosphate, which is needed for cellular sodium-potassium pump. Energy requirements are significantly decreased in the setting of hypothermia. Successful performance of bench surgery has been reported in small series of patients with bilateral Wilms tumor.[15,16] Ex vivo perfusion with organ preservation solution may make it difficult for the surgeon and the pathologist to distinguish between normal renal tissue, nephroblastomatosis, and tumor.[16]

TESTIS-SPARING SURGERY
Introduction

Prepubertal testis tumors are relatively uncommon, accounting for approximately 1% of all pediatric solid tumors, and occur in 0.5 to 2 per 100,000 boys.[17] In contrast to adult testicular neoplasms, most prepubertal testis tumors are benign and have biologic characteristics that make them amenable to local treatment. The abilities to distinguish malignant from benign neoplasms fairly reliably preoperatively and confirm the histopathologic diagnosis with intraoperative frozen pathology have promoted the practice of testis-sparing surgery for select prepubertal testis tumors.

In 1980, the American Academy of Pediatrics Section on Urology established the Prepubertal Testis Tumor Registry. At that time, little was known about the incidence or biologic behavior of prepubertal testis tumors. Treatment recommendations for testicular neoplasms in this age group were drawn largely from adult data. From that registry, it was concluded that most prepubertal testis tumors were yolk sac tumors; other identified tumors included (in decreasing order of incidence) teratoma, unspecified stromal tumors, epidermoid cysts, juvenile granulosa cell tumors, Sertoli cell tumors, Leydig cell tumors, and gonadoblastoma.[18] A more recent multicenter report suggests that the vast majority of prepubertal testis tumors are benign, with yolk sac tumors accounting for only 15% of such tumors. In this report, teratoma was the most prevalent prepubertal testis tumor, representing 48% of tumors in this cohort of patients younger than 12 years with primary testis tumors; overall, 74% of tumors were benign.[19] Several single-institution series confirm the observation that most prepubertal testis tumors are benign.[20–22] The discrepancy between rates of malignancy in the Prepubertal Testis Tumor Registry and these reports is likely attributable to underreporting of benign lesions

to the registry. In addition, the vast majority of prepubertal testis tumors (in contrast to adult testicular neoplasms) have a single rather than mixed histopathology.[19]

The concept of testis-sparing surgery for prepubertal testis tumors emerged in the early 1980s, when it was first applied to primary testicular teratoma[23] and then to excision of benign testicular cysts.[24] Previously, the approach to prepubertal testis tumors was radical orchiectomy. Elegant histopathologic and clinical analysis of prepubertal testicular teratoma demonstrated that these tumors were uniformly unifocal and were not associated with intratubular germ cell neoplasia (carcinoma in situ).[25] The benign nature of most prepubertal testis tumors has expanded application of testis-sparing surgery to several prepubertal testicular neoplasms.

Prepubertal testis tumors in which testis-sparing surgery has been described
- Germ Cell Tumors
  - Epidermoid cyst
  - Teratoma
- Gonadal Stromal Tumors
  - Sertoli cell tumor
  - Leydig cell tumor
  - Juvenile granulosa cell tumor
- Cystic Lesions
  - Simple intratesticular cyst
  - Tubular ectasia of the rete testis
- Miscellaneous
  - Testicular adrenal rest tumor/adrenogenital syndrome refractory to medical management.

Preoperative Evaluation

The vast majority of boys with prepubertal testis tumors present with a painless scrotal mass. Other presenting signs and symptoms include pain; trauma, hernia or hydrocele, or cryptorchidism, which leads to testicular imaging; gynecomastia or precocious puberty; or incidental discovery.[20–22,26] A thorough history and physical examination should be performed. In addition to the presence of a palpable testicular mass, the presence of signs of precocious puberty should raise suspicion for a Leydig cell tumor,[26] a Sertoli cell tumor, or the adrenogenital syndrome.[27] In boys with gynecomastia and a testicular mass, Leydig or Sertoli cell tumor should be considered.[28]

Testicular sonography is routinely performed in patients with suspicion for testicular neoplasm. Scrotal sonography can effectively distinguish testicular from extratesticular lesions and can provide insight as to whether an intratesticular lesion is benign or malignant.[29] Sonographic findings suggestive of a benign lesion include unifocality, anechoic or hypoechoic lesions, distinct demarcation, and hypovascularity.[30–33] Sonographic demonstration of hypoechoic cystic areas with adjacent hyperechoic areas within a well-circumscribed lesion and surrounding tissue with normal testicular echotexture are suggestive of testicular teratoma (**Fig. 7**).[25] Color Doppler sonography is likely to demonstrate hypervascularity in testicular malignancies.[34] When considering testis-sparing surgery, it is important to recognize that scrotal sonography often underestimates the volume of residual normal testicular parenchyma. Therefore, the decision to perform testis-sparing surgery should not be based on sonographic estimation of normal testicular parenchymal volume.[35]

Preoperative laboratory evaluation is typically limited to measurement of serum α-fetoprotein (AFP) for most prepubertal testis tumors. AFP is a single polypeptide chain produced by the fetal yolk sac, the liver, and the gastrointestinal tract. The consistent production of AFP by yolk sac tumors makes it a useful marker to distinguish malignant from benign prepubertal testis tumors.[36] AFP is elevated in infant boys, with elevations up to 10,000 times the normal adult levels. AFP is unreliable as a tumor marker until the age of 8 months, at which point values reach the normal adult range.[37] Human chorionic gonadotropin levels are not typically elevated in prepubertal testis tumors.

Prepubertal patients with virilization in the presence of a testicular tumor should undergo further biochemical evaluation including serum testosterone, follicle-stimulating hormone, luteinizing hormone, androstenediol, 17-hydroxyprogesterone, and urinary 17-ketosteroids. Virilization resulting from a Leydig cell neoplasm will reveal normal follicle-stimulating hormone and luteinizing hormone with elevated testosterone, androstenediol, 17-hydroxyprogesterone, and urinary 17-ketosteroids.[17]

In prepubertal patients with a testicular mass who have normal preoperative AFP levels and testicular sonography that reveals the presence of normal testicular parenchyma in the ipsilateral testis, testis-sparing surgery should be considered as the initial treatment of choice. Patients 6 to 12 months of age with AFP levels greater than 100 and patients older than 1 year with elevated AFP levels are not ideal candidates for testis-sparing surgery.[18]

Surgical Technique

For patients scheduled to undergo testis-sparing surgery, parents should be counseled regarding the potential for radical orchiectomy. Preoperative communication with Pathology should take place to coordinate intraoperative frozen section. If the tumor is not palpable preoperatively, intraoperative sonography should be available.

The testicle is approached initially through an inguinal incision, as in radical orchiectomy, and early vascular control of the spermatic cord is achieved with a vessel loop or Penrose drain. The testicle is delivered through the scrotal incision and the tunica vaginalis is incised to expose the testicle. With lesions involving or immediately adjacent to the tunica albuginea, an elliptical incision beyond the tumor margins should be made in the tunica albuginea (**Fig. 8**A). With deeper lesions, an equatorial incision typically suffices. In patients with nonpalpable lesions, the authors have used intraoperative sonography for localization, a technique that is reported in the adult literatature.[38] Ice may be applied to reduce warm

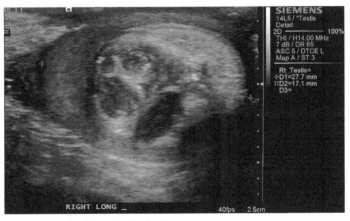

Fig. 7. Sonographic appearance of primary testicular teratoma.

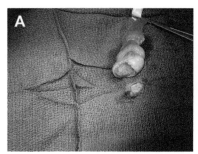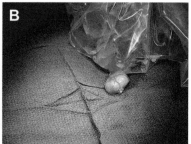

Fig. 8. Technique of testis-sparing surgery. (*A*) After early spermatic cord control with a Penrose drain, an elliptical incision is made in the tunica albuginea and the tumor is enucleated. (*B*) Testis after closure.

ischemia time. Benign prepubertal testis tumors are enucleated bluntly, which typically leaves an attached margin of normal parenchyma. While awaiting intraoperative frozen pathology, the tunica albuginea may be reapproximated with 5-0 running interlocked polydioxanone suture (see **Fig. 8**B). Intraoperative considerations for testis-sparing surgery include the presence of sufficient normal parenchyma to facilitate closure of the testis and intraoperative frozen pathology that confirms a benign lesion.[20] Ideally, histopathology should be reviewed by the operating surgeon with the pathologist. If intraoperative frozen pathology confirms a benign diagnosis, vascular control of the spermatic cord is reduced, the testicle is returned to the scrotum, and the inguinal incision is closed. If intraoperative frozen pathology reveals malignancy, radical orchiectomy is completed.

Intraoperative frozen section has been shown to correlate with final pathologic diagnosis in the vast majority of cases and has been able to distinguish malignant from benign lesions accurately,[39] which is critical for intraoperative decision-making. To the authors' knowledge, no reports document a malignant diagnosis on final pathology when intraoperative frozen pathology revealed a benign diagnosis.

TUMOR-SPECIFIC CONSIDERATIONS
Teratoma

Teratoma is the most common prepubertal testis tumor, representing nearly half of these tumors and has a uniformly benign course.[19–21] The diagnosis of testicular teratoma in prepubertal boys can be made presumptively with ultrasonographic examination and a normal AFP. Although ultrasonography cannot ultimately distinguish between benign and malignant testicular lesions in prepubertal boys, the characteristic findings of cystic components with intervening septa and solid components suggests the diagnosis.[25]

Histopathologic analysis must be performed to confirm the diagnosis. In peripubertal boys, pathologic examination of the surrounding testicular parenchyma should also be performed intraoperatively. It has been recommended that the presence of pubertal testicular histology should preclude testis-sparing surgery.[18]

Testis-sparing surgery is the treatment of choice for prepubertal testis teratoma.[18,20–22,40–42] Because of the uniformly benign tumor biology of prepubertal testis teratoma, metastatic evaluation is not warranted.

Immature teratoma represents a subset of testicular tumors which, although benign, may have the propensity to recur, especially in tumors with foci of malignancy. Specifically in the presence of elevated AFP or yolk sac tumor on pathology, recurrence of yolk sac tumors may be seen. Salvage with platinum-based chemotherapy can be achieved in most patients, so observation alone is recommended for follow-up.[43,44]

Epidermoid Cyst

Epidermoid cysts account for 1% to 3% of all prepubertal testis tumors.[33,45] Histolopathologically, they are monophasic teratomas that demonstrate epidermal differentiation.[46,47] Sonographically, epidermoid cysts are characteristically well demarcated with a hyperechoic border and contain predominately cystic components and a mixed echogenic center.[48,49] Definitive treatment is accomplished through enucleation via a testis-sparing approach.[33,50]

Leydig Cell Tumor

Leydig cell tumors represent approximately 5% to 10% of all prepubertal testis tumors.[17,19,28] Patients with precocious puberty should be evaluated biochemically (as previously discussed) to differentiate between pituitary lesions, Leydig cell tumors, Sertoli cell tumors, adrenal carcinoma, and uncontrolled congenital adrenal hyperplasia associated with adrenogenital syndrome. There have been no reported cases of malignant unilateral Leydig cell tumors in prepubertal patients. However, one case of malignancy has been reported in a 9-year-old boy presenting with bilateral Leydig cell tumors who was treated with bilateral radical orchiectomy. The patient developed pulmonary metastasis 2 years after initial intervention.[51] Although radical orchiectomy has been the preferred historical treatment of Leydig cell tumors, testis-sparing approaches have been increasingly employed.[22,26,52] An unusual complication of testis-sparing enucleation has been reported in association with Leydig cell tumor: namely, growth arrest and persistence of a circumscribed hypoechoic lesion in the ipsilateral testis with 7 years of follow-up.[53]

Sertoli Cell Tumor

Sertoli cell tumors represent 0.4% to 1.5% of testicular tumors. Although malignancy is thought to be much more common in adult patients, both histopathologic evidence of malignancy and metastatic disease have been reported in prepubertal Sertoli cell tumors.[54–56] Although the feasibility of testis-sparing surgery for Sertoli cell tumors has been demonstrated,[22] the potential for malignancy must be considered. Treatment by radical orchiectomy should be considered and metastatic evaluation should be performed.

Juvenile Granulosa Cell Tumor

Juvenile granulosa cell tumors are rare, accounting for approximately 1% of prepubertal testis tumors.[57] These tumors are most commonly diagnosed in infancy and have a uniformly benign course.[28] Patients typically have a palpable testicular mass and sonographic imaging revealing multicystic, circumscribed masses. Although generally treated by radical orchiectomy, successful testis-sparing surgery has been reported for juvenile granulosa cell tumor without evidence of recurrence or testicular atrophy on 5-year follow-up.[57]

Testicular Adrenal Rest Tumors or Adrenogenital Syndrome

In male children with congenital adrenal hyperplasia, the presence of testicular adrenal rest tumors (TART, also referred to as adrenogenital syndrome) is estimated to be 24%.[58] TART is generally a bilateral process. In patients with a long history of TART, destruction of normal testicular parenchyma can occur. Therefore, early intervention for TART has been proposed to maximize future fertility potential.[27,59] Patients with poorly controlled congenital adrenal hyperplasia will typically demonstrate regression with administration of mineralocorticoids.[60] However, some patients are refractory to medical management. Successful treatment of TART lesions using a testis-sparing approach without recurrence and preserving normal testicular parenchyma has been reported.[27,60]

SUMMARY

Technological advances in imaging as well as increased knowledge of tumor-specific biology have promoted the role of organ-sparing approaches to pediatric renal and testicular tumors. Application of these techniques continues to evolve as data on long-term follow-up becomes available and as protocol-guided investigation provides answers to therapeutic outcomes of these approaches. Optimally, organ-sparing surgery will continue to provide increased potential for preservation of both renal function and fertility.

REFERENCES

1. Ritchey ML, Green DM, Thomas PR, et al. Renal failure in Wilms' tumor patients: a report from the National Wilms' Tumor Study Group. Med Pediatr Oncol 1996;26:75.
2. Blute ML, Kelalis PP, Offord KP, et al. Bilateral Wilms tumor. J Urol 1987;138:968.
3. Horwitz JR, Ritchey ML, Moksness J, et al. Renal salvage procedures in patients with synchronous bilateral Wilms' tumors: a report from the National Wilms' Tumor Study Group. J Pediatr Surg 1996; 31:1020.
4. Shamberger RC, Guthrie KA, Ritchey ML, et al. Surgery-related factors and local recurrence of Wilms tumor in National Wilms Tumor Study 4. Ann Surg 1999;229:292.
5. Hamilton TE, Green DM, Perlman EJ, et al. Bilateral Wilms' tumor with anaplasia: lessons from the National Wilms' Tumor Study. J Pediatr Surg 2006; 41:1641.
6. Shamberger RC, Haase GM, Argani P, et al. Bilateral Wilms' tumors with progressive or nonresponsive disease. J Pediatr Surg 2006;41:652.
7. Breslow NE, Takashima JR, Ritchey ML, et al. Renal failure in the Denys-Drash and Wilms' tumor-aniridia syndromes. Cancer Res 2000;60:4030.
8. Haecker FM, von Schweinitz D, Harms D, et al. Partial nephrectomy for unilateral Wilms tumor: results of study SIOP 93-01/GPOH. J Urol 2003; 170:939.
9. Zani A, Schiavetti A, Gambino M, et al. Long-term outcome of nephron sparing surgery and simple

nephrectomy for unilateral localized Wilms tumor. J Urol 2005;173:946.

10. Moorman-Voestermans CG, Aronson DC, Staalman CR, et al. Is partial nephrectomy appropriate treatment for unilateral Wilms' tumor? J Pediatr Surg 1998;33:165.

11. Beckwith JB. Nephrogenic rests and the pathogenesis of Wilms tumor: developmental and clinical considerations. Am J Med Genet 1998;79:268.

12. Lonergan GJ, Martinez-Leon MI, Agrons GA, et al. Nephrogenic rests, nephroblastomatosis, and associated lesions of the kidney. Radiographics 1998;18:947.

13. Rohrschneider WK, Weirich A, Rieden K, et al. US, CT and MR imaging characteristics of nephroblastomatosis. Pediatr Radiol 1998;28:435.

14. Lilly JR, Pfister RR, Putnam CW, et al. Bench surgery and renal autotransplantation in the pediatric patient. J Pediatr Surg 1975;10:623.

15. Desai D, Nicholls G, Duffy PG. Bench surgery with autotransplantation for bilateral synchronous Wilms' tumor: a report of three cases. J Pediatr Surg 1999;34:632.

16. Millar AJ, Davidson A, Rode H, et al. Bilateral Wilms' tumors: a single-center experience with 19 cases. J Pediatr Surg 2005;40:1289.

17. Brosman SA. Testicular tumors in prepubertal children. Urology 1979;13:581.

18. Ross JH, Rybicki L, Kay R. Clinical behavior and a contemporary management algorithm for prepubertal testis tumors: a summary of the Prepubertal Testis Tumor Registry. J Urol 2002;168:1675.

19. Pohl HG, Shukla AR, Metcalf PD, et al. Prepubertal testis tumors: actual prevalence rate of histological types. J Urol 2004;172:2370.

20. Metcalfe PD, Farivar-Mohseni H, Farhat W, et al. Pediatric testicular tumors: contemporary incidence and efficacy of testicular preserving surgery. J Urol 2003;170:2412.

21. Shukla AR, Woodard C, Carr MC, et al. Experience with testis sparing surgery for testicular teratoma. J Urol 2004;171:161.

22. Valla J. Testis-sparing surgery for benign testicular tumors in children. J Urol 2001;165:2280.

23. Weissbach L, Altwein JE, Stiens R. Germinal testicular tumors in childhood. Report of observations and literature review. Eur Urol 1984;10:73.

24. Altadonna V, Snyder HM 3rd, Rosenberg HK, et al. Simple cysts of the testis in children: preoperative diagnosis by ultrasound and excision with testicular preservation. J Urol 1988;140:1505.

25. Rushton HG, Belman AB, Sesterhenn I, et al. Testicular sparing surgery for prepubertal teratoma of the testis: a clinical and pathological study. J Urol 1990;144:726.

26. Henderson CG, Ahmed AA, Sesterhenn I, et al. Enucleation for prepubertal Leydig cell tumor. J Urol 2006;176:703.

27. Walker BR, Skoog SJ, Winslow BH, et al. Testis sparing surgery for steroid unresponsive testicular tumors of the adrenogenital syndrome. J Urol 1997;157:1460.

28. Thomas JC, Ross JH, Kay R. Stromal testis tumors in children: a report from the prepubertal testis tumor registry. J Urol 2001;166:2338.

29. Rifkin MD, Kurtz AB, Pasto ME, et al. Diagnostic capabilities of high-resolution scrotal ultrasonography: prospective evaluation. J Ultrasound Med 1985;4:13.

30. Dieckmann KP, Loy V. Epidermoid cyst of the testis: a review of clinical and histogenetic considerations. Br J Urol 1994;73:436.

31. Neumann DP, Abrams GS, Hight DW. Testicular epidermoid cysts in prepubertal children: case report and review of the world literature. J Pediatr Surg 1997;32:1786.

32. Peretsman SJ, Maldazys JD. Infantile testicular cyst: diagnosis and conservative surgical management. J Pediatr Surg 1995;30:1488.

33. Ross JH, Kay R, Elder J. Testis sparing surgery for pediatric epidermoid cysts of the testis. J Urol 1993;149:353.

34. Luker GD, Siegel MJ. Pediatric testicular tumors: evaluation with gray-scale and color Doppler US. Radiology 1994;191:561.

35. Patel AS, Coley BD, Jayanthi VR. Ultrasonography underestimates the volume of normal parenchyma in benign testicular masses. J Urol 2007;178:1730.

36. Huddart SN, Mann JR, Gornall P, et al. The UK Children's Cancer Study Group: testicular malignant germ cell tumours 1979-1988. J Pediatr Surg 1990; 25:406.

37. Wu JT, Book L, Sudar K. Serum alpha fetoprotein (AFP) levels in normal infants. Pediatr Res 1981;15:50.

38. Hopps CV, Goldstein M. Ultrasound guided needle localization and microsurgical exploration for incidental nonpalpable testicular tumors. J Urol 2002; 168:1084.

39. Tokuc R, Sakr W, Pontes JE, et al. Accuracy of frozen section examination of testicular tumors. Urology 1992;40:512.

40. Grady RW, Ross JH, Kay R. Epidemiological features of testicular teratoma in a prepubertal population. J Urol 1997;158:1191.

41. Marshall S, Lyon RP, Scott MP. A conservative approach to testicular tumors in children: 12 cases and their management. J Urol 1983;129:350.

42. Pearse I, Glick RD, Abramson SJ, et al. Testicular-sparing surgery for benign testicular tumors. J Pediatr Surg 1999;34:1000.

43. Mann JR, Raafat F, Robinson K, et al. The United Kingdom Children's Cancer Study Group's second germ cell tumor study: carboplatin, etoposide, and

bleomycin are effective treatment for children with malignant extracranial germ cell tumors, with acceptable toxicity. J Clin Oncol 2000;18:3809.

44. Marina NM, Cushing B, Giller R, et al. Complete surgical excision is effective treatment for children with immature teratomas with or without malignant elements: a Pediatric Oncology Group/Children's Cancer Group Intergroup Study. J Clin Oncol 1999;17:2137.

45. Shah KH, Maxted WC, Chun B. Epidermoid cysts of the testis: a report of three cases and an analysis of 141 cases from the world literature. Cancer 1981;47:577.

46. Price EB Jr. Epidermoid cysts of the testis: a clinical and pathologic analysis of 69 cases from the testicular tumor registry. J Urol 1969;102:708.

47. Reinberg Y, Manivel JC, Llerena J, et al. Epidermoid cyst (monodermal teratoma) of the testis. Br J Urol 1990;66:648.

48. Bahnson RR, Slasky BS, Ernstoff MS, et al. Sonographic characteristics of epidermoid cyst of testicle. Urology 1990;35:508.

49. Shapeero LG, Vordermark JS. Epidermoid cysts of testes and role of sonography. Urology 1993;41:75.

50. Heidenreich A, Engelmann UH, Vietsch HV, et al. Organ preserving surgery in testicular epidermoid cysts. J Urol 1995;153:1147.

51. Slama A, Elleuch A, Yacoubi MT, et al. [Malignant bilateral Leydig cell tumor of the testis in children: about one case]. Ann Urol (Paris) 2003;37:213 [in French].

52. Konrad D, Schoenle EJ. Ten-year follow-up in a boy with Leydig cell tumor after selective surgery. Horm Res 1999;51:96.

53. Trobs RB, Hoepffner W, Friedrich T, et al. Growth-arrest and inhomogenous echotexture of the affected testis after tumor enucleation for unilateral Leydig cell tumor. J Pediatr Surg 2001;36:E20.

54. Kolon TF, Hochman HI. Malignant Sertoli cell tumor in a prepubescent boy. J Urol 1997;158:608.

55. Rosvoll RV, Woodard JR. Malignant Sertoli cell tumor of the testis. Cancer 1968;22:8.

56. Sharma S, Seam RK, Kapoor HL. Malignant Sertoli cell tumour of the testis in a child. J Surg Oncol 1990;44:129.

57. Shukla AR, Huff DS, Canning DA, et al. Juvenile granulosa cell tumor of the testis: contemporary clinical management and pathological diagnosis. J Urol 2004;171:1900.

58. Claahsen-van der Grinten HL, Sweep FC, Blickman JG, et al. Prevalence of testicular adrenal rest tumours in male children with congenital adrenal hyperplasia due to 21-hydroxylase deficiency. Eur J Endocrinol 2007;157:339.

59. Claahsen-van der Grinten HL, Otten BJ, Hermus AR, et al. Testicular adrenal rest tumors in patients with congenital adrenal hyperplasia can cause severe testicular damage. Fertil Steril 2008;89:597.

60. Srikanth MS, West BR, Ishitani M, et al. Benign testicular tumors in children with congenital adrenal hyperplasia. J Pediatr Surg 1992;27:639.

Pediatric Psychology in Genitourinary Anomalies

Aileen P. Schast, PhD[a],*, William G. Reiner, MD[b,c]

KEYWORDS

- Psychosocial • Urology • Pediatric
- Genitourinary • Adjustment

Over the past 30 years, the importance of considering "the whole" patient has gradually become a major focus of medicine across the spectrum. Health is now viewed as an interactive process between physical, emotional, and behavioral well-being. In pediatrics, this has been exemplified by the increase in emphasis on family-centered care, the *medical home*, and the recognition that children are not just small adults—they have physical and emotional issues that are specific to their age and developmental level. In addition, working with children always requires working with the adults, the parents, who care for them.

In adult urology practices, it is not uncommon to collaborate with mental health providers who work with patients with prostate cancer, infertility, or sexual dysfunction associated with urological disease. Pediatric medical services, including oncology, nephrology, endocrinology, and rheumatology, have incorporated psychological care for the patient and family into standard practice for many years. Pediatric surgical practices have been slower to include mental health services as part of the continuum of care. In this article, the authors propose that pediatric urologists and mental health providers can work together to provide complementary services that benefit patient care.

MENTAL HEALTH PROVIDERS AS TEAM MEMBERS

"Pediatric Psychology" as first described in 1967 by Logan Wright[1] involves "dealing primarily with children in a medical setting which is nonpsychiatric in nature." The focus of the field is working with children whose primary concerns are medical or physical but who may also manifest emotional or behavioral concerns. Pediatric psychology recognizes the *bidirectional* relationships between medical issues and psychological factors, with the goal of maximizing physical and emotional health.

There are several ways in which psychological factors can affect a child's medical condition generally

- The psychological factors influence the course of the medical condition (eg, an oppositional child refuses to comply with care while a well-adjusted child can focus on their ability to participate).
- The psychological factors interfere with the treatment of the medical condition (eg, a depressed child does not perform clean intermittent catheterization [CIC] as directed, while an adjusted child follows the protocol).

[a] Division of Urology, The Children's Hospital of Philadelphia, Richard D Wood Center, 3rd Floor, 34th Street and Civic Center Boulevard, Philadelphia, PA 19104, USA
[b] Pediatric Urology and Child and Adolescent Psychiatry, University of Oklahoma Health Sciences Center, WP 3150, 920 Stanton L Young Boulevard, Oklahoma City, OK 73104, USA
[c] Psychosexual Development Clinic, Division of Pediatric Urology, Department of Urology, University of Oklahoma Health Sciences Center, WP 3150, 920 Stanton L Young Boulevard, Oklahoma City, OK 73104, USA
* Corresponding author.
E-mail address: schast@email.chop.edu

Urol Clin N Am 37 (2010) 299–305
doi:10.1016/j.ucl.2010.03.013

- The psychological factors cause additional health risks (eg, an anxious child is afraid to ask to be excused to use the bathroom at school, so increases her risk of urinary tract infections while a less wary child can ask for what she needs).

Similarly, medical conditions can affect the psychological well-being of children and their families. Mental health providers can address issues such as depression, suicidality, anxiety, behavior problems, and problematic family dynamics that emerge in the context of managing the medical condition. These issues may present during the medical appointment, but few medical providers have the time or training to address them in this context. The adjustment to complex genitourinary (GU) anomalies has condition-specific developmental implications as well. Thus, psychological factors can influence a child's condition generally and can be influenced by that condition more specifically. A collaborative relationship with a mental health provider can facilitate treatment by helping parents and the child adjust to the medical protocols within their specific capacities to do so, so that the child's medical care is optimal. Indeed, when mental health and medical providers collaborate, there is an increased opportunity to help identify barriers to implementation of recommended treatments and to develop interventions to ameliorate challenges.[2]

These goals are most effectively reached when the mental health provider is embedded in the settings where patients get their care.[3] Successful collaboration requires that (1) the psychologist have expertise in the application of clinical knowledge, (2) there be significant shared knowledge and expertise where collaboration is necessary, and (3) there be a commitment to ongoing exchanges of information.[2] These requirements are best achieved when the psychologist is entrenched in the urological clinic and can learn about urological needs in particular while applying accepted psychological principles and interventions. For example, a psychologist is going to be less well equipped to help new parents cope with the diagnosis of exstrophy without an understanding of the complexity of the condition. Similarly, recommendations about a child's readiness for bladder augmentation will be less effective if the reasons for augmentation, the challenges of CIC, and the possible surgical complications are not understood and taken into account.

DEVELOPMENTAL PERSPECTIVE

An understanding of the cognitive and emotional development of the child with GU disorders is essential to the medical practitioner. Although patients with relatively minor GU disorders may have no psychological sequelae, those with complex or chronic conditions are at greater risk for emotional and developmental challenges. Deviation from the more typical child developmental trajectories should be monitored in these groups. However, such departures may not necessarily be easily recognized or understood. Mental health providers, therefore, become central to this recognition and understanding and to engaging the child and the family with prevention and intervention, from the child's infancy through adulthood. For example, the authors have worked with families who did not want their toddler attending preschool programs for fear that their GU condition would be discovered. Although protecting the child's privacy is important, this need has to be balanced against the child's developmental tasks of gaining independence, learning to separate from the parents, and socializing with peers. A similar problem may develop in adolescence and young adulthood, as patients avoid dating and other social circumstances as a way of evading questions about their condition.

Whether the condition represents a new diagnosis or a congenital anomaly, the child's understanding of the medical condition depends on the developmental level. For children with chronic medical conditions such as exstrophy, spina bifida, hypospadias, or posterior urethral valves, their understanding of the condition changes as their level of development changes.

Infants and Toddlers

A major goal of this period is learning to trust and develop a sense of security. Children at this age generally have very little understanding of their medical condition. They experience pain, restriction of motion, and separation from parents as challenges to developing trust and security.

Preschool Children

This time is marked by an increasing desire for independence and autonomy. Children at this age understand what it is to feel sick, but they may not understand the cause-and-effect nature of illness. The child may try to counter lack of control over their world by challenging limits set by parents (and doctors).

School-aged Children

Children at this age are developing a sense of mastery over their environment. They can describe reasons for illness, but because they often engage in "magical thinking," especially in the early school years, these reasons may not be wholly logical. Throughout this period, children start to develop a sense of self and how they are similar to, or different from, their peers.

Adolescents

Teens begin to develop an individual identity that is separate from their family. Self-image becomes extremely important during the teenage years, which can be a problem when the teen's appearance is altered by illness or medication. This can be especially problematic for children with urological disorders that affect the genitals. A particular challenge for this age is balancing their desire for independence with the irresponsibility that can accompany a sense of immortality. Many teens go through times of denial of their illness when they may neglect to take medications or follow catheterization schedules.

It is also important to consider the context provided by the presenting medical issue. For example, short-term anxiety problems are common with procedures and can often be addressed with simple, short-term pharmacologic anxiolytics. Long-term problems pose greater challenges. Children with GU disorders may experience cognitive and emotional development that is mismatched with their physical or behavioral development (eg, school-aged children who are still incontinent because of a neuropathic bladder). This mismatch, especially as children become more aware of it, has the potential to lead to feelings of stress, low self-esteem, and shame.

SCOPE OF PRACTICE

The roles for a mental health provider within the urology department are varied and include work with patients with chronic and acute conditions. This work can be grouped into 3 overall categories: assessment, intervention, and prevention.

Assessment

Psychologists can address 2 different assessment needs in urology practices. The first involves screening urology patients with suspected comorbidities, and the second is evaluating patients for readiness for complex reconstruction.

Comorbid urological and behavioral health problems

Links have been established between some mental health diagnoses and urological problems. For example, there is a known association between attention-deficit/hyperactivity disorder and enuresis.[4,5] Similarly, children with autism typically have challenges with toilet training and

may struggle with constipation and incontinence far longer than their nonaffected peers. The psychological and behavioral issues do not cause the urological problem, but they must be considered during treatment, as interventions may need to be adjusted to account for these additional challenges.

Readiness for reconstruction

Undertaking a complex genital or bladder reconstruction demands a lot from the patient and family, as well as the physician. It is critical that families understand the procedure and its risks and implications, not only from the medical side, as discussed during the consent process, but also from the practical and emotional side. It is here that psychologists can be helpful. Being ready for a big procedure, such as augmentation cystoplasty with closure of the bladder neck, encompasses several things: an understanding of how life will change (eg, no longer being wet from the urethra), the new behaviors and burdens that accompany that change (eg, routine catheterization and irrigation of the bladder), and the potential complications and what they mean for the patient and family (eg, fistulas that leak afterward, need for redo surgery). Often, patients are so focused on the primary goal (being dry) that they minimize what is actually involved with reaching and maintaining that goal. Psychologists can support their physician colleagues by ensuring that the child and family's expectations are reasonable and that any barriers to the family's full participation in care have been identified and addressed and by identifying areas of child and family strength on which the medical team can draw during challenging periods in the patient's care.

Intervention

Chronic physical disorders in children, fairly common in urology, affect both child and family adjustment and can be sources of chronic strain for the child in the family. As Wallander and Varni[6] have stated, "Chronic strains are defined as persistent objective conditions requiring continued readjustment and repeatedly interfering with the performance of ordinary role-related activities." Psychological intervention with GU patients may be appropriate in specific areas as described in the following sections.

Coping with procedures

Pediatric patients may present with acute cases of anxiety in anticipation of surgery or procedures. Common examples in urology include voiding cystourethrograms (VCUGs) or video urodynamic studies, postoperative stent or tube removal, and venipuncture. Concerns may also develop as patients transition to new phases of treatment, such as the initiation of CIC. Mental health providers are uniquely suited to intervene to help patients and their families cope with anxiety, reduce distress, and increase cooperation with necessary procedures.

Research has shown that children with high levels of preoperative anxiety experience more pain, sleep, and other problems in the postoperative period.[7] In a review of treatments for procedure-related pain, cognitive-behavioral therapy was identified as a well-established treatment according to the Chambless criteria.[8] Similarly, an intervention that taught specific coping strategies to children preparing for a VCUG resulted in decreased distress, increased coping, and improved cooperativeness with the procedure when compared with children who had not received the intervention.[9]

Pain

Although chronic pain is not common with most urological disorders, patients with recurrent stone disease are often challenged with sudden, unpredictable, episodic pain that can interrupt their daily functioning.[10] The unpredictable nature of the recurrence is similar to that experienced by patients with other pain disorders. For example, in a study of patients with fibromyalgia (similar in its episodic nature), when illness uncertainty was high, any increase in pain was associated with increased difficulty in coping.[11] Further, increases in coping difficulty were associated with a decrease in coping efficacy. That is, when patients most needed their coping skills, they were the least equipped to use them effectively. Mental health providers are trained to work with these kinds of patients to build coping skills and to provide additional support and intervention during the time of a pain crisis. Cognitive-behavioral protocols for treating coping with episodic pain have been found to be efficacious in other disorders[12] and could easily be adapted for work with patients with stone disease.

Adjustment to diagnosis

Children with chronic conditions, who commonly make up a fairly large part of the pediatric urologist's practice, pose a special set of problems for the parents as well as for the child. The diagnosis of a serious medical condition in the child is scary and unsettling for parents. Parents go through a mourning process: in case of congenital problems, they mourn the loss of the "hoped for" child and in case of later-diagnosed issues, the loss of

the life they had before.[13] Some parents continue to struggle even years after the diagnosis. Research has shown that failure to come to terms with the child's diagnosis affects not only parent's state of mind but also the actual care that they provide.[14] In his follow-up study of children discharged from the neonatal intensive care unit, Minde[15] found that babies who had successfully recovered were still treated as gravely ill by their mothers after 6 months.

The adjustment process is not simple, and it follows no predetermined timeline. The recognition of a GU anomaly can be an emotional shock to the mother, the father, and the entire family. Research on other medical conditions has shown that failure to come to terms with the child's diagnosis can have long-term effects on the parents, emotionally and in terms of their relationship with their child.[14,16] Parents often blame themselves for causing the condition, although they may never say that to their physician. The nature of GU anomalies may also make it difficult for many parents to seek support from friends and families. Many parents have never heard of epispadias, congenital adrenal hyperplasia, posterior urethral valves, or any of the other myriad GU disorders before receiving their child's diagnosis. The unfamiliarity of a diagnosis adds additional challenges to the coping process.[17] Parents of children with GU disorders may feel more isolated than parents of children with other conditions. The unfamiliarity of the diagnosis is one component of this, but a combination of wanting to protect their child's privacy and a discomfort discussing such intimate information likely also play roles. Such isolation has been shown to interfere with long-term coping in other pediatric conditions.[18] These issues are particularly salient for families of children with a disorder of sex development. The unfamiliar conditions, the genital ambiguity, and concerns about gender of rearing, all come together in a perfect storm to leave families feeling confused, isolated, and overwhelmed. Psychologists can work best with these families as partners with the urologists, ensuring that consistent messages are given and that parents feel less isolated by having a sounding board and place to obtain support and helping them to come to hard decisions about the best ways to raise these children.

Children, too, go through a process of coming to terms with their own medical condition. Three crucial principles of living things are the patterns of self-organization, self-maintenance, and self-transcendency (the central theme of evolution). For the child, self-transcendency is the potential to change in relationship to dynamic changes inherent within life experiences. Thus, a child's understanding changes as their development changes, and the impact of the condition on their day-to-day life varies as well. Children affected by conditions that have a lifelong impact may struggle with accepting the implications of their diagnosis at each new developmental stage when their understanding of the permanence and the impact of the condition changes. And it is not just the children who suffer. Parents, too, may grieve anew as their children reach new developmental stages and the differences between them and their peers are evident.

The adaptations that a child makes, the adjustments, to changing circumstances around their diagnosis are the hallmark of understanding the psychology of pediatric urology. Specific adjustments are peculiar to and intertwined with a given child's personality, temperament, cognitive functions, parental influence, and other social and environmental factors. Interventions for these children, therefore, should include recognizing potential adjustment problems across the lifespan of the child. In early childhood, parents may worry about incontinence and their child having to wear diapers to school. In middle childhood, the worry may turn to teasing by peers and how to handle that. Adolescence may be fraught with concerns about how to manage changing for gym class and approaching dating relationships. All are variations on the same theme, but developmentally distinct. The perceptions and fears of the child, as well as of the parents, must be explored to help a family have a satisfactory adjustment, a useful behavioral and emotional adaptation.

Body image and self-esteem

Self-esteem is a significant factor in GU disorders. Body image likely has a different effect on self-esteem, and adjustment issues to such body image may become more problematic as the child develops through school-age, early adolescence, and into mid and late adolescence, as well as emerging adulthood. The psychosocial work with these patients tends to focus on the emotional aspect (accepting ones body for what it is) and the practical aspect (how to handle fears about how the body will be perceived by others).

Genital anomalies can destabilize the sense of self as a male or female. That is, knowing that the genitalia, the hallmark differentiators between men and women, are not normal can influence a developing child's sense of gender identity and competence, particularly in areas of sexual functioning. These disorders are particularly challenging because they are not usually obvious to others. The authors find that it is common for patients with genital anomalies to develop a sense of shame about their genitals and a fear that their secret will be revealed. A recent review of the literature on the adjustment of boys with hypospadias indicated that boys with hypospadias commonly view their genitals negatively and suffer from sexual inhibition as they get older.[19] Patients must be made to understand that there is a problem with the body's *plumbing* and not with *them*, just as the mother may have trouble with digestion, the grandmother with heart disease, and so on. The important point is that the patient is not *bad* but he is living in an imperfect machine: his body.

Self-esteem issues also come into play for patients with more obvious disabilities. A meta-analysis of studies examining self-concept in patients with spina bifida found that, in comparison to their typical peers, these patients suffered from significantly lower global self-worth and saw themselves deficient in physical appearance, athletic competence, social acceptance, and scholastic competence.[20]

The psychosocial needs and surgical recommendations for our patients may sometimes be at odds. Surgeons have expertise in making bodies look and work better. For the child with GU anomalies, that expertise is a double-edged sword. On one hand, the surgeon can correct the GU defects, but on the other, it is a clear signal to the child that they are defective. This tension is a challenge to overcome, as all involved with the child want optimal function and appearance, primarily to help the child feel as normal as possible. When multiple surgeries are involved (eg, repeated hypospadias repairs), the benefit of the repair may become subjugated to the trauma the child perceives to the body's integrity.[21] For some, the scarring after multiple procedures feels, at that time, more disfiguring than the original defect. Physical (or sexual) disfigurement, real or perceived, is typically associated with significant emotional vulnerability. Congenital conditions with physical disfigurement often lead to progressive anxiety with increasing age. This anxiety tends to peak in adolescence and is often followed by depression.[22] The authors recommend basic psychosocial screening for all children undergoing any kind of genital reconstruction beyond early childhood, and especially for those who have needed or will need several procedures.

Adherence to treatment

Adherence to treatment in the urology clinics is an issue for simple diagnoses like day and nighttime wetting, as well as for more complex problems like posterior urethral valves and spina bifida. The reasons for nonadherence are varied, but most issues of nonadherence can be remedied with good behavioral intervention.

It is often frustrating when children seen for day and night wetting do not get better, given that the interventions (eg, the moisture sensing alarm, timed voiding) seem so simple. Research has shown that the biggest factor in failure to achieve nighttime dryness using the bedwetting alarm is failure to use it correctly or to discontinue use prematurely.[23] Clinically, many families struggle to implement the most basic voiding routine. Mental health providers are well equipped to work with these families to identify the barriers to implementing the recommended treatment and devising a treatment plan to help the child improve.[24]

In children with more complex disorders, one commonly sees nonadherence in the areas of taking medication (eg, antibiotic prophylaxis) and catheterization schedules. These issues are particularly problematic in adolescence, when overall adherence with medical recommendations typically drops off.[25] The pediatric psychology literature is rich with research on adherence to medical regimens across numerous chronic conditions. Although there is little information on adherence to catheterization regimens in the pediatric urology literature, the methods and interventions created for insulin administration, medication compliance, and other behaviors associated with pediatric medical care could easily be exported and applied to the adolescent urology patient.

Prevention

Mental health providers are probably most useful in the urology clinic if they can help to prevent the development of long-term coping and adjustment problems. Many children and families do well throughout treatment, but others need support. It can be difficult to tell into which group families will fall during regular medical visits, until that time the crisis hits. Having psychosocial services available as part of the continuum of care within the clinic may encourage families to participate in mental health treatment when problems are germinating, as there may be less stigma attached to working with a mental health provider who is just another member on their health care team. The authors encourage parents of all children born with complex anomalies in their clinic to meet with the psychologist in the child's infancy and then to have psychosocial check-ins as part of their ongoing care at times of transition or development (ie, toilet training, entry to school, transition to middle school/puberty, high school, and transition out of high school). Sometimes these check-ins are quick; sometimes developing challenges are discussed and strategies for ameliorating them are identified.

SUMMARY

Children with GU anomalies are at risk for several developmental and adjustmental challenges. Surgical teams and their patients can benefit from complementary behavioral health services. A collaborative relationship with a mental health provider can provide surgical teams with resources to help manage challenging patients. Likewise, patient care will be optimized, as the services necessary to help children and families cope and adapt will be easily accessible.

REFERENCES

1. Wright L. The pediatric psychologist: a role model. Am Psychol 1967;22(4):323–5.
2. Aylward BS, Bender JA, Graves M, et al. Historical developments and trends in pediatric psychology. In: Roberts M, Steele R, editors. Handbook of Pediatric Psychology. New York: The Guilford Press; 2009. p. 3–18.
3. Grant M, Economou D. The evolving paradigm of adult cancer survivor care. Oncology (Williston Park, N.Y.) 2008;22(Suppl 4 Nurse Ed):13–22, 27.
4. Baeyens D, Roeyers H, D'Haese L, et al. The prevalence of ADHD in children with enuresis: comparison between a tertiary and non-tertiary care sample. Acta Paediatr 2006;95(3):347–52.
5. Baeyens D, Roeyers H, Van Erdeghem S, et al. The prevalence of attention deficit-hyperactivity disorder in children with nonmonosymptomatic nocturnal enuresis: a 4-year followup study. J Urol 2007; 178(6):2616–20.
6. Wallander JL, Varni JW. Effects of pediatric chronic physical disorders on child and family adjustment. J Child Psychol Psychiatry 1998;39(1):29–46.
7. Kain ZN, Mayes LC, Caldwell-Andrews AA, et al. Preoperative anxiety, postoperative pain, and behavioral recovery in young children undergoing surgery. Pediatrics 2006;118(2):651–8.
8. Powers SW. Empirically supported treatments in pediatric psychology: procedure-related pain. J Pediatr Psychol 1999;24(2):131–45.
9. Zelikovsky N, Rodrigue Jr, Gidycz CA, et al. Cognitive behavioral and behavioral interventions help young children cope during a voiding cystourethrogram. J Pediatr Psychol 2000;25(8):535–43.
10. Polito C, Manna AL, Signoriello G, et al. Recurrent abdominal pain in childhood urolithiasis. Pediatrics 2009;124(6):e1088–94.
11. Johnson LM, Zautra AJ, Davis MC. The role of illness uncertainty on coping with fibromyalgia symptoms. Health Psychol 2006;25(6):696–703.

12. Thieme K, Flor H, Turk D. Psychological pain treatment in fibromyalgia syndrome: efficacy of operant behavioural and cognitive behavioural treatments. Arthritis Res Ther 2006;8(4):R121.

13. Bowlby J. Attachment and loss, vol. 3. New York: Basic Books; 1980.

14. Pianta RC, Marvin RS, Britner PA, et al. Mothers' resolution of their children's diagnosis: organized patterns of caregiving representations. Infant Ment Health J 1996;17(3):239–56.

15. Minde K. Mediating attachment patterns during a serious medical illness. Infant Ment Health J 1999;20(1):105–22.

16. Robinson KE, Gerhardt CA, Vannatta K, et al. Parent and family factors associated with child adjustment to pediatric cancer. J Pediatr Psychol 2007;32(4):400–10.

17. Speltz ML, Armsden GC, Clarren SS. Effects of craniofacial birth defects on maternal functioning postinfancy. J Pediatr Psychol 1990;15(2):177–96.

18. Chibbaro P. Understanding and managing stressors facing the pediatric craniofacial patient and family. Plast Surg Nurs 1994;14(2):86–91.

19. Schonbucher VB, Weber DM, Landolt MA. Psychosocial adjustment, health-related quality of life, and psychosexual development of boys with hypospadias: a systematic review. J Pediatr Psychol 2008;33(5):520–35.

20. Shields N, Taylor NF, Dodd KJ. Self-concept in children with spina bifida compared with typically developing children. Dev Med Child Neurol 2008;50(10): 733–43.

21. Sandberg DE, Meyer-Bahlburg HF, Hensle TW, et al. Psychosocial adaptation of middle childhood boys with hypospadias after genital surgery. J Pediatr Psychol 2001;26(8): 465–75.

22. Breslau N, Marshall IA. Psychological disturbance in children with physical disabilities: continuity and change in a 5-year follow-up. J Abnorm Child Psychol 1985;13(2):199–214.

23. Glazener CM, Evans JH, Peto RE. Treating nocturnal enuresis in children: review of evidence. J Wound Ostomy Continence Nurs 2004;31(4):223–34.

24. Wiener JS, Scales MT, Hampton J, et al. Long-term efficacy of simple behavioral therapy for daytime wetting in children. J Urol 2000;164(3 Pt 1):786–90.

25. Quittner AL, Modi AC, Lemanek KL, et al. Evidence-based assessment of adherence to medical treatments in pediatric psychology. J Pediatr Psychol 2008;33(9):916–36.

Pediatric Urologic Advanced Imaging: Techniques and Applications

Pooja Renjen, MD[a],*, Richard Bellah, MD[b],
Jeffrey C. Hellinger, MD[b], Kassa Darge, MD, PhD[b]

KEYWORDS
- MR Urography (MRU) • Voiding Urosonography (VUS)
- CT Angiography (CTA) • CT Urography (CTU)

Diagnostic imaging of pediatric urologic disorders is continuously changing as technological advances are made. Although the backbone of pediatric urologic imaging has been ultrasound (US), voiding cystourethrography (VCUG), and radionuclide scintigraphy, newer and advanced modalities are increasingly becoming important. The aim of this review is to discuss the techniques and clinical applications of 3 such imaging modalities as they pertain to pediatric urologic disorders: MR urography (MRU), advanced US (harmonic imaging, 3-dimensional [3D], voiding urosonography [VUS]), and CT angiography (CTA).

MAGNETIC RESONANCE UROGRAPHY

MRU is a powerful examination that has the distinct advantage of providing both anatomic *and* functional information in one examination. MRU allows a one-stop-shop evaluation of the renal parenchyma, collecting system, vasculature, bladder, and surrounding structures. MRU has intrinsic high soft tissue contrast resolution and multiplanar 3D reconstruction capabilities, without the use of radiation. Additionally, MRU allows quantification of numerous renal functional parameters including transit times, an index of glomerular filtration rate (GFR), and differential renal functions. To date, MRU may serve as the most comprehensive and definitive study in the evaluation of urinary tract obstruction, complex genitourinary anomalies, and infection. The following sections discuss patient preparation, technique, clinical applications, and limitations of MRU as it pertains to the evaluation of pediatric urologic disorders.[1–5]

Patient Preparations

Patient preparation is a crucial part of the successful MRU examination. The examination begins with discussion with the family as to the purpose and operations of the study. The patient preparation portion of the MRU examination typically takes approximately 1 hour, which includes sedation, hydration, and catheterization. Patients younger than 7 years are typically sedated to eliminate patient motion artifact. Although sedation protocols must be adapted according to the experience of each center, at our institution, a combination of versed, fentanyl, and phenobarbital is typically used. All children undergoing sedation are under continuous close electrocardiogram (ECG) and pulse oximetry monitoring under the control of an appropriately trained member of the sedation unit. Older nonsedated children are asked to breathe quietly, or if they are able to cooperate, breath hold imaging is performed.

[a] Department of Radiology, The Children's Hospital of Philadelphia (CHOP), 34th Street and Civic Center Boulevard, Philadelphia, PA 19104, USA
[b] Division of Body Imaging, Department of Radiology, The Children's Hospital of Philadelphia (CHOP), University of Pennsylvania, 34th Street and Civic Center Boulevard, Philadelphia, PA 19104, USA
* Corresponding author.
E-mail address: renjenp1@email.chop.edu

Urol Clin N Am 37 (2010) 307–318
doi:10.1016/j.ucl.2010.03.007
0094-0143/10/$ – see front matter © 2010 Elsevier Inc. All rights reserved.

Provided no contraindications (eg, fluid restriction, congestive heart failure) exist, patients are given 20 mL/kg (maximum of 1 L) of normal saline or Ringer's solution intravenously over the course of 30 to 60 minutes before the start of imaging. To minimize the need for additional manipulations during the scan, the infusion is stopped before entering the MR scanner room. The administration of intravenous (IV) fluid helps to reduce the MR contrast concentration and thus decrease the potential of T2* effect, making a linear relationship of the gadolinium concentration to the signal intensity possible. It also improves the visualization of the pelvicalyceal system and ureter and optimizes the baseline for subsequent furosemide (Lasix) administration.[6]

A bladder catheter without inflatable balloon is placed. In a patient with planned sedation, this is done after sedation. The catheter helps to decompress the bladder. A decompressed bladder is important, as it ensures that the contrast washout is not disturbed by full bladder effect and/or reflux. The catheter may also serve as a urethral marker in cases of possible ureteral ectopy.

The patient is positioned in the MRI scanner supine with the arms above the head. Patients with dilated pelvicalyceal system and without contrast in the ipsilateral ureter need to be turned to the prone position for the acquisition of additional delayed sequences.

Once the patient is appropriately positioned, before the start of imaging, furosemide is administered intravenously with a dose of 1 mg/kg up to a maximum dose of 20 mg. The purpose of the furosemide injection is several-fold.[6] furosemide increases urine flow and ensures the urinary tract is distended without increasing GFR. This increased distension of the urinary tract allows improved visualization of nondilated collecting systems. It serves to reduce the gadolinium concentration for the same reasons as discussed under hydration. Furosemide results in a more uniform distribution of gadolinium-based contrast, which reduces susceptibility artifacts. It is necessary for the evaluation of the excretory function under diuresis. Finally, furosemide administration shortens the examination time. Contraindications to furosemide administration include anuria, electrolyte imbalance, and hypotension. Patients with sulfonamide allergies may also be allergic to furosemide.[7]

The imaging portion of the examination can be expected to take between 30 to 60 minutes, depending on the need of delayed images including after repositioning the patient to the prone position.

Technique

A comprehensive MRU protocol is a 2-part imaging technique composed of precontrast sequences (static MRU) and postcontrast sequences (dynamic or excretory MRU).

Part 1—static MRU (precontrast imaging)

Static MRU uses heavily T2-weighted fluid-sensitive sequences in which urine-containing structures are bright (**Fig. 1**A, B). These T2-weighted images serve to delineate the anatomy of the renal

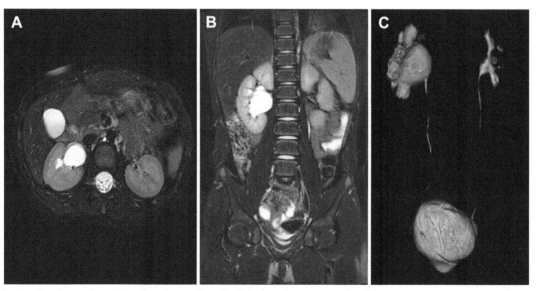

Fig. 1. UPJ obstruction. MRU showing a dilated pelvicalyceal system on the right: precontrast T2-weighted axial (*A*) and coronal (*B*) images and postcontrast MIP (*C*).

collecting systems and ureters. Unlike the postcontrast excretory MRU images, these T2-weighted images are not dependent on renal function and excretion of contrast material into the collecting systems to outline the anatomy of the urinary tract. Therefore, the T2-weighted sequences prove to be of greatest value in delineating the anatomy of the collecting system of a poorly or nonfunctioning renal moiety or kidney. These sequences become particularly important in identifying ureteral ectopy, for example in the case of the girl with constant wetting. Three-dimensional respiratory triggered T2 sequences can be reconstructed to create maximum intensity projections (MIP) and volume rendered images of the entire collecting system. Additional high-quality axial T2 sequences are also obtained to provide a high-resolution view of the renal parenchyma.

Part 2—dynamic MR urography (postcontrast imaging)

Dynamic MRU not only provides anatomic information including that of the vascular system, but it also offers functional information, which is in many ways analogous to a nuclear medicine study (**Fig. 2**A, B). Intravenous gadolinium is administered and sequential 3D dynamic sequences of the whole urinary tract are acquired. These images can be presented as a MIP and a cine loop. The former provides morphologic information (see **Fig. 1**C). The dynamic sequences are the basis of the functional calculation, assess renal perfusion, evaluate renal transit and excretion, and allow generation of signal intensity versus time curves. The images are transferred and postprocessed on an external computer using a freely available custom-made software package (www.chop-fmru.com).[8] The software package is used to calculate a number of functional parameters including calyceal and renal transit times, differential renal functions (DRF) based on renal parenchymal volume and Patlak number (an index of GFR), and both parenchymal volume and Patlak number. Moreover, the software package provides time-signal intensity curves of the renal parenchyma and contrasted part of the pelvicalyceal system corresponding to the renal enhancement and excretion (washout) curves, respectively (**Fig. 3**).

Calyceal transit time (CTT) and renal transit time (RTT) refer to the time period between the appearance of contrast in the aorta and just before its appearance in the calyces and proximal ureter, respectively. CTT is the more reliable parameter, as RTT can vary according to the volume of the renal pelvis and the morphology of uretero-pelvic junction (UPJ); the RTT value alone may not always differentiate between stasis and obstruction. CTT and RTT should be interpreted only in conjunction with both the static and dynamic images. The influence of parenchymal disease on these values should not be underestimated. The cut-off points for normal and abnormal RTT as published in one study do not seem to be universally reliable in classifying UPJ obstruction as compensated and decompensated.[9]

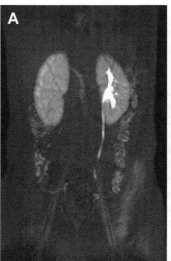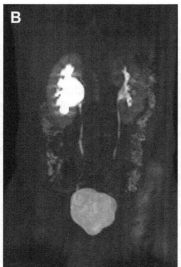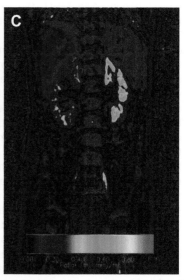

Fig. 2. UPJ obstruction. MRU postcontrast dynamic series (*A, B*) shows delayed dense nephrogram (*A*) and dilated pelvicalyceal system on the right. The functional map (Patlak map) (*C*) reveals significant decrease of function on the right compared with the left. DRF values were: vDRF: Right 46%, Left 56%.

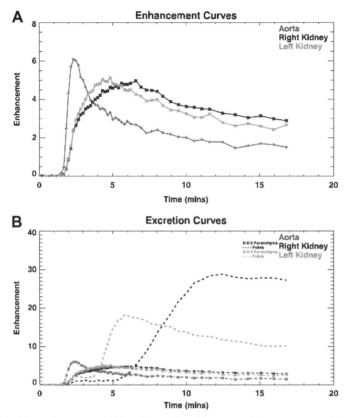

Fig. 3. UPJ obstruction. The enhancement (*A*) and excretion (*B*) curves of the case presented in **Figs. 1** and **2**. The enhancement curve appears to be symmetric but the excretion curve demonstrates a normal curve on the left but a climbing one on the right. RTT was 3 times longer on the right than on the left (Right, 9 minutes vs Left, 3 minutes).

DRF remains the most widely used measure of renal function. With MRU, the differential renal function is calculated using 2 distinct methods. The first method is referred to as the *volumetric differential renal function* (vDRF) and is based on the volume of enhancing renal parenchyma, which essentially represents functional renal mass. The vDRF is calculated by measuring the volume of enhancing renal parenchyma at the time point of homogeneous renal enhancement before contrast excretion in the calyces as determined by viewing the dynamic series. This method of calculation makes a distinction between functioning enhancing tissue and nonfunctional dysplastic or scarred tissue. This method also allows for the calculation of the individual contributions from upper and lower pole moieties in duplex kidneys. The second method is referred to as the *Patlak differential renal function* (pDRF), and is an index of GFR. The pDRF is calculated using the Patlak model. The same enhancing parenchyma that determines vDRF is the basis for calculating pDRF, but takes the contrast concentration over time in the aorta into consideration. After the injection of gadolinium, sequential intensity values of the aorta and renal parenchyma are obtained and subsequently entered automatically in the Patlak equation; this generates the Patlak plot and Patlak numbers.[1] The vDRF is a relatively stable number, whereas the pDRF tends to change with acute changes in GFR. This change in pDRF may reflect a measure of renal function recoverability. Comparatively speaking, vDRF is thought to correlate with the DRF measured by dimercaptosuccinic acid (DMSA) scintigraphy, whereas pDRF is thought to correlate with mercaptotriglycylglycine (MAG3) scintigraphy. When the percentage of the renal parenchyma is taken into consideration with the pDRF, a volumetric pDRF (vpDRF) can be calculated.

Comparison with Renal Scintigraphy

MRU has been shown to be superior to renal scintigraphy in many regards.[10] MRU has superior contrast and temporal and spatial resolution, and can provide precise anatomic information, which radionuclide studies cannot. MRU has also been shown to be superior to renal scintigraphy in distinguishing between pyelonephritis and scar.[1,11] The functional analysis of MRU also provides more comprehensive functional information.

Limitations

Although MRU is a powerful study with numerous advantages, few limitations do exist. MRU can have relatively long imaging times and is sensitive to motion artifact, which necessitates sedation for young children. This may be considered a minor limitation by some, as MRU can provide both anatomic and functional information in one examination.

Although, in an effort to avoid ionizing radiation, MRU may be used to follow children with bigger recurrent stone disease, CT remains the gold standard for the detection of small urinary tract calculi that are not always necessarily resolvable on MR.

The postcontrast dynamic images and interpretation of time-signal intensity curves can be used to assess for the possibility of vesicoureteral reflux. However, MR VCUG is unlikely to replace conventional VCUG because of technical limitations including the inability of sedated patients to completely empty their bladder.

An important limitation of the dynamic postcontrast part of the MRU is that it can be contraindicated in patients with moderate renal insufficiency. As stated, excretory MRU involves the administration of intravenous gadolinium and requires excretion into the collecting systems. Although it was previously thought that gadolinium could be safely administered in patients with renal insufficiency/failure in an effort to avoid iodinated contrast material, relatively recent reports have linked the disorder nephrogenic systemic fibrosis (NSF) to gadolinium administration.[12,13] New recommendations are to make every effort to avoid administering gadolinium-based contrast material in patients with moderate to severe renal insufficiency (GFR <30 mL/min). However, this issue remains a topic of investigation and recommendations may change in the future.

Clinical Applications

MRU can be used in the evaluation of congenital genitourinary (GU) anomalies, urinary tract obstruction, infection versus scarring, renal transplantation, hematuria, and surgically altered anatomy. The 2 most common indications for MRU in the pediatric population include complex congenital anatomic anomalies of the GU tract and hydronephrosis.

Congenital GU Anomalies

Congenital anomalies of the GU tract are more common than those of any other organ system, with a frequency of between 1:650 and 1:1000. Urinary tract anomalies predispose the child to a variety of complications, including infection, obstruction, wetting, stasis, and stone disease. At present, US is still most often used to provide anatomic information and renal scintigraphy to obtain functional information. MRU has the potential to replace multimodality imaging by providing both the 3D anatomic evaluation of the entire urinary tract and the renal functional information that will aid in management decisions. For example, in the evaluation of the girl who is "wet all the time," MRU has been shown to be superior to US both in the detection of occult upper pole moieties and in demonstrating ureteral ectopy.[3,14,15] In this instance, excretory function of the kidney is not a limiting factor in diagnosing an ectopic ureter because the static-fluid MRU images are sufficient. This is also true for the detection of dysplastic ectopic kidneys that are very difficult to see with other imaging modalities. MRU can also clarify the anatomy and complications related to complex urinary tract anomalies, such as crossed fused renal ectopia and horseshoe kidney.

Hydronephrosis/Obstruction

Hydronephrosis is the most common abnormality seen in the kidney on both prenatal and postnatal imaging. UPJ obstruction is the most common cause of hydronephrosis in childhood. In neonates, UPJ obstruction is most often attributable to intrinsic narrowing of the proximal ureter; however, in older children it is often attributable to a crossing vessel causing extrinsic compression and kinking of the ureter. Prognosis and need for surgical intervention is best predicted on the basis of renal function.

MRU can provide both the anatomic and functional information necessary to guide management.[16,17] Obstruction is suggested morphologically by dilation of the renal pelvis and narrowing of the ureter (see **Fig. 2**A, B). MRU can depict the site of ureteral narrowing, assess for a possible crossing vessel, and evaluate for possible obstructing urothelial mass. Obstruction is suggested functionally by non- or delayed excretion of contrast material.

Dynamic MRU can also be used to assess the success of pyeloplasty. Prepyeloplasty parameters, vDRF, pDRF, and RTT can be compared with those obtained postpyeloplasty to ascertain the effect of surgery.[18]

Pyelonephritis Versus Scar

MRU can demonstrate pyelonephritis but may also distinguish acute pyelonephritis from renal scarring, which is a distinct advantage compared with renal scintigraphy.[1,3,11] MRU has also been shown to be more sensitive in detecting renal scarring when compared with US, a finding of clinical importance when deciding if a Deflux procedure should be performed.[19] The normal renal cortex demonstrates homogeneous low signal intensity on T2-weighted images. Acute pyelonephritis will appear as areas of abnormal T2 signal hyperintensity in the renal cortex and will also demonstrate a striated or patchy nephrogram on postcontrast imaging similar to that seen with CT. Unlike acute pyelonephritis, renal scarring will appear as focal area(s) of parenchymal volume loss with deformity of the renal contour, with or without associated deformity of the underlying calyx.

Renal Transplantation

Renal transplant complications can be categorized as prerenal (vascular), renal (intrinsic parenchymal disease), and postrenal (obstruction). MRU has the ability to evaluate and distinguish among these complications in a single comprehensive examination. Because gadolinium is being administered for the dynamic portion of the MRU, MR angiography (MRA) can also be performed during the first pass of contrast material through the aorta and renal arteries. As such, evaluation for possible renal artery stenosis can be made. Additionally, delayed images will allow assessment for patency of the renal veins. Intrinsic parenchymal disease can be suggested on the T2-weighted images if increased cortical T2 signal and loss of corticomedullary differentiation are seen. The T2-weighted sequences can also be used to depict hydronephrosis, ureteral stenosis/kinks, lymphoceles, and urinomas. The dynamic

MRU can provide functional information of the transplant kidney such as GFR. Decreased transplant function may provide an earlier clue to acute or chronic rejection and potentially reduce the need for biopsy.[4]

Hematuria

MR urography can evaluate for possible renal parenchymal lesions, vascular lesions, and urothelial abnormalities as an etiology for hematuria. Additionally, MRU can be used to follow children with large recurrent urinary tract calculi in an effort to avoid ionizing radiation.[4,5] Urinary tract calculi will appear as filling defects in the collecting systems on both the static-fluid urography images and excretory MRU images. Secondary signs of stone disease such as perirenal edema, renal enlargement, and urothelial thickening can be demonstrated.

ADVANCED ULTRASONOGRAPHY
Harmonic Imaging

Harmonic imaging is a technical method that has proven to be useful in urosonography based on nonlinear properties of US that provide clearer and sharper US images more than does fundamental US.[20–22] Harmonic imaging constructs images based on higher frequencies than conventional US and also reduces US artifacts. Harmonic imaging improves border recognition and tissue differentiation, particularly of fluid-filled structures (**Fig. 4**). Additionally, it improves the conspicuity of even a small amount of echo-enhancing agents.[23] It has been shown to improve the detection of renal stones, renal parenchymal lesions, and the overall US scan of the urinary tract in children.[24,25] However, the improved border recognition may create artifacts that have to be recognized; specifically, harmonic imaging

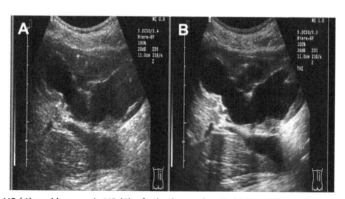

Fig. 4. Conventional US (A) and harmonic US (B) of a hydronephrotic kidney. The US image with harmonic image is clearer without artifacts and the different structures are better delineated.

exaggerates the normal corticomedullary differentiation and may falsely mimic nephrocalcinosis.

Three-Dimensional Ultrasound

Three-dimensional US combines conventional 2D ultrasound with position information to provide a 3D data set. Three-dimensional US has numerous advantages.[21,22,26] First, 3D ultrasound can create multiplanar views, similar to MR and CT. This multiplanar capability provides greater anatomic information. For example, it may help in distinguishing a renal cyst from a calyceal diverticulum. Three-dimensional US also allows for better evaluation of surfaces and curved structures and, as such, may better delineate the collecting system of a complex duplex kidney, or a dilated, hydronephrotic kidney. Three-dimensional US has been shown to have increased accuracy in the calculation of renal parenchymal volumes and, thereby, improve standardization of renal measurements, particularly of hydronephrotic and scarred kidneys. It also provides more exact bladder volume measurement.

Voiding Urosonography Technique, Clinical Application, and Limitations

VUS is a relatively new modality in the detection of vesicoureteral reflux (VUR) in children. Although VCUG and radionuclide cystography (RNC) are currently the 2 methods most commonly used to evaluate for VUR, recent developments of commercially available echo-enhancing agents have significantly improved the sonographic detection of fluid movement within the urinary tract (**Fig. 5**). The most commonly used echo-enhancing agent is Levovist (Bayer-Schering, Berlin, Germany), which is composed of 99.9% microcrystalline galactose particles and 0.1% palmitic acid. This introduces stabilized microbubbles, which allow improved visualization of fluid movement. More recently, a newer-generation US contrast agent, namely SonoVue (Bracco, Milan, Italy), with distinctly more practical advantages than Levovist is starting to be used.[27–29] These US contrast agents have made VUS a reliable alternative to VCUG and RNC with the distinct advantage of avoiding ionizing radiation and, at the same time, increasing the detection rate of VUR. Given that radiation exposures continue to be a concern in the pediatric population, strong consideration to performing VUS over conventional methods can be given. In the following sections, patient preparation, technique, and clinical applications and limitations of VUS will be discussed.[27,28,30,31]

Overall, the VUS examination consists of scanning the patient before, during, and after the intravesical administration of US contrast agent, as well as during voiding. First, the patient will be placed in the supine position on the examination table for a baseline US examination of the urinary tract. Subsequently, a bladder catheter will be inserted under aseptic conditions and urine will be allowed to drain. The bladder will then be slowly filled with a warmed saline solution under physiologic pressure until the predicted bladder volume is reached ([age + 2] × 30) or the patient feels an urge to void. The saline infusion is warmed to minimize patient discomfort. The US contrast agent is intravesically administered during the early filling phase. The kidneys, ureter, and bladder are then imaged to assess for possible VUR, which is diagnosed by the presence of echogenic microbubbles

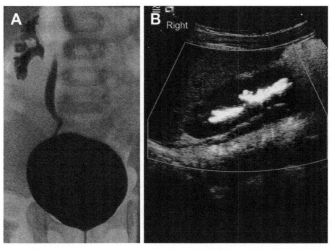

Fig. 5. VCUG (*A*) and VUS (*B*) in the same patient during the same study session. The right-sided grade II reflux is equally well demonstrated with both modalities.

in either the ureters or the renal pelves. The patient is then asked to void around the catheter and additional sonographic images of the kidneys, ureters, and bladder are obtained during voiding. Although most patients are able to void in the supine, prone, or decubitus position, if the child is older a potty or urine bottle may be offered to the child and the child may be scanned from the back while seated or standing. If desired, cyclic filling may also be performed with the procedure repeated under the same conditions using the same filling volume and the same catheter, which needs to be left in place after the first cycle.

VUS can be used in workup of urinary tract infections, follow-up of known VUR, and in the evaluation of reflux in renal transplant patients. Comparative studies have shown that VUS depicts not only more refluxing units but also higher-grade refluxes than does VCUG. Most VUR labeled Grade I on VCUG actually are Grade II or higher on VUS. A reflux grading system similar to the one used in VCUG is used in VUS, as follows: Grade I, microbubbles reaching the ureter only; Grade II, microbubbles reaching the nondilated renal pelves; Grade III, microbubbles reaching the moderately dilated pyelocalyceal system; Grade IV, microbubbles reaching the significantly dilated pyelocalyceal system; Grade V, microbubbles reaching the significantly dilated pyelocalyceal system with loss of the normal renal pelvic contour and with a dilated, tortuous ureter.

The main limitation of VUS is the evaluation of the urethra, although this may be less of a consideration in female patients. This limitation may potentially be overcome by attempting to incorporate transperineal US with the examination. Like RNC, VUS is an excellent technique for screening patients and for follow-up of known VUR in patients of both sexes.

A second minor limitation is that the examination is longer than VCUG. Specifically, the examination may take up to 30 minutes to perform including catheterization, whereas a VCUG may only take approximately 15 minutes. However, the examination time can be decreased with the use of harmonic imaging or newer contrast-specific modalities and if a baseline US does not need to be performed. The 10% increase in reflux detection rate combined with the absence of radiation compensates for the longer duration of the study.

COMPUTED TOMOGRAPHY

State-of-the-art CT technology offers 2 advanced imaging protocols for pediatric urological applications: CT angiography (CTA) (**Fig. 6**) and CT urography (CTU) (**Fig. 7**). For each of these methods,

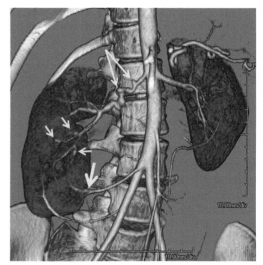

Fig. 6. A 14-year-old female with neurofibromatosis type 1 and progressively worsening hypertension underwent renal CTA. Coronal volume-rendered (VR) image shows 3 right and 1 left renal arteries. Advanced extraparenchymal (postostial, *long arrows*) and intraparenchymal (second to third order, *short arrows*) beading and irregularity involve the main right renal artery distribution. Note intraparenchymal collateral flow from the first accessory right renal artery (*thick arrow*). No disease was identified in the left renal arteries.

workstation visualization techniques are essential. Among many technical factors, CTA and CTU require precise synchronization between contrast medium delivery and the scan acquisition. For CTA, synchronization is to the arterial or venous phase, whereas for CTU, synchronization is to the delayed excretory renal phase. Although inherently dependent on radiation and iodinated contrast medium, CTA and CTU can be performed safely in pediatric patients using low radiation and contrast medium dose strategies. To facilitate patient and family counseling before CT, it is recommended that the pediatric urologist is familiar with some of these essential strategies as well as key patient preparations and clinical applications.

Technical Considerations

Current state-of-the-art scanners offer 64- to 320-channel multidetector-row CT (MDCT) technology. Both isotropic (0.50–0.75-mm-thick images) and high-resolution (1.25–1.50-mm-thick images) datasets can be generated. In most instances, however, a high-resolution acquisition provides sufficient detail for accurate CTA and CTU diagnoses and subsequent treatment planning. In selecting this mode, patients are exposed to less radiation, as MDCT collimation will not be

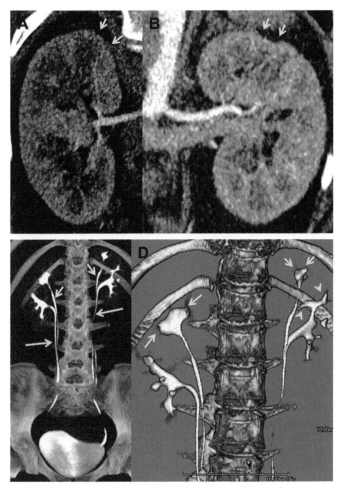

Fig. 7. CTA was performed in a 16-year-old female with hypertension. Single bilateral renal arteries were patent; however, preliminary review of the renal parenchyma demonstrated right (*A*) and left (*B*) upper pole mild focal cortical thinning (*arrows*) prompting a delayed urographic acquisition. CTU revealed bilateral duplex configurations (*C*, maximum-intensity projection image; *arrows*) with calyceal blunting involving the bilateral upper pole moieties (*D*, VR; *arrows*), consistent with reflux nephropathy. Mild calyceal blunting was also noted to involve the superior portion of the left lower pole moiety (*D, arrowheads*).

submillimeter. Additional strategies and acquisition parameters to control radiation exposure include restricting coverage to the anatomy of interest and using the lowest possible voltage (kVp) and amperage (mA). Coverage, voltage, and amperage all have direct relationships with the amount of patient radiation exposure. Regarding CTA coverage, when targeting the renal vasculature, the minimum scan volume extends from the supraceliac aorta to the upper pelvis, to account for anomalous arteries that may arise from the celiac artery and iliac arteries, respectively. If the examination is to assess pre- or post-renal transplant vasculature, coverage is limited to the pelvis and lower abdomen. Regarding CTU coverage, the scan volume includes the abdomen and pelvis, from the suprarenal regions through the bladder. Voltage options include 80, 100, 120, and 140 kVp; 80 kVp is recommended until 50 kg, 100 kVp from 50 to 90 kg, and 120 kVp greater than 90 kg. Amperage is typically prescribed using an automated dose algorithm, which delivers a variable range of amperage over the length of the coverage, based on prescan-determined body density and a targeted threshold value for acceptable noise.

In our experience, using a 64-channel MDCT scanner for abdominal CTA and abdominal–pelvis CTU in neonates to adolescent patients, average radiation exposures are approximately 1 to 2 mSv with scan times of 1.5 to 4.0 seconds. This radiation dose is equivalent to that of approximately 50 to 100 chest radiographs.[32] Room time is on average 10 to 15 minutes for both types of examinations, and may be slightly longer depending on whether sedation or anesthesia is required. Sub-mSv exposure is possible using 64-channel scanners, with the tradeoff being higher image noise and decreased image quality. The 128- to 320-channel systems offer the potential for routine sub-mSv exposure without compromise in image quality. In addition, subsecond scan times will be possible with these MDCT scanners, reducing or obviating the need for sedation and anesthesia.

As with 3D MRI-MRA and 3D US, CTA, and CTU, datasets are transferred to a server-based thin client or independent thick client workstation for real-time display and review using a combination of multiplanar and curved planar reconstructions, 3D volume rendering, and maximum intensity projections. Alternatively, static postprocessed images are generated on the workstation per established protocols, and transferred to a Picture Archive and Communications System (PACS) for subsequent review along with the source images. Thin client workstations offer the urologist the advantage of being able to review studies volumetrically from any location at any time of day and perform advanced quantitative analysis for treatment planning. Select images can be captured and transmitted electronically, directly from the workstation, for examination communication with colleagues, families, and patients. The system can also be accessed for clinical consultations with patients and for patient conferences with the urology team. Virtual group conferences are possible, with remote sharing of the workstation screen and interactive 2D and 3D display options. The most recent thin client technology streams data over the Internet from a server with a Web-based interface that does not require additional executable software. Web client workstation technology is available on select handheld devices, which has the potential to further enhance care of the pediatric urology patient.

Clinical Considerations

Pediatric CTA and CTU are considered only after US and MRI have been exhausted or when CT is considered superior for clinical imaging objectives. Emphasizing the advantages of CT, appropriate primary indications for CTA or CTU include the presence of metallic hardware and implantable devices; the requirement for higher spatial resolution; and the need for rapid scan time, such as in emergent imaging or in the high-risk sedation/anesthesia patient. If MRI or US is nondiagnostic or negative and clinical requirements remain for additional imaging, CTA and CTU should be considered before conventional catheter angiograms and intravenous pyelograms (IVP), respectively.

Once there is a decision to proceed forward with CT, the pediatric urology patient should be screened to confirm normal renal function and an absence of contrast allergies. The patient should also be assessed to determine if sedation or anesthesia is required. It is recommended to counsel the family and patient on risks and benefits for CT. Following appropriate discussions with the imaging department and review of their pediatric CTA and CTU protocols, the urology team may also choose to emphasize that CTA or CTU protocols will use pediatric-safe parameters. Examinations for neonates, infants, and toddlers should be scheduled with consideration to feeding schedules, as most imaging departments have 2- to 4-hour food restrictions before a contrast-enhanced CT. On the day of the examination, a suitable-size peripheral vein is accessed for optimized contrast delivery. This is often in the hand for the neonate or infant and the forearm or antecubital fossa for the toddler, young child, or adolescent. In a neonate, a 24-gauge (g) IV catheter is placed, whereas in an infant, a 22 g or 24 g is used. Beyond this age, a 20 g or 22 g is recommended.

CTA applications for the pediatric urology patient include evaluation of suspected or known renovascular hypertension (see **Fig. 6**), crossing renal hilar vessels (in the setting of UPJ obstruction), renal aneurysms (commonly syndromic related), small-vessel vasculitis, renal venous occlusive disease (ie, tumor invasion), vascular malformations (in the setting of hematuria), and traumatic renovascular injury. Additional indications include preoperative vascular mapping (ie, before resection of vascular renal and adrenal tumors) and if involved with hemodialysis access care, assessment of upper or lower extremity dysfunctional grafts and fistulas. Diagnostic-quality pediatric renal CT arteriograms are motion free, achieving robust enhancement of extraparenchymal renal arteries through to at least the third- to fourth-order intraparenchymal segments, with the goal of depicting the subcapsular fourth- to fifth-order arteries. This is particularly important in the setting of renovascular hypertension secondary to fibromuscular dysplasia, as it is not uncommon to have isolated intraparenchymal arterial disease. As with conventional angiography, assessment addresses the number, caliber, contour, course, and patency of native and anomalous renal arteries and veins. Although arterial flow is not directly evaluated, global and regional enhancement patterns provide indirect measures of flow and parenchymal perfusion; global and regional kidney size and cortical thickness serve as means to assess renal function and potential sequelae from vascular or, alternatively, nonvascular pathology.

CTU applications include the evaluation of suspected or known congenital anomalies, obstructive uropathy, traumatic nephroureteral injury, reflux nephropathy (see **Fig. 7**), and papillary necrosis. Acquisitions may be performed as a single dedicated urographic 8- to 10-minute delay acquisition or as a second series following a routine CT or CTA acquisition. In our experience, given the dominant role for MRU in the diagnosis and surveillance of pediatric renal parenchymal and nephroureteral disease, CTU is most commonly performed following the first pass arteriogram. In this instance, if preliminary review of the CTA images reveals parenchymal abnormalities, with or without vascular abnormalities, the monitoring physician determines whether an 8- to 10-minute delayed urographic series is warranted, which might elucidate the cause for the patient's symptoms (see **Fig. 7**). Diagnostic-quality CT urograms are motion free, achieving dense enhancement of the upper and lower collecting systems and the bladder, while maintaining enhancement in the renal parenchyma. As with MRU or conventional IVP, evaluation addresses the number, caliber, contour, course, and patency of native and anomalous upper and lower collecting systems. Renal pelvis, infundibular, and calyceal abnormalities are assessed with regard to feeding arteries and draining veins as well as regional parenchymal abnormalities. Normal ipsilateral and contralateral segments are used as internal normative references, applying flexible visualization techniques. Although urographic flow is not directly evaluated, delayed hyperenhanced renal parenchyma provides an indirect measure of urinary flow. As with the vascular phase, global and regional kidney size and cortical thickness serve as means to assess nephron function.

REFERENCES

1. Grattan-Smith JD, Jones RA. MR urography in children. Pediatr Radiol 2006;36:1119–32.
2. Grattan-Smith JD, Little SB, Jones RA. MR urography in children: how we do it. Pediatr Radiol 2008; 38(Suppl 1):S3–17.
3. Cerwinka WH, Grattan-Smith JD, Kirsch AJ. Magnetic resonance urography in pediatric urology. J Pediatr Urol 2008;4:74–83.
4. Kalb B, Votaw JR, Salman K, et al. Magnetic resonance nephrourography: current and developing techniques. Radiol Clin North Am 2008;46:11–24.
5. Leyendecker JR, Barnes CE, Zagoria RJ. MR urography: techniques and clinical applications. Radiographics 2008;28:23–48.
6. Grattan-Smith JD, Perez-Bayfield MR, Jones RA, et al. MR imaging of kidneys: functional evaluation using F-15 perfusion imaging. Pediatr Radiol 2003; 33:293–304.
7. Healy R, Jankowski TA. Which diuretics are safe and effective for patients with a sulfa allergy? J Fam Pract 2007;56:488–90.
8. Khrichenko D, Darge K. Functional MR urography—made simple. Pediatr Radiol 2009;Doi:10.1007/s00247-009-1458-4.
9. Grattan-Smith JD, Little SB, Jones RA. MR urography evaluation of obstructive uropathy. Pediatr Radiol 2008;38(Suppl 1):S49–69.
10. Perez-Brayfield MR, Kirsch AJ, Jones RA, et al. A prospective study comparing ultrasound, nuclear scintigraphy and dynamic contrast enhanced magnetic resonance imaging in the evaluation of hydronephrosis. J Urol 2003;170:1330–4.
11. Kavanagh EC, Ryan S, Awan A, et al. Can MRI replace DMSA in the detection of renal parenchymal defects in children with urinary tract infections? Pediatr Radiol 2005;35:275–81.
12. Grobner T. Gadolinium—a specific trigger for the development of nephrogenic fibrosing dermopathy and nephrogenic systemic fibrosis? Nephrol Dial Transplant 2006;21:1104–8.
13. Thomsen HS, Morcos SK, Dawson P. Is there a causal relation between the administration of gadolinium based contrast media and the development of nephrogenic systemic fibrosis (NSF)? Clin Radiol 2006;61:905–6.
14. Avni FE, Nicaise N, Hall M, et al. The role of MR imaging for the assessment of complicated duplex kidneys in children: preliminary report. Pediatr Radiol 2001;31:215–23.
15. Staatz G, Rohrmann D, Nolte-Ernsting CC, et al. Magnetic resonance urography in children: evaluation of suspected ureteral ectopia in duplex systems. J Urol 2001;166:2346–50.
16. Rohrschneider WK, Haufe S, Wiesel M, et al. Functional and morphologic evaluation of congenital urinary tract dilatation by using combined static-dynamic MR urography: findings in kidneys with a single collecting system. Radiology 2002;224:683–94.
17. Jones RA, Easley K, Little SB, et al. Dynamic contrast-enhanced MR urography in the evaluation of pediatric hydronephrosis: part I, functional assessment. AJR Am J Roentgenol 2005;185:1598–607.
18. Kirsch AJ, McMann LP, Jones RA, et al. Magnetic resonance urography for evaluating outcomes after pediatric pyeloplasty. J Urol 2006;176:1755–61.
19. Rodriguez, Larissa V, Spielman D, et al. Magnetic resonance imaging for the evaluation of

hydronephrosis, reflux, and renal scarring in children. J Urol 2001;166:1023–7.

20. Tranquart F, Grenier N, Eder V, et al. Clinical use of ultrasound tissue harmonic imaging. Ultrasound Med Biol 1999;25:889–94.

21. Riccabona M. Modern pediatric ultrasound: potential applications and clinical significance. A review. Clin Imaging 2006;30:77–86.

22. Riccabona M. Potential of modern sonographic techniques in pediatric uroradiology. Eur J Radiol 2002;43:110–21.

23. Darge K, Zeiger B, Rohrschneider W, et al. Contrast-enhanced harmonic imaging for the diagnosis of vesicoureteral reflux in pediatric patients. AJR Am J Roentgenol 2001;177:1411–5.

24. Kim B, Lim HK, Choi MH, et al. Detection of parenchymal abnormalities in acute pyelonephritis by pulse inversion harmonic imaging with or without microbubble ultrasonographic contrast agent: correlation with computed tomography. J Ultrasound Med 2001;20:5–14.

25. Bartnam U, Darge K. Harmonic versus conventional ultrasound imaging of the urinary tract in children. Pediatr Radiol 2005;35:655–60.

26. Riccabona M, Fritz G, Ring E. Potential applications of three-dimensional ultrasound in the pediatric urinary tract: pictorial demonstration based on preliminary results. Eur Radiol 2003; 13:2680–7.

27. Darge K. Voiding urosonography with ultrasound contrast agents for the diagnosis of vesicoureteral reflux in children. I. Procedure. Pediatr Radiol 2008;38:40–53.

28. Darge K. Voiding urosonography with US contrast agents for the diagnosis of vesicoureteric reflux in children. II. Comparison with radiological examinations. Pediatr Radiol 2008;38:54–63.

29. Robrecht J, Darge K. In-vitro comparison of a 1st and 2nd generation US contrast agent for reflux diagnosis. Rofo 2007;179:818–25.

30. Giordano M, Marzolla R, Puteo F, et al. Voiding urosonography as first step in diagnosis of vesicoureteral reflux in children: a clinical experience. Pediatr Radiol 2007;37(7):674–7.

31. Darge K, Troeger D, Duetting T, et al. Reflux in young patients: comparison of voiding US of the bladder and retrovesical space with echo enhancement versus voiding cystourethrography for diagnosis. Radiology 1999;210:201–7.

32. Brody AS, Frush DP, Huda W, et al. Radiation risk to children from computed tomography. Pediatrics 2007;120:677–82.

Index

Note: Page numbers of article titles are in **boldface** type.

A

Ablation, percutaneous varicocele, 275

Abscesses, renal, urinary tract infections in children related to, 233

Adherence, to treatment, in pediatric genitourinary anomalies, 303–304

Adolescents, pediatric psychology for genitourinary anomalies in, 301
    treatment strategy for varicocele in, **269–278**

Adrenal hyperplasia, congenital, in neonates with ambiguous genitalia, 195

Adrenal metabolites, reflux of as mechanism of varicocele in adolescents, 271

Adrenogenital syndrome, testis-sparing surgery in, 296

Age, effect on resolution of vesicoureteral reflux, 246–247

Ambiguous genitalia, practical approach in the newborn, **195–205**
    diagnosis, 195–200
    genetic tests, 200–203
    history and physical examination, 200
    multidisciplinary team, 203
    nomenclature, 195
    patient evaluation, 200
    radiographic tests, 203

Anatomic anomalies, of urinary tract, UTIs in children related to, 234–235
    See also Congenital anomalies.

Androgen biosynthesis, hypospadias and, 160

Androgen insensitivity syndrome, resulting in ambiguous genitalia, 198

Androgen receptor signaling, in pathogenesis of cryptorchidism, 184

Anorchia, congenital, resulting in ambiguous genitalia, 198

Antibiotic use, for UTIs in children, 231
    perioperative, in management of pediatric urolithiasis, 254–255

Appendicovesicostomy, robotically assisted, 284–285

Artificial urinary sphincter, in children with neurogenic bladder, 210–211

ATF3 gene, in etiology of hypospadias, 161

Augmentation, bladder, laparoscopic and robotic, 284–285
    with neurogenic bladder, 211–212

Autotransplantation, in pediatric urologic oncology, 292–293

B

Behavioral health problems, comorbid with pediatric genitourinary anomalies, 301

Biofeedback, in treatment of pediatric lower urinary tract dysfunction, 221–223

Bladder, laparoscopic and robotic augmentation in children, 284–285
    neurogenic, in children, urologic care of, **207–214**
        changes in bladder pressure after outlet procedures, 209–210
        current protocol at Texas Scottish Rite Hospital, 207–208
        initial management, 207
        lessons from artificial urinary sphincter, 210–211
        management at toilet training age, 208
        slings and augments, 211–212
        sphincteric insufficiency, 208–209

Bladder control, development of in children, 215–216

Bladder dynamics, effects on vesicoureteral reflux resolution, 248–249

Body image, in pediatric genitourinary anomalies, 303

C

Catheterization, clean intermittent, in treatment of pediatric lower urinary tract dysfunction, 225

Chordee, with hypospadias, 169–170, 172

Clean intermittent catheterization, in treatment of pediatric lower urinary tract dysfunction, 225

Computed tomography, advanced, of pediatric urologic disorders, 314–317
    clinical considerations, 316–317
    technical considerations, 314–316

Computed tomography angiography, of pediatric urologic disorders, 314–317

Computed tomography urography, of pediatric urologic disorders, 314–317

Computer models, predicting vesicoureteral reflux resolution, 249–250

Congenital anomalies, ambiguous genitalia, **195–205**
    of the genitourinary tract, magnetic resonance urography of, 311
    prenatal management of, **149–158**

Constipation, in pediatric lower urinary tract dysfunction, 218

Coping procedures, in pediatric genitourinary anomalies, 301–302

Urol Clin N Am 37 (2010) 319–326
doi:10.1016/S0094-0143(10)00045-5

urologic.theclinics.com

Printed and bound by CPI Group (UK) Ltd, Croydon, CR0 4YY

03/10/2024

02:04:55-0016

Moving?

Make sure your subscription moves with you!

To notify us of your new address, find your **Clinics Account Number** (located on your mailing label above your name), and contact customer service at:

Email: journalscustomerservice-usa@elsevier.com

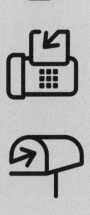

800-654-2452 (subscribers in the U.S. & Canada)
314-447-8871 (subscribers outside of the U.S. & Canada)

Fax number: 314-447-8029

Elsevier Health Sciences Division
Subscription Customer Service
3251 Riverport Lane
Maryland Heights, MO 63043